# PRAISE FOR EVIDENCE-BASED PR[...] COMPREHENSIVE STRATEGIES, TOOL[...], [...] TIPS FROM THE UNIVERSITY OF IOWA HOSPITALS AND CLINICS

"Anyone involved in implementing and sustaining evidence-based practice (EBP) has no doubt utilized the Iowa Model. Since its inception in 1994, the model has been one of the most widely used EBP models. In this book, readers will find the Iowa Model explained and demonstrated in practical situations that are intuitive to practitioners, with application-oriented tools and resources included in every step. This comprehensive resource will be valuable to everyone engaged in this work."

–Kathy Oman, PhD, RN, FAEN, FAAN, Caritas Coach
Children's Hospital Colorado Chair in Pediatric Nursing
Professor, UC Denver College of Nursing

"In fast-paced, dynamic healthcare settings, we are challenged to provide high-quality evidence-based care. This book, written by the experts in evidence-based practice, concisely summarizes strategies and tools supported by translational science and validated in practice. If you are ready to integrate high-quality evidence into practice and sustain these initiatives, this is the book for you."

–Elizabeth Bridges, PhD, RN, CCNS, FCCM, FAAN
Professor/Clinical Nurse Researcher, University of Washington

"Laura Cullen and colleagues provide a highly pragmatic framework for organizations wishing to enhance the evidentiary basis for creating practice policy. This innovative text provides a comprehensive reference list for each step of the EBP process as conceived by the University of Iowa Hospitals and Clinics (UIHC). Each phase is accompanied by specific steps of what to do and how to do it. Learning from the extensive experiences of UIHC will facilitate the EBP journey for novice EBP practitioners."

–Sheila Cox Sullivan, PhD, RN
Director/Research, EBP, & Analytics
Office of Nursing Services
Department of Veterans Affairs
Washington, DC

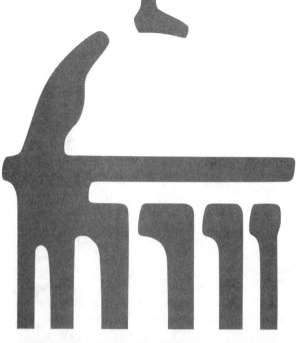

# EVIDENCE-BASED PRACTICE IN ACTION

Comprehensive Strategies, Tools, and Tips From the
University of Iowa Hospitals and Clinics

Laura Cullen, DNP, RN, FAAN
Kirsten Hanrahan, DNP, ARNP, CPNP-PC
Michele Farrington, BSN, RN, CPHON
Jennifer DeBerg, OT, MLS
Sharon Tucker, PhD, RN, PMHCNS-BC, FAAN
Charmaine Kleiber, PhD, RN, FAAN

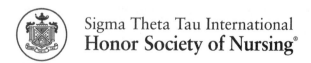

Sigma Theta Tau International
**Honor Society of Nursing**®

*The Honor Society of Nursing, Sigma Theta Tau International (STTI) is a nonprofit organization whose mission is advancing world health and celebrating nursing excellence in scholarship, leadership, and service. Founded in 1922, STTI has more than 135,000 active members in over 90 countries and territories. Members include practicing nurses, instructors, researchers, policymakers, entrepreneurs, and others. STTI's 530 chapters are located at more than 700 institutions of higher education throughout Armenia, Australia, Botswana, Brazil, Canada, Colombia, England, Ghana, Hong Kong, Japan, Jordan, Kenya, Lebanon, Malawi, Mexico, the Netherlands, Pakistan, Philippines, Portugal, Singapore, South Africa, South Korea, Swaziland, Sweden, Taiwan, Tanzania, Thailand, the United States, and Wales. Learn more at www.nursingsociety.org*

**Sigma Theta Tau International**
**550 West North Street**
**Indianapolis, IN, USA 46202**

To order additional books, buy in bulk, or order for corporate use, contact Nursing Knowledge International at 888. NKI.4YOU (888.654.4968/US and Canada) or +1.317.634.8171 (outside US and Canada).

To request a review copy for course adoption, email solutions@nursingknowledge.org or call 888.NKI.4YOU (888.654.4968/US and Canada) or +1.317.634.8171 (outside US and Canada).

**Suggested citation:**

Cullen, L., Hanrahan, K., Farrington, M., DeBerg, J., Tucker, S., & Kleiber, C. (2018). *Evidence-based practice in action: Comprehensive strategies, tools, and tips from the University of Iowa Hospitals and Clinics.* Indianapolis, IN: Sigma Theta Tau International.

To request author information, or for speaker or other media requests, contact Marketing, Honor Society of Nursing, Sigma Theta Tau International at 888.634.7575 (US and Canada) or +1.317.634.8171 (outside US and Canada).

| | |
|---|---|
| **ISBN:** | 9781940446936 |
| **EPUB ISBN:** | 9781940446943 |
| **PDF ISBN:** | 9781940446950 |
| **MOBI ISBN:** | 9781940446967 |

Library of Congress Cataloging-in-Publication Data

Names: Cullen, Laura, author. | Sigma Theta Tau International, publisher.

Title: Evidence-based practice in action : comprehensive strategies, tools, and tips from the University of Iowa Hospitals and Clinics / Laura Cullen, Kirsten Hanrahan, Michele Farrington, Jennifer DeBerg, Sharon Tucker, Charmaine Kleiber.

Description: Indianapolis, IN : Sigma Theta Tau International, [2017] | Includes index.

Identifiers: LCCN 2017021355 (print) | LCCN 2017021692 (ebook) | ISBN 9781940446943 (Epub) | ISBN 9781940446950 (Pdf) | ISBN 9781940446967 (Mobi) | ISBN 9781940446936 (alk. paper) | ISBN 9781940446967 (mobi)

Subjects: | MESH: University of Iowa. Hospitals and Clinics. | Evidence-Based Nursing | Models, Nursing

Classification: LCC RT51 (ebook) | LCC RT51 (print) | NLM WY 100.7 | DDC 610.73--dc23

LC record available at https://lccn.loc.gov/2017021355

**First Printing, 2017**

**Publisher:** Dustin Sullivan
**Acquisitions Editor:** Emily Hatch
**Editorial Coordinator:** Paula Jeffers
**Cover Designer:** Michael Tanamachi
**Page Design & Composition:** Tricia Bronkella
**Indexer:** Larry Sweazy

**Principal Book Editor:** Carla Hall
**Project Editor:** Kevin Kent
**Copy Editor:** Becky Whitney
**Proofreader:** Todd Lothery
**Illustrator:** Laura Robbins

# Acknowledgments

The authors wish to thank their colleagues at the University of Iowa (UI) Hospitals and Clinics for their partnership and continued commitment to the provision of evidence-based healthcare. We have learned a lot from their creativity, open discussions, and strong commitment to improving patient care. This work builds upon many years of partnership between visionary legends in nursing at the UI Hospitals and Clinics and the UI College of Nursing (CON). The very first evidence-based practice (EBP) improvement was led by Dr. Marita Titler in the mid-1980s. The formal partnership with the CON followed in 1989 under the leadership of Dr. Toni Tripp-Reimer, Dr. Kathleen Buckwalter, and Dr. Geraldine Felton, and Sally Mathis from the UI Hospitals and Clinics' Department of Nursing. We sincerely appreciate the many nurse leaders who have played key roles in building the culture, assisted our learning, and offered mentoring that made this book possible. We also thank the many point-of-care clinicians who question practice and use EBP to improve outcomes.

Kristen Rempel has been steadfast in her commitment to shepherd this book through the many growing pains of development and revision. We are indebted to you and your creative problem-solving skills.

We would also like to thank Kimberly Jordan and Grace Rempel for their invaluable assistance in making the original publication a reality. This work paved the way for the expanded and updated content.

We thank Robert Anderson, Elijah Olivas, Rosanna Seabold, and Emily Wiitanen for providing behind-the-scenes support and assistance that made writing and editing easier.

A number of nurses made contributions and provided leadership; in particular, we would like to acknowledge Cindy Dawson, BJ Hannon, Grace Matthews, and Michele Wagner, who provided creative answers to challenges inherent in implementing new practices.

The following nurses participated in optional coursework creating early drafts of select implementation strategies. We thank them for their work.

| | | |
|---|---|---|
| Michelle Cline | Dan Howlett | Catherine Odum |
| Tia Cloke | Katie Huether | Thoa Phan |
| Sarah Cole | Alexcia James | Amanda Pitts |
| Meghan Cooley | Kayla Kellogg | Kylea Ryther |
| Tara Cunnane | Samantha Mikota | Nathan Scadlock |
| Alicia L. Duyvejonck | Colleen Mohr | Reed Underwood |
| Anne Gentil-Archer | Megan Mortensen | |
| Julie Hoegger | Larry Newman | |

And finally, we could not have completed this work without our families and friends. Their love and support helped us find time and energy when we needed it most. How precious you are to us.

# About the Authors

## LAURA CULLEN, DNP, RN, FAAN

Laura Cullen is an Evidence-Based Practice Scientist at the University of Iowa (UI) Hospitals and Clinics. Cullen is known for her innovative educational programs and for supporting adoption of evidence-based practice (EBP) by point-of-care clinicians and teams. Her work has led to the adoption of innovative practices; improved patient safety; improved patient, family, and clinician satisfaction; reduced hospital length of stay and costs; and transformation of many organizations' infrastructures to support EBP. She has numerous publications and national and international presentations and has received multiple awards for her work. Cullen is Adjunct Faculty at the UI College of Nursing and has served as the U.S. representative on an international panel for the Honor Society of Nursing, Sigma Theta Tau International. Cullen co-authors a regular EBP column in the *Journal of PeriAnesthesia Nursing*, is a member of the editorial board of the *American Journal of Nursing*, and participates on the grant review panel for the DAISY Foundation™. She is a Fellow in the American Academy of Nursing and has been named one of Iowa's 100 Great Nurses. Cullen is the first author, overseeing the writing team, and the primary author for the following chapters: "Identify Triggering Issues/Opportunities" (Chapter 1), "Is This Topic a Priority?" (Chapter 3), "Implementation" (Chapter 8), and "Integrate and Sustain the Practice Change" (Chapter 11), as well as the majority of strategies in "Implementation" (Chapter 8).

## KIRSTEN HANRAHAN, DNP, ARNP, CPNP-PC

Kirsten Hanrahan is the Interim Director of Nursing Research, Evidence-Based Practice, and Quality at the UI Hospitals and Clinics and a Pediatric Nurse Practitioner transitioning neonatal intensive care unit infants to home from the UI Stead Family Children's Hospital. She is Adjunct Faculty at the UI College of Nursing and is well-versed in EBP and clinical research. Her research interests include pediatric IV management and pain. She has consulted for a National Institutes of Health multi-site study and is co-founder of the Distraction in Action© tool that helps parents learn to be a distraction coach for their child during medical procedures. She is currently the principal investigator for studies related to pediatric intensive care unit pain management, parent distraction for procedural pain, and evaluation of a children's hospital healing environment. Hanrahan has authored evidence-based guidelines and implemented multiple EBP changes in the clinical setting. She has numerous publications and national and international presentations and has been named one of Iowa's 100 Great Nurses. Hanrahan is the primary author of the following chapters: "Assemble, Appraise, and Synthesize Body of Evidence" (Chapter 5), "Is There Sufficient Evidence?" (Chapter 6), "Is Change Appropriate for Adoption in Practice?" (Chapter 10), and various strategies in "Implementation" (Chapter 8).

## MICHELE FARRINGTON, BSN, RN, CPHON

Michele Farrington is a Clinical Healthcare Research Associate at the UI Hospitals and Clinics and is certified in pediatric hematology oncology nursing. She serves as a study coordinator and EBP mentor. Previously, she served as a staff nurse in pediatrics and has tremendous experience and expertise in pediatric oncology and EBP, leading or co-leading initiatives since 2003. Her work has been awarded extramural funding, validating the strength of the projects and impact on nursing care. Moreover, she has numerous publications related to EBP projects and has given multiple local, national, and international presentations. Farrington is *ORL – Head and Neck Nursing* Media Review Column Department Editor; AAO-HNSF Guideline Task Force member; Chair of the SOHN Nursing Practice and Research Committee; SOHN National Education Committee member; SOHN Congress Planning Committee member (2016–2019); *EBP to Go®: Accelerating Evidence-Based Practice* Series Editor; and she is actively involved in multiple professional organizations. She is a past recipient of the Nursing Excellence in Clinical Education Award, 100 Great Iowa Nurses Award, and ENT-NF Literary Awards. Farrington is the primary author of "Evaluation" (Chapter 9) and "Disseminate Results" (Chapter 12) and wrote a significant number of new strategies in "Implementation" (Chapter 8).

## JENNIFER DEBERG, OT, MLS

Jennifer DeBerg is a User Services Librarian at the Hardin Library for the Health Sciences at the UI Libraries. She provides information management instruction and services to clinicians, students, faculty, and staff from various health science disciplines. She is Adjunct Lecturer with the UI College of Nursing, where she collaborates with faculty in undergraduate and graduate courses pertaining to research and EBP. Because of previous experience as an occupational therapist, she has a passion for providing support to clinicians related to EBP and quality care. DeBerg is active in several professional organizations, has been a presenter at numerous regional and national conferences, and is a regular contributor to articles published in both library and health sciences journals. She served as primary author for "State the Question or Purpose" (Chapter 2), provided editorial assistance for all chapters, and conducted literature searches to find evidence support for many of the chapters.

## SHARON TUCKER, PHD, RN, PMHCNS-BC, FAAN

Sharon Tucker is the Grayce Sills Endowed Professor in Psychiatric-Mental Health Nursing and Director of the Translational Research Core of the new Helene Fuld Health Trust National Institute for Evidence-Based Practice in the College of Nursing at The Ohio State University (OSU). She assumed this position in 2017 after serving 6 years as the Director of Nursing Research, Evidence-Based Practice, and Quality at the UI Hospitals and Clinics and held a joint appointment at the UI College of Nursing. Tucker's research program relates to understanding and motivating human behaviors through interventions that promote health and reduce health risks, with a particular focus on working mothers and their children. She brings this behavioral expertise to the adoption and translation of evidence-based nursing practices among clinicians. Tucker has extensive clinical, teaching, and research experiences in mental and behavioral health. Through her research, she partners with colleagues from across OSU, UI,

Mayo Clinic, Iowa State University, and Johns Hopkins University. She has extramural funding and support, has published extensively, and actively participates in parent and child wellness initiatives at the local, state, and national levels. Tucker is an author of "Is This Topic a Priority?" (Chapter 3) and several strategies in "Implementation" (Chapter 8).

## CHARMAINE KLEIBER, PHD, RN, FAAN

Charmaine Kleiber is an Associate Research Scientist at the UI Hospitals and Clinics and Associate Professor Emeritus at the UI College of Nursing. Kleiber's clinical career focused on pediatrics and intensive care. Her research focus is the management of children's pain, especially during medical procedures. Kleiber is co-founder of the Distraction in Action© tool that helps parents learn to be a distraction coach for their child during medical procedures. While on faculty at the UI College of Nursing, Kleiber developed and taught undergraduate and graduate courses for nurses on the conduct of research and EBP. She has been honored by the American Academy of Nursing as an "Edgerunner" for innovative pain management research and by the Midwest Nursing Research Society Pain and Symptom Management Research Interest Groups for "Advancing the Science." She also had a key role in the development and publication of the original Iowa Model and both published revisions. Kleiber is the primary author for "Overview," "Form a Team" (Chapter 4), "Design and Pilot the Practice Change" (Chapter 7), and several strategies in "Implementation" (Chapter 8).

# Table of Contents

# Foreword

There has never been a time in history when the need for evidence-based practice (EBP) in the clinical arena has been greater to guide patient, clinician, and health-system decisions. Building on the seminal work of the Iowa Model (Titler et al., 1994), *Evidence-Based Practice in Action: Comprehensive Strategies, Tools, and Tips From the University of Iowa Hospitals and Clinics* delivers exactly what nurses and leaders have told me they need for EBP success. Supporting EBP within healthcare settings requires 1) a process that is clear, logical, and usable in practice settings; 2) tools and examples to support each step of the process; 3) links to available resources; and 4) mentors.

This book starts with an introduction of a clear, logical EBP process framed by the Iowa Model—which many of us are familiar with or have used in the past. The process originates with identifying problem triggers and then moves through the steps of formulating actionable questions, determining if the topic is a priority, and forming a team. The process of acquiring and appraising the evidence follows, which then forms the basis for the practice recommendation. Next, the authors describe how to design and pilot the practice change before implementing and evaluating. Change, sustainability, and dissemination strategies are also included. Contemporary issues are raised, such as engaging patients in decisions related to patient-centered practices.

Tools and examples to guide the EBP process aligned with each step are very important to foster the work of EBP teams. Not only are tools prevalent in supporting the EBP process, they are also provided for implementing recommendations to practice. Examples are particularly helpful for nurses who are new to the EBP process to help them understand what the final product will look like. The chapters are replete with pertinent and timely examples (e.g., oral mucositis and management of pain after surgery) that include policy, procedures, templates, communication strategies, slides, and flow diagrams.

Available resources that allow teams or settings to access and tailor their processes to meet the needs of their own organizational context are also imperative. Links are provided for EBP guidelines; search databases (e.g., PubMed); evidence assessment instruments for critical appraisal of research, guidelines, and systematic reviews; and tools for rating evidence. The approach to available resources is nonprescriptive, so readers can choose the resources that best meet their needs.

Experienced mentors are essential to teach and support the EBP process, verify professional development outcomes of teams (knowledge, skills, and attitudes), and foster a supportive infrastructure for the process and evidence translation. Mentors in clinical practice or academia can use the book to teach the process and will find benefit in the tips and tools.

Nurses and leaders in clinical environments need EBP models with clinical usability and utility for their setting. *Evidence-Based Practice in Action: Comprehensive Strategies, Tools, and Tips From the University of*

*Iowa Hospitals and Clinics* provides a systematic process with the tools, examples, and links to resources that both novice and experienced teams in clinical and academic settings need.

–Robin P. Newhouse, PhD, RN, NEA-BC, FAAN
Dean and Distinguished Professor
Indiana University School of Nursing
Deputy Chair, University Clinical Affairs Cabinet
Associate Vice President for Academic Affairs, IU Health

## Reference

Titler, M. G., Kleiber, C., Steelman, V., Goode, C., Rakel, B., Barry-Walker, J., . . . Buckwalter, K. (1994). Infusing research into practice to promote quality care. *Nursing Research, 43*(5), 307–313.

# The Iowa Model Revised: Evidence-Based Practice to Promote Excellence in Health Care

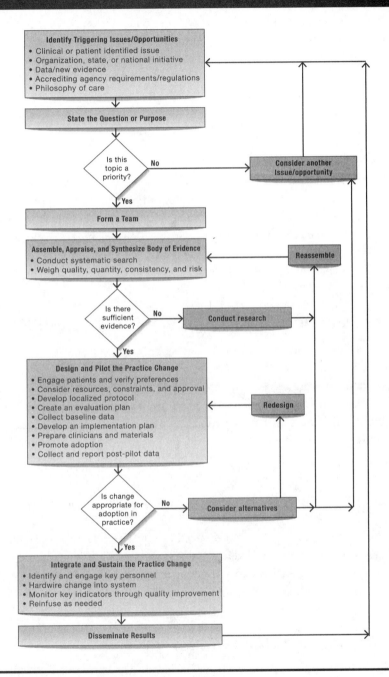

Iowa Model Collaborative. (2017). Iowa Model of Evidence-Based Practice: Revisions and validation. *Worldviews on Evidence-Based Nursing, 14*(3), 175–182. doi:10.1111/wvh.12223

# Overview

Welcome to *Evidence-Based Practice in Action: Comprehensive Strategies, Tools, and Tips From the University of Iowa Hospitals and Clinics*. This book uses the newly modified Iowa Model Revised: Evidence-Based Practice to Promote Excellence in Health Care (Iowa Model Collaborative, 2017). The original Iowa Model (Titler et al., 1994) was an outgrowth of the Quality Assurance Model Using Research (Watson, Bulechek, & McCloskey, 1987). As the importance of including different levels of evidence became clear, it was modified as the Iowa Model of Evidence-Based Practice to Promote Quality Care (Titler et al., 2001). Each version of the Iowa Model was designed to provide guidance for nurses and other clinicians to make decisions about day-to-day practices that affect patient outcomes. Select published project reports that used the Iowa Model are located in Appendix C.

Changes to the Iowa Model were made based upon new knowledge about the EBP process and recommendations from over 600 users of the model (Iowa Model Collaborative, 2017). Major refinements to the model are expansion of the sections on (1) designing and pilot testing the practice change and (2) integrating and sustaining the practice change. The implementation strategies included in this book were created to provide specific guidance for implementing and sustaining change. An additional companion workbook (*Evidence-Based Practice in Action: Workbook*) was developed to enhance EBP planning and implementation. It offers a selection of practical tools that correspond to each chapter of this book.

## A Word About Evidence-Based Practice Process Models

Selecting an EBP model is an important first step for any organization (Gawlinski & Rutledge, 2008; Schaffer, Sandau, & Diedrick, 2013). Various models have been developed to guide organizational and project leaders through the EBP process (see Appendix D). Most EBP process models include similar overarching steps such as identifying a problem, critiquing the evidence, selecting and implementing interventions recommended from research, evaluating the change, and disseminating results. Because EBP process models use the same basic problem-solving process, this book will be useful regardless of the EBP model.

## Using This Book

The Institute of Medicine (IOM) goal is that 90% of healthcare will be evidence-based by 2020 (2010a). In order to achieve this goal, resources are needed to promote adoption of evidence-based clinical practice recommendations. This book was developed to assist clinicians and those responsible for leading EBP to work through the EBP process with associated strategies, tools, and tips.

### Chapter 1: Identify Triggering Issues/Opportunities

EBP begins when clinicians identify practice issues, challenges, or desired changes in outcome metrics. In the Iowa Model, an issue or "trigger" is identified from a clinical problem, organizational initiative, or new knowledge. The purpose of EBP is to solve the problem or compare new knowledge to current practice. Identification of triggers may originate from any member of the healthcare team but often comes from clinicians questioning current practice.

## Chapter 2: State the Question or Purpose

This is a new formal step in the Iowa Model. The chapter explains how to formulate actionable questions using the PICO (P = patient/problem/population, I = intervention, C = comparison, O = outcome) framework (Schardt, Adams, Owens, Keitz, & Fontelo, 2007). The PICO components are used to develop the project's purpose statement, which helps set boundaries around project work.

## Chapter 3: Is This Topic a Priority?

Identification of priority topics is essential as not every clinical question can be addressed through the EBP process. Higher priority may be given to topics that address high volume, high risk, or high cost issues; those that are closely aligned with the institution's strategic plan; or other institutional or market forces (e.g., patient or clinician safety, changing reimbursement). If the topic is not an organizational priority, clinicians may want to consider a different focus, different project outcomes, or other opportunities for improving practice. This and similar feedback loops within the Iowa Model highlight that the work is not linear, so feedback loops are suggested.

## Chapter 4: Form a Team

Once there is commitment to address the topic, an EBP team should be formed to develop, implement, and evaluate the practice change. EBP team membership requires several considerations to ensure the correct clinicians are involved and to maximize use of the team members' skills and organizational linkages. This chapter provides an example of team formation and tips for successfully leading a team.

## Chapter 5: Assemble, Appraise, and Synthesize Body of Evidence

The EBP team selects, critiques, and synthesizes the best available evidence. A comprehensive literature search must be completed before all the available evidence is critically reviewed and synthesized to make a recommendation for practice. A step-by-step guide with numerous resources is provided.

## Chapter 6: Is There Sufficient Evidence?

At this point, the entire body of evidence—including research, case studies, quality data, expert opinions, and patient input—is synthesized. This chapter covers the steps to take to determine when the evidence is considered sufficient, or not sufficient, for pilot testing.

## Chapter 7: Design and Pilot the Practice Change

Piloting is an essential step in the EBP process. Outcomes achieved in a controlled research environment may result in different outcomes than those found when EBP is used in a real-world clinical setting. Piloting the EBP change is essential for identifying issues with the intervention, implementation, and rollout to multiple clinical areas. An overview of pilot testing activities is provided in this chapter, with more in-depth information on implementation and evaluation in Chapters 8 and 9.

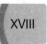 

## Chapter 8: Implementation

Implementation is fluid, complex, and highly interactive, and it changes over the course of the pilot period. Multiple implementation strategies are selected and used cumulatively (see Appendix B) to create a comprehensive plan based on the four phases of implementation: creating awareness and interest, building knowledge and commitment, promoting action and adoption, and pursuing integration and sustainability (Cullen & Adams, 2012).

## Chapter 9: Evaluation

Evaluation of the pilot must focus on select key indicators related specifically to the practice change and for input to guide implementation. Both process and outcome indicators are collected before and after implementation of the practice change. This chapter provides suggestions on data to collect and data analysis.

## Chapter 10: Is Change Appropriate for Adoption in Practice?

This decision point requires the EBP team to either recommend adoption of the practice change or pursue other courses of action. This chapter outlines the key issues that should be addressed when making this decision and describes possible actions to take.

## Chapter 11: Integrate and Sustain the Practice Change

This step promotes integration and sustainability of the practice change over time and prevents regression to previous practices. The importance of "hardwiring" the change into the system, tracking and evaluating data over time, and planning for periodic reinfusion is emphasized.

## Chapter 12: Disseminate Results

Dissemination of project results is a key step in the EBP process to promote the adoption of EBPs within the larger healthcare community (Sigma Theta Tau International 2005–2007 Research and Scholarship Advisory Committee [STTI], 2008). Sharing project reports within and outside the organization through presentation and publication supports the growth of an EBP culture in the organization, expands nursing knowledge, and encourages EBP updates in other settings.

# Conclusion

Steps in the EBP process build progressively to inform subsequent actions. The Iowa Model and other EBP process models provide direction, yet adoption in practice remains challenging. Application of EBP achieves improvements for patients, their families, clinicians, and healthcare organizations. This book is designed as a guide with application-oriented tools and resources for the journey.

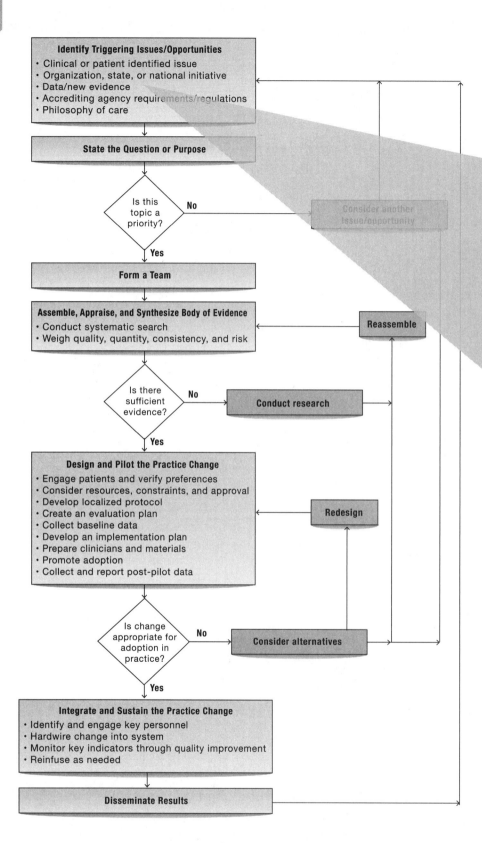

**Identify Triggering Issues/Opportunities**
- Clinical or patient identified issue
- Organization, state, or national initiative
- Data/new evidence
- Accrediting agency requirements/regulations
- Philosophy of care

**State the Question or Purpose**

Is this topic a priority?
**No** → Consider another issue/opportunity

**Yes**

**Form a Team**

**Assemble, Appraise, and Synthesize Body of Evidence**
- Conduct systematic search
- Weigh quality, quantity, consistency, and risk

**Reassemble**

Is there sufficient evidence?
**No** → **Conduct research**

**Yes**

**Design and Pilot the Practice Change**
- Engage patients and verify preferences
- Consider resources, constraints, and approval
- Develop localized protocol
- Create an evaluation plan
- Collect baseline data
- Develop an implementation plan
- Prepare clinicians and materials
- Promote adoption
- Collect and report post-pilot data

**Redesign**

Is change appropriate for adoption in practice?
**No** → **Consider alternatives**

**Yes**

**Integrate and Sustain the Practice Change**
- Identify and engage key personnel
- Hardwire change into system
- Monitor key indicators through quality improvement
- Reinfuse as needed

**Disseminate Results**

# IDENTIFY TRIGGERING ISSUES/OPPORTUNITIES

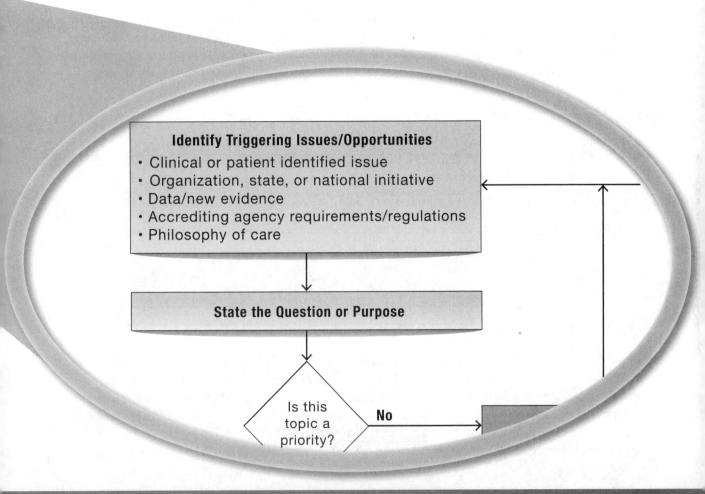

**Identify Triggering Issues/Opportunities**
- Clinical or patient identified issue
- Organization, state, or national initiative
- Data/new evidence
- Accrediting agency requirements/regulations
- Philosophy of care

**State the Question or Purpose**

Is this topic a priority?

No

*"If I have ever made any valuable discoveries, it has been owing more to patient attention than to any other talent."*

–Isaac Newton

High-quality healthcare for patients and families, as well as clinicians, demands a culture of inquiry and continuous improvement. This mindset leads to identification of many practice questions that can be addressed through evidence-based practice (EBP). EBP is the process of shared decision-making between practitioner, patient, and others significant to them based on research evidence, the patient's experiences and preferences, clinical expertise or know-how, and other available robust sources of information (Sackett, Rosenberg, Gray, Haynes, & Richardson, 1996; Sigma Theta Tau International 2005–2007 Research and Scholarship Advisory Committee [STTI], 2008). Point-of-care clinicians are in a key position to ask and answer clinical questions to promote quality and safety. Shared governance committee members and organizational leaders also generate clinical or operational questions (Cullen, Wagner, Matthews, & Farrington, 2017). Identifying a question initiates or triggers the EBP process (Iowa Model Collaborative, 2017). Questioning practice creates a culture of inquiry and is the foundation to developing a learning healthcare system (Wilson, Sleutel, et al., 2015). Identifying triggering issues or opportunities for improvement is the first step in the Iowa Model and EBP process, which is described in the remaining chapters.

The triggering issue or opportunity for improvement may be generated in a variety of ways. Potential sources are:

- Clinical or patient identified issue

- Organization, state, or national initiative

- Data or new evidence

- Accrediting agency requirements or regulations

- Philosophy of care

## Clinical or Patient Identified Issue

Doing the right thing for patients is always a priority. Staying focused on meeting patient and family needs and continuous improvement leads to practice questions and a culture of inquiry. Clinicians are able to identify triggering issues by considering common patient symptoms or experiences, frequent assessments or interventions, and questions from patients and their families. By partnering with patients and families, clinicians can also identify EBP opportunities that promote shared decision-making so people can manage their own health (Agency for Healthcare Research and Quality [AHRQ], 2017).

## Organization, State, or National Initiative

Triggering issues and opportunities can also be generated when considering organization, state, or national initiatives. Consider the organization's strategic plan, messages from senior leaders, or discussion with other leaders to identify opportunities for EBP. High-volume patient and quality care issues may be the target of some organizational initiatives. However, low volume, highly specialized procedures with their own unique set of practice implications also need to be considered. Organizations are always interested in topics supporting recognition for excellence (e.g., American Nurses Credentialing Center, 2017).

Healthcare settings are often influenced by activities happening within the state or territory in which they reside. Health systems increasingly cross boundaries and must be responsive to additional regulations. State level initiatives may be identified through changes in state funding (e.g., mental healthcare), legislative agendas, or board of nursing announcements.

National initiatives and the national quality agenda are also drivers of local practice. Look for topics being explored by healthcare organizations, upcoming changes in reimbursement (e.g., value-based purchasing [Centers for Medicare & Medicaid Services, 2017]), or turn to organizations such as Choosing Wisely® (http://www.choosingwisely.org/) for ideas. National or international initiatives continually evolve.

## RESOURCES: Agencies and Organizations

The following list includes influential organizations and federally funded initiatives that continue to influence the current healthcare agenda or updates:

| Resource | Source |
|---|---|
| Agency for Healthcare Research and Quality (AHRQ) | https://www.ahrq.gov/ |
| American Nurses Association | http://www.nursingworld.org/ |
| Centers for Medicare & Medicaid Services | https://www.cms.gov/ |
| Honor Society of Nursing, Sigma Theta Tau International | https://www.nursingsociety.org/ |
| Institute for Healthcare Improvement | http://www.ihi.org/Pages/default.aspx |
| National Academy of Medicine | https://nam.edu/ |
| National Institute of Health and Care Excellence | https://www.nice.org.uk/ |
| Press Ganey (U.S. database of nursing quality indicators) | http://www.pressganey.com/ |
| Registered Nurses' Association of Ontario | http://rnao.ca/ or http://rnao.ca/bpg |
| United States Department of Health and Human Services | https://www.hhs.gov/ |

Operational issues, just as clinical topics, make good questions to address through the EBP process. Leaders may be interested in operational issues such as teamwork (Chapman, Rahman, Courtney, & Chalmers, 2017), transformational leadership practices (Kouzes & Posner, 2012), or application of human factors principles (Carayon, Xie, & Kianfar, 2014; Hopkinson & Jennings, 2013).

## Data or New Evidence

A topic that stems from existing data within the healthcare system makes it a priority to address. Data may be available from epidemiology, hospital quality, billing, utilization review, reports from patient health records, informatics, or other offices. If data already exist, organizational commitment and potential resources to address the problem may be available. Obtaining relevant and convincing data may be helpful to gain support and generate interest in the topic by reporting a practice gap (see Strategy 2-12).

A topic is also a trigger if it is generated from new information, scientific findings, or reports. Clinicians or leaders can obtain new knowledge from

- New research or other literature
- Conferences
- Updates from professional specialty organizations

One way to stay current is by reading professional and scholarly literature. Reading literature from a variety of fields can stimulate interesting and innovative ways to consider old problems that may lend themselves to EBP solutions. Staying current also requires clinicians to identify reversal of practice recommendations requiring de-implementation, to keep practice current, but at the same time creating additional EBP opportunities (van Bodegom-Vos, Davidoff, & Marang-van de Mheen, 2016).

## Accrediting Agency Requirements or Regulations

Healthcare organizations and clinicians in all settings work with many accrediting and regulatory agencies that influence practice. National patient safety goals, certification program standards, and other accrediting agencies are evidence-based (AABB, 2017; National Cancer Institute, n.d.; The Joint Commission, 2017a, 2017b). While benefit from meeting regulatory standards may need additional research (Flodgren, Gonçalves-Bradley, & Pomey, 2016), regulatory standards remain priorities for organizations. The process for developing standards is increasingly applying EBP, creating new opportunities for evidence-based improvements in care. Organizational leaders are in an ideal position to identify upcoming practice standards to address through the EBP process.

## Philosophy of Care

Nurses have a long history of putting patients and families first, and as such may identify other issues to be addressed. Clinicians connect with patients and their families, and through those interactions identify issues or opportunities to address that fit their underlying philosophy of care (Lau et al., 2016; Shoemaker & Fischer, 2011). Nurses' commitment to provide care across the continuum, from health promotion through end-of-life care, creates vast opportunities for EBP. For example, care for the dying remains a philosophical priority and may trigger an opportunity to improve care at the end of life. In which case, symptom management and bereavement become opportunities to address through EBP. Other nurses might identify missed nursing care, such as ambulation (Bragadóttir, Kalisch, & Tryggvadóttir, 2017), as important issues based on their philosophy of care.

To achieve the Institute of Medicine (IOM) goal of providing evidence-based healthcare greater than 90% of the time (IOM, 2010a; IOM, 2015b), there are gaps to address. Opportunities come from identifying clinical or patient identified issues; organization, state, or national initiatives; data and new evidence; standards set by accrediting and regulatory agencies; and a philosophy of high quality patient care that triggers the EBP process (see Tool 1.1). Once a trigger is identified, it is important to consider potential stake-holders to partner with for the next steps in the EBP process. These colleagues may be helpful in clarifying priority issues and opportunities in order to develop a clear, specific purpose statement (see Chapter 2).

## TIPS: Topics and Triggers

■ Remain open to new ideas and opportunities to improve care.

■ Basic care and fundamental values provide a starting point for developing an idea.

■ Time and thought may be required to develop a practice question.

■ Patient or family questions or concerns provide a new perspective to consider as potential EBP topics.

■ Clinicians new to a clinical area can identify questions that create a new perspective on current practices.

■ Practice updates and reversals are expected as the science continues to develop.

■ As you begin, stay focused on the desired goal or outcome; starting with the intervention too early may slow progress.

■ The topic of interest is likely to evolve as you work through the next steps in the EBP process.

■ Some triggering issues may have data supporting need for the EBP, which may provide a rationale for garnering organizational resources for project work.

## Tool 1.1   Potential EBP Topics

**INSTRUCTIONS:** Read the questions below and record your responses. Skip questions that do not apply and proceed to the next question. Take these ideas to a leader and discuss each to identify a topic of interest.

### Clinical or Patient Identified Issue

What are the procedures you spend a lot of time doing or do frequently?

What questions are patients and families asking?

Who are the high volume patients?

Who are the patients with highest risk for a poor outcome?

### Organization, State, or National Initiative

Is there a new practice in the organization (e.g., policy) that needs to be implemented?

Are there benchmarks for new practices that you would like to try?

Do you know of a new protocol (i.e., policy, procedure, or standard) that could improve practice?

What is interesting to you among the current organizational initiatives?

Are there clinical practices that can be linked to the strategic plan?

Where could cost savings be achieved?

## Data/New Evidence

Are there quality data that you want to improve?

What did you learn at the last conference or program you attended?

When you read journals, which articles are you drawn toward first?

Is your professional organization publishing on topics of interest (e.g., guidelines, position statements)?

Are you aware of research findings that might apply to your practice?

## Accrediting Agency Requirements/Regulations

Which regulatory standards would you be interested in addressing through a practice improvement?

What are National Patient Safety Goals for improving quality care?

Are there anticipated or new reimbursement structures (e.g., revisions to value-based purchasing)?

## Philosophy of Care

Where is care missing in daily practice (e.g., holistic or comfort interventions)?

What common patient/family experiences could be improved?

Has patient/family shared their experience in a way you had not anticipated?

EXAMPLES

TOOLS

10

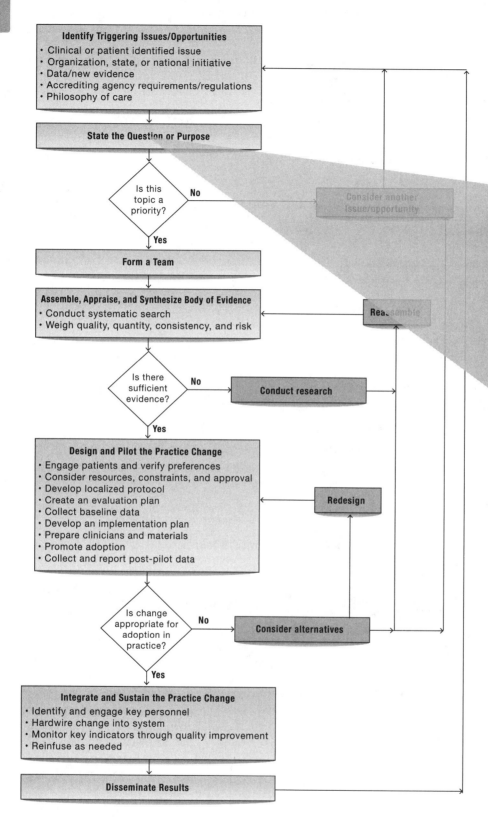

**Identify Triggering Issues/Opportunities**
- Clinical or patient identified issue
- Organization, state, or national initiative
- Data/new evidence
- Accrediting agency requirements/regulations
- Philosophy of care

**State the Question or Purpose**

Is this topic a priority?  **No** → Consider another issue/opportunity

**Yes**

**Form a Team**

**Assemble, Appraise, and Synthesize Body of Evidence**
- Conduct systematic search
- Weigh quality, quantity, consistency, and risk

Reassemble

Is there sufficient evidence?  **No** → **Conduct research**

**Yes**

**Design and Pilot the Practice Change**
- Engage patients and verify preferences
- Consider resources, constraints, and approval
- Develop localized protocol
- Create an evaluation plan
- Collect baseline data
- Develop an implementation plan
- Prepare clinicians and materials
- Promote adoption
- Collect and report post-pilot data

**Redesign**

Is change appropriate for adoption in practice?  **No** → **Consider alternatives**

**Yes**

**Integrate and Sustain the Practice Change**
- Identify and engage key personnel
- Hardwire change into system
- Monitor key indicators through quality improvement
- Reinfuse as needed

**Disseminate Results**

# STATE THE QUESTION OR PURPOSE

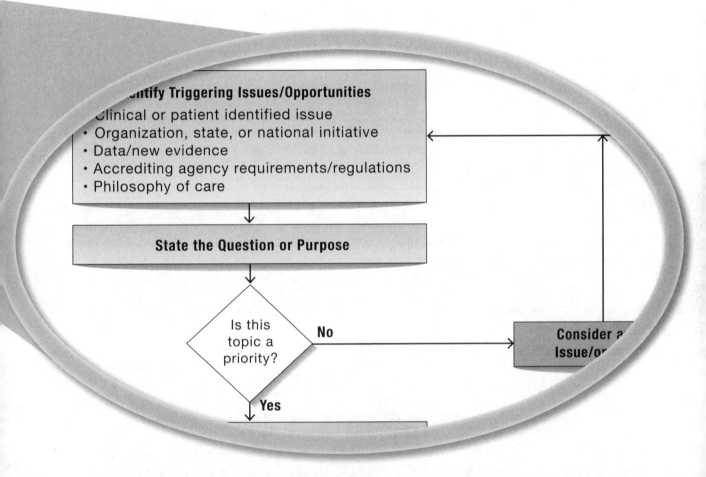

M ost disciplines in health-related fields find that using a consistent method for structuring clinical questions is an important component of evidence-based practice (EBP), whether the use is to guide clinical or research inquiries. In the early 1990s, PICO (P = patient/problem/population, I = intervention, C = comparison, O = outcome) was developed as a means of focusing a broad need for clinical information to a narrower and more focused query (Oxman, Sackett, & Guyatt, 1993; Richardson, Wilson, Nishikawa, & Hayward, 1995). Adaptations to PICO have appeared in the literature to customize it for different needs (see Table 2.1). For example, in this book we use the P to mean patient population/problem/ pilot area, and the term PICOT employs the same elements as PICO with the addition of T = time frame, which can be useful when creating a timeline for short-term projects. Using PICO to identify components of a purpose statement helps articulate important points to include and guides formulation of a focused and clear purpose statement (Rice, 2010; Rios, Ye, & Thabane, 2010).

# Using PICO: When and How

Identifying PICO elements serves two key steps in the EBP process. First is for development of the purpose statement or question. Second is as a guide for the search for evidence. Including PICO elements in a purpose statement creates a comprehensive yet clear intent. Once the team's purpose is agreed upon, the purpose statement becomes the charge to the team for work to accomplish. This statement sets boundaries around the work to accomplish and related issues to avoid. For example, the purpose may be to implement and evaluate use of an evidence-based pain scale for older adults with cognitive impairment. In that case, interventions for pain management are not included in the work to accomplish. Interventions, as an important clinical issue, may be addressed by cycling back to the top of the Iowa Model with an additional EBP improvement that becomes a program for pain management for older adults with cognitive impairment. Use of PICO helps clinicians focus their questions.

Building on PICO elements and using a tool will help to create a purpose statement and plan for an EBP project. Having a clear and focused purpose statement guides all the work that follows and sets boundaries around the charge to the work group (Rice, 2010; Rios et al., 2010). When developing an EBP project plan, it will be helpful to focus your efforts. See Example 2.1 and Tools 2.1 and 2.2 for an example and a worksheet.

The impact of employing PICO or a similar tool on the identification of evidence is somewhat inconsistent, and there may be a need for additional research in this area (Eldredge, Carr, Broudy, & Voorhees, 2008; Hoogendam, de Vries Robbe, & Overbeke, 2012; Schardt et al., 2007). However, the use of the PICO method or an adaptation of it is now advised by many EBP leaders to guide a project purpose, to direct the search process, and to guide project work (McKibbon & Marks, 2001; Schardt et al., 2007; Stillwell, Fineout-Overholt, Melnyk, & Williamson, 2010).

## Table 2.1    Clinical Questions and Domains

| Question Domain | Purpose | Elements | Example | Best Primary Sources of Evidence** |
|---|---|---|---|---|
| Therapy | To determine efficacy of a therapy or an intervention | **P** = patient population/problem/ pilot area<br><br>**I** = intervention<br><br>**C** = comparison with another intervention, no intervention, placebo, usual care<br><br>**O** = outcomes | In older, community-dwelling adults, how effective are assistive devices, compared with usual care, at reducing the frequency of falls? | Randomized controlled trials |
| Etiology* | To identify risk factors/causes of a condition | **P** = patient population/problem/ pilot area<br><br>**I** = intervention or factors<br><br>**O** = outcomes | Are children of mothers with long-standing bipolar disorder at an increased risk of psychological conditions? | Cohort studies |
| Diagnosis | To identify the most effective method for diagnosis | **P** = patient population/problem/ pilot area<br><br>**I** = intervention or test<br><br>**C** = comparison or gold standard<br><br>**O** = outcomes | In preschool-age children with suspected autism, how does the *Autism Diagnostic Observation Schedule* compare with the *Childhood Autism Rating Scale* for accurate diagnosis? | Randomized controlled trials or other controlled experimental studies |
| Prognosis* | To determine the impact of a specific factor on the course of a condition | **P** = patient population/problem/ pilot area<br><br>**I** = intervention or factors<br><br>**O** = outcomes | For individuals with multiple sclerosis, does living in a warm climate affect the number of condition exacerbations? | Cohort studies |
| Meaning* | To understand the experiences of an individual or group | **P** = patients, individuals, communities<br><br>**I** = experiences<br><br>**O** = perceptions | How do parents of physically disabled children believe they can best promote their child's well-being? | Qualitative studies |

* The elements of these question domains may lack a comparison, or "C."
** When available, secondary sources such as high-quality systematic reviews and guidelines may be the strongest level.

Having PICO elements in a purpose statement gives direction to find answers more quickly because it:

- Keeps the team focused

- Defines the scope of the change to the group

- Directs evidence search to best resources

- Helps focus reading

- Assists with developing appropriate implementation and evaluation plan

- Focuses attention on identified learning needs

## TIPS: State the Question or Purpose

- Use the PICO method to configure clinical questions.

- Try regularly putting clinical questions into PICO—it is an excellent EBP habit.

- Use the PICO worksheet or a similar tool *before* you begin other steps in the EBP process.

- Use the PICO method (see Tool 2.2) for focusing the project aim and purpose.

- Be patient. A purpose statement may require time and thought to develop.

- The purpose statement provides direction and boundaries for the team.

## Example 2.1     EBP Purpose Using PICO

### PICO for Falls

| Patient population | ▪ Medical oncology |
|---|---|
| | ▪ In hospital |
| | ▪ Older adults |

| Problem | ▪ Falls |
|---|---|
| | ▪ Fall injury |

| Pilot area | ▪ 4 North Nursing Unit |
|---|---|

| Interventions | ▪ Regular toileting | ▪ Nursing rounds |
|---|---|---|
| | ▪ Ambulation promotion | ▪ Sitters |
| | ▪ Sleep promotion at night | ▪ Q-foam chair |
| | ▪ Safe handling | |

| Comparison | ▪ Pre-/post-implementation groups comparing usual care with EBP |
|---|---|

| Anticipated outcomes | ▪ Better identification of at-risk patients |
|---|---|
| | ▪ Reduced fall rate |
| | ▪ Reduced number of injuries |
| | ▪ Reduced severity of injuries |

### Purpose Statement

The purpose of this evidence-based practice project is to reduce falls on 4 North through implementation of an ambulation and toileting program for older adults with cancer. Fall rates will be compared before and after implementation of the evidence-based ambulation and toileting programs.

### Keywords or Concepts for Identifying and Organizing Literature

| Concept 1: Assistive devices | Concept 2: Falls | Concept 3: Elderly |
|---|---|---|
| Assistive device | Fall | Elderly |
| Ambulation aid | Accident | Older adults |
| Walker | Accidental falls | Seniors |
| Cane | | Aged |

### Inclusion and Exclusion Criteria

▪ Occupational falls/hazards

*continues*

EXAMPLES

TOOLS

## Example 2.1   EBP Purpose Using PICO (Continued)

### Concepts for Organizing Literature

| | |
|---|---|
| Fall risk tools | Toileting |
| Fall risk factor | Ambulation |
| Fall injury risk | Sleep |
| Interventions/preventions | Safe handling |
| Interventions/after a fall | Rounds |
| Interventions/fall injury | Sitters |
| Fall programs | Equipment/chair |
| Older adult | Cancer |

## Tool 2.1   PICO Concepts for Developing a Purpose Statement

**INSTRUCTIONS:** Use this worksheet to explore concepts of interest for your EBP work. Organize using the PICO elements. Begin by identifying a goal or outcome first. Identify potential interventions last; interventions may evolve after reading the evidence. Use all PICO elements to write a purpose statement in one to two sentences. Use PICO elements to identify potential keywords related to the purpose statement.

Patient Population

Clinical Problem or Condition

Pilot Area

Interventions

Comparison

Anticipated Outcomes

### EBP Purpose Statement

### Keywords or Concepts for Identifying and Organizing Literature

## Tool 2.2    PICO Elements for a Purpose Statement and Evidence Search

**INSTRUCTIONS:** Use this worksheet to develop a purpose statement or question. Describe each PICO element addressing the topic of interest. Identify the outcome before considering interventions; interventions may evolve after reading the evidence. Write a purpose statement and determine the kind of question. Use Table 2.1 to identify study designs most likely to answer this question. List related concepts, inclusion and exclusion criteria, and keywords or concepts for organizing evidence.

**Step 1: Define elements or clinical question using PICO:**

P = Patients or population to target: _____

Problem or condition to address: _____

Pilot area (e.g., unit/clinic): _____

I = Intervention (assessment or treatment): _____

C = Comparison: _____

O = Outcomes: _____

T = Time frame (optional): _____

**Step 2: Purpose statement:** _____

_____

**Step 3: Determine what your question is about (circle one):**

Therapy                Diagnosis                Etiology                Prognosis                Meaning

**Step 4: Identify study types that best address your question (circle one or more):**

Experimental studies                Observational studies                Qualitative studies

Systematic review or meta-analysis                Case reports                Other

**Step 5: List the main terms and synonyms for your purpose statement. Typical number of concepts per question is two to three.**

| Concept 1: | Concept 2: | Concept 3: |
|---|---|---|
| | | |

**Step 6: List inclusion and exclusion criteria:** _____

_____

**Step 7: Keywords or concepts for organizing literature:** _____

_____

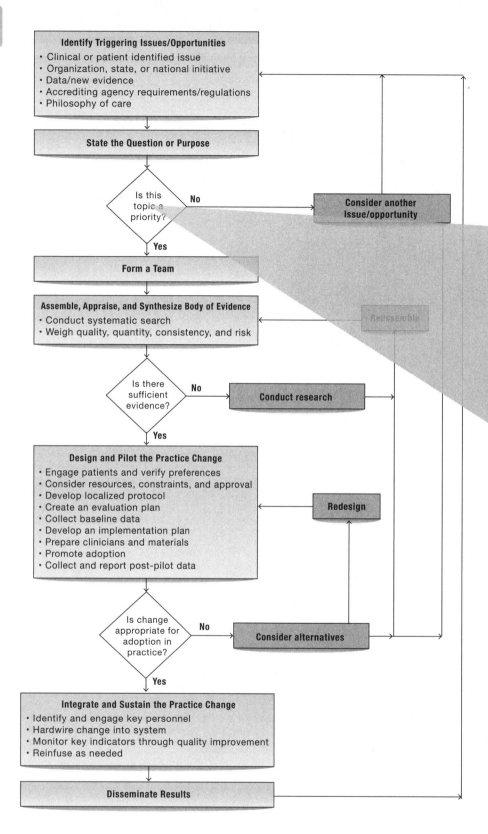

**Identify Triggering Issues/Opportunities**
- Clinical or patient identified issue
- Organization, state, or national initiative
- Data/new evidence
- Accrediting agency requirements/regulations
- Philosophy of care

**State the Question or Purpose**

Is this topic a priority?

**No** → **Consider another Issue/opportunity**

**Yes**

**Form a Team**

**Assemble, Appraise, and Synthesize Body of Evidence**
- Conduct systematic search
- Weigh quality, quantity, consistency, and risk

Reassemble

Is there sufficient evidence?

**No** → **Conduct research**

**Yes**

**Design and Pilot the Practice Change**
- Engage patients and verify preferences
- Consider resources, constraints, and approval
- Develop localized protocol
- Create an evaluation plan
- Collect baseline data
- Develop an implementation plan
- Prepare clinicians and materials
- Promote adoption
- Collect and report post-pilot data

**Redesign**

Is change appropriate for adoption in practice?

**No** → **Consider alternatives**

**Yes**

**Integrate and Sustain the Practice Change**
- Identify and engage key personnel
- Hardwire change into system
- Monitor key indicators through quality improvement
- Reinfuse as needed

**Disseminate Results**

# IS THIS TOPIC A PRIORITY?

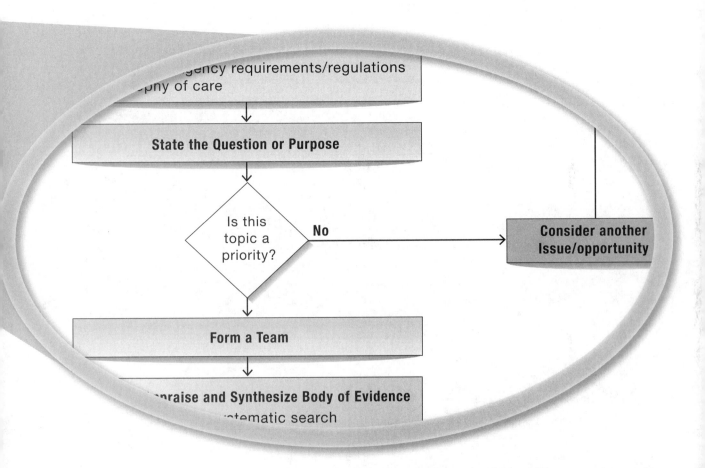

...gency requirements/regulations
...phy of care

**State the Question or Purpose**

Is this topic a priority?

**No** → **Consider another Issue/opportunity**

**Form a Team**

...praise and Synthesize Body of Evidence
...tematic search

*"Often he who does too much does too little."*

–Italian proverb

When a culture of inquiry supports evidence-based practice (EBP), many triggering issues and opportunities will be identified. In fact, it is often the case that there are far more questions than resources available to address them. A number of criteria can be used to determine whether the purpose of the EBP project matches organizational priorities (see Figure 3.1). Considering departmental priorities, the existing infrastructure, and available resources may be helpful (Braithwaite, Marks, & Taylor, 2014; Clay-Williams, Nosrati, Cunningham, Hillman, & Braithwaite, 2014; Fleiszer, Semenic, Ritchie, Richer, & Denis, 2016a).

**Figure 3.1**    Indications for Deciding: Is This Topic a Priority?

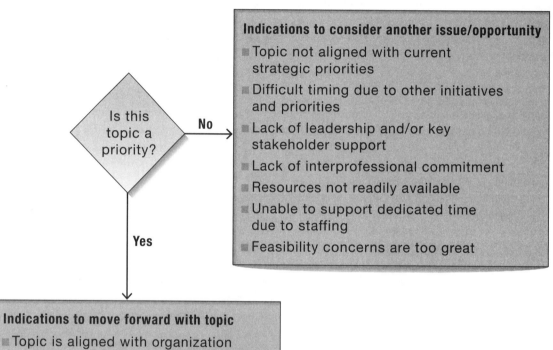

Is this topic a priority?

**No**

**Indications to consider another issue/opportunity**
- Topic not aligned with current strategic priorities
- Difficult timing due to other initiatives and priorities
- Lack of leadership and/or key stakeholder support
- Lack of interprofessional commitment
- Resources not readily available
- Unable to support dedicated time due to staffing
- Feasibility concerns are too great

**Yes**

**Indications to move forward with topic**
- Topic is aligned with organization strategic priorities
- Topic relates to safety issue
- Leadership support exists
- Interprofessional commitment and engagement
- Resources available
- Patient volume and staffing level support clinician time and involvement
- Project is feasible to implement
- Data are available to evaluate the topic

Clinicians can identify organizational priorities in a number of ways (see Tool 3.1). The nursing and organizational strategic plans identify priorities, responsibilities, strategies for achieving them, and metrics for evaluating progress (Hauck, Winsett, & Kuric, 2013). Executive announcements and annual reports provide insight into priorities of organizational leaders. Core metrics, national patient safety goals, and publicly reported quality and safety data are an ongoing priority with resources, expertise, and an infrastructure to support continuous improvement (Centers for Medicare & Medicaid Services, 2017; The Joint Commission, 2017a). Additional organizational initiatives (e.g., facility or program expansion) have an associated investment that makes them priorities with implications for EBP (Sandström, Borglin, Nilsson, & Willman, 2011). However, other priorities may develop as healthcare needs, standards, and funding evolve (Centers for Disease Control and Prevention [CDC], 2017b; CDC, 2017c).

After developing a clear purpose statement for the EBP initiative, consider how to link to existing and emerging priorities. When developing a link between the EBP purpose and key priorities, consider:

- Scope of the problem described in research

- Impact on patient quality of life or health disparity

- Economic burden (e.g., lost work days, related disability, quality adjusted life-year, length of stay, readmission)

- Relevance to current practice or setting

This step in the EBP process supports early partnering with key stakeholders and eventual sustainment of the resulting practice improvement (Ellen et al., 2013; Fleiszer et al., 2016a). Talking points or a brief EBP project proposal could be developed to share with key stakeholders (see Tool 3.2). For example, use elements of a business case to clearly describe the EBP as a priority to garner senior leadership support (Williams, Perillo, & Brown, 2015).

## RESOURCES: Creating a Business Case

| Description | Source |
|---|---|
| How to write a business proposal in 5 easy steps | http://fitsmallbusiness.com/how-to-write-a-business-proposal/ |
| Making a business case for change management | https://www.prosci.com/change-management/thought-leadership-library/making-a-business-case-for-change-management |
| Write your way to a win: Business proposal 101 | https://www.business.com/articles/write-your-way-to-a-win-business-proposal-101/ |

Project work will benefit from taking the time to match the purpose of the EBP work with organizational priorities (see Tool 3.3). These early partnerships with key stakeholders about the practice change may build links within the system (Hauck et al., 2013; Lavoie-Tremblay et al., 2015; Lowson et al., 2015). Team leaders can benefit from the planning for this step by identification of team members, committees, and infrastructure that will facilitate project work (see Chapter 4).

If the topic is not a priority, a feedback loop provides guidance for moving forward. At this point, consider another issue or opportunity that is a better match for the setting. Consider revising the business case and revisiting stakeholders.

### TIPS: Determining Organizational Priorities

- Identify key criteria or reports for determining organizational priorities (for example, strategic plan).
- Identify how priorities are determined.
- Involve key stakeholders.
- Work with the EBP committee to identify local stakeholders or for assistance with establishing the topic priority.
- Maintain a transparent selection process.

## Tool 3.1   Determining if Topic Is a Priority

**INSTRUCTIONS:** This worksheet is designed to help you determine whether a new clinical or operational question is a priority for your setting or organization. Use it individually, in groups, or as a point for discussion when reviewing the EBP purpose statement.

1. To what extent do you agree that this topic:

| | | Strongly Agree | Agree | Disagree | Strongly Disagree |
|---|---|---|---|---|---|
| a) | Addresses a common or high-priority problem in our practice or setting | 1 | 2 | 3 | 4 |
| b) | Is relevant to patients' preferences for care and/or quality of life | 1 | 2 | 3 | 4 |
| c) | Has an economic burden associated with it (e.g., readmission, lost work time) | 1 | 2 | 3 | 4 |
| d) | Is likely to improve processes or patient outcomes in our practice or setting | 1 | 2 | 3 | 4 |
| e) | Would improve safety for our patients, their families, clinicians, or other staff | 1 | 2 | 3 | 4 |
| f) | Has new evidence or quality data that identify a need to change | 1 | 2 | 3 | 4 |
| g) | Provides an opportunity for innovative practice improvement | 1 | 2 | 3 | 4 |

2. To what extent would this be a priority based on:

| | | Low | | High | | Don't Know |
|---|---|---|---|---|---|---|
| a) | Matches organizational or department strategic plan | 1 | 2 | 3 | 4 | |
| b) | Matches messages from executives | 1 | 2 | 3 | 4 | |
| c) | Is linked to an established core metric | 1 | 2 | 3 | 4 | |
| d) | Is part of a new initiative | 1 | 2 | 3 | 4 | |
| e) | Is a publicly reported measure | 1 | 2 | 3 | 4 | |
| f) | Addresses an accreditation or regulatory standard | 1 | 2 | 3 | 4 | |
| g) | Has an established sponsor or is part of a supported training program (e.g., EBP internship, leadership training) | 1 | 2 | 3 | 4 | |

3. Are there any other considerations for determining the priority for this topic?

_____

_____

## Tool 3.2    Linking EBP Topic With Organizational Priorities

**INSTRUCTIONS:** Write the purpose statement at the top. Identify the scope of the problem (e.g., consider patient volume), using data where possible. Identify where the topic and scope of the problem match elements in the next sections. Identify the sponsor or sponsoring program, as an additional indication the topic matches stakeholder priorities.

### EBP Purpose Statement or Goal

### Scope of the Problem

### Organizational Considerations

☐    Links to organization mission/vision/values or initiatives (specify):

☐    Existing data–data source:

☐    Gap analysis or organizational assessment:

### Impact for Patient and/or Family

☐    Matches patient preferences:

☐    Impact on quality of life:

☐    Other:

### Economic Considerations

☐    Hospital costs (e.g., readmission, length of stay):

☐    Patient and/or family costs (e.g., lost work time):

☐    Resource requirements:

☐    Other:

### Established Sponsorship

☐    Sponsor:

☐    Program:

## Tool 3.3  EBP Topic Selection

**INSTRUCTIONS:** Identify topics of interest to patients or families, clinicians, or teams. Use more than one sheet if many topics have been identified. Individually review the topics and select a rating; rate each topic using a 0–10 scale (0 = Not at all; 10 = Exceptional). Tally a total score for each topic. Share scores as a group. Discuss the rationale for selecting highest scoring topics. Make a selection as a group.

| Review Criteria | Criteria Met/ Points | Topic 1 | Topic 2 | Topic 3 |
|---|---|---|---|---|
| Topic addresses a departmental or organizational priority | 0–10 | | | |
| Priority for the patient population or the unit | 0–10 | | | |
| Topic is an issue that is amenable to being addressed through the EBP process (versus research) and addresses quality or safety | 0–10 | | | |
| Magnitude of the problem for the population (e.g., high risk or high volume) | 0–10 | | | |
| Sufficient evidence available to guide practice | 0–10 | | | |
| Likelihood of improving patient, family, clinician, or fiscal outcomes | 0–10 | | | |
| Sufficient team/interprofessional support or is linked to the work of an existing committee or work group | 0–10 | | | |
| Sufficient resources (e.g., patient health record data, data management for evaluation, reporting, equipment, purchase mailing list, clinical expertise) | 0–10 | | | |
| Other criteria: | 0–10 | | | |
| Rating scale: 0 = Not at all; 10 = Exceptional | Total score(s): | | | |

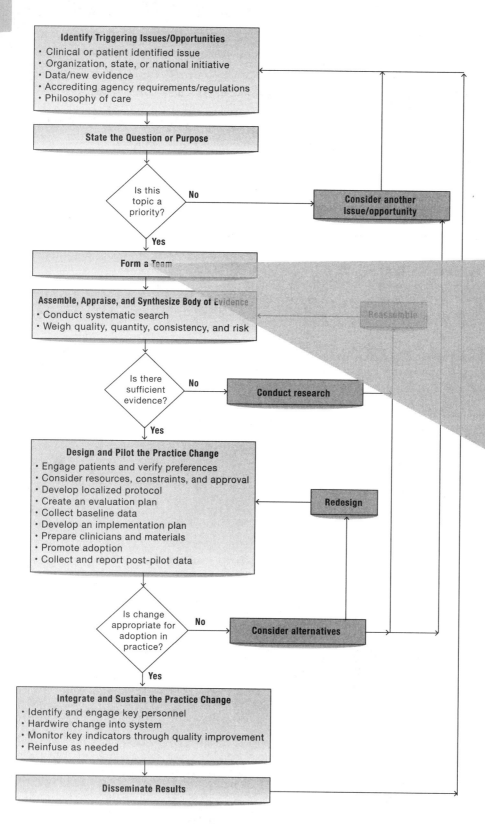

**Identify Triggering Issues/Opportunities**
- Clinical or patient identified issue
- Organization, state, or national initiative
- Data/new evidence
- Accrediting agency requirements/regulations
- Philosophy of care

**State the Question or Purpose**

Is this topic a priority?

**No** → **Consider another issue/opportunity**

**Yes**

**Form a Team**

**Assemble, Appraise, and Synthesize Body of Evidence**
- Conduct systematic search
- Weigh quality, quantity, consistency, and risk

Reassemble

Is there sufficient evidence?

**No** → **Conduct research**

**Yes**

**Design and Pilot the Practice Change**
- Engage patients and verify preferences
- Consider resources, constraints, and approval
- Develop localized protocol
- Create an evaluation plan
- Collect baseline data
- Develop an implementation plan
- Prepare clinicians and materials
- Promote adoption
- Collect and report post-pilot data

**Redesign**

Is change appropriate for adoption in practice?

**No** → **Consider alternatives**

**Yes**

**Integrate and Sustain the Practice Change**
- Identify and engage key personnel
- Hardwire change into system
- Monitor key indicators through quality improvement
- Reinfuse as needed

**Disseminate Results**

# FORM A TEAM

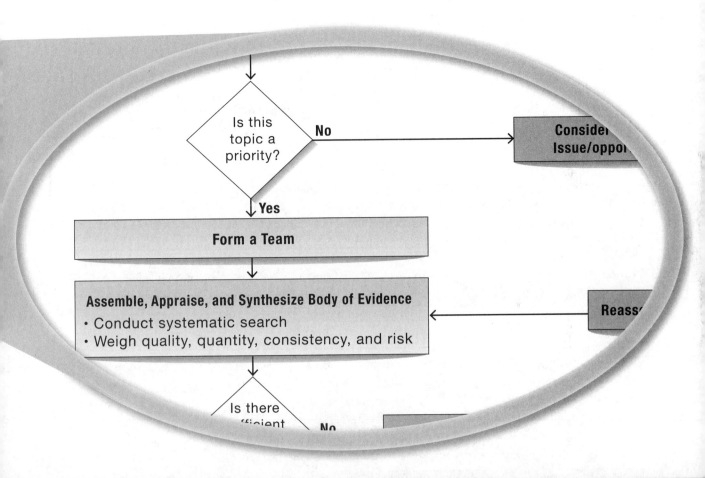

"*I am a member of a team, and I rely on the team, I defer to it and sacrifice for it, because the team, not the individual, is the ultimate champion.*"

—Mia Hamm

The importance of forming a carefully constructed team early in the evidence-based practice (EBP) process cannot be overstated. We all recognize that healthcare is provided by teams. Failing to include key players at the beginning of the EBP process can slow progress. These team-structure factors have an impact on success (Xyrichis & Lowton, 2008):

- Location: People who work near each other may find it easier to attend meetings and stay up to date with communications.

- Size of the team: Smaller teams are more efficient than teams that are too large. This is a balancing act between having every stakeholder involved and keeping the team size manageable.

- Composition: Interprofessional diversity and skill mix are important.

- Communication: All members need to feel safe in expressing their views, regardless of their position in the organization.

- Stability: EBP projects can take a long time to organize, roll out, and sustain. It is important to have team members who will stay the course and commit to the project in the long run.

- Leadership: Appoint a leader or project director who will keep projects on track and keep members accountable.

When developing the team, think about disciplines to involve (for example, physical therapy, social services); representation across roles (nursing assistants, radiology technicians); services impacted by a practice change (pharmacy, housekeeping); and relevant committee members within the governance structure (quality improvement, information technology). Keep the team balanced with skills and the ability to influence. Look for members having a positive effect on colleagues who can influence their peers. Clinicians who are opinion leaders (see Strategy 2-6) can bring important energy to promote adoption of EBP. Your choice of participants will affect how the team functions as a whole (Porter-O'Grady, Alexander, Baylock, Minkara, & Surel, 2006). A team communication wheel may be useful for planning membership and coordinating efforts within the infrastructure (see Example 4.1).

Identify strategies for building collaboration with and support from key stakeholders (Issel, 2014) who are invested in the practice and may contribute resources for the EBP (*Harvard Business Review*, 2004). Stakeholders will have varying involvement with project work, yet all will want progress reports so they can stay up to date. The amount of influence and support from stakeholders will vary. Strategies to build a team including different stakeholders may be developed based on their level of influence and support (AHRQ, n.d.-b; Registered Nurses' Association of Ontario, 2012).

EBP team members can divide the workload associated with the EBP process. They will need to have an understanding of the evidence supporting the practice change and their roles and responsibilities to support implementation (Gifford, Davies, Tourangeau, & Lefebre, 2011). Effective communication and coordination strategies are needed to keep team meetings focused on the purpose and to use time effectively (Taylor, Clay-Williams, Hogden, Braithwaite, & Groene, 2015). Timelines and action plans (see Tools 4.1, 4.2, and Example 4.2) help the team move through the steps of the EBP process. A useful example of a fully developed action plan was published by Clutter, Reed, Cornett, and Parsons (2009).

The plan specifies:

- What needs to be done

- Step-by-step action needed to complete it

- Who is responsible for each action

- When the action needs to be completed

- Activities (e.g., inservices) that will be done

- Criteria used to judge the success of the action

Action plans are an effective way to improve coordination and divide the work.

Attention to coordination and collaboration is critical for creating the most effective team (Bosch et al., 2009). It is important to establish expectations or ground rules for teams (see Example 4.3). Enhancing the expertise of clinicians within the system is an investment in future EBP work and integration of the practice change (Forsner et al., 2010). Combining clinical and process experts or teams with characteristics of change agents leads to continuous improvement in patient care and healthcare outcomes (Driessen et al., 2010).

Teamwork can be quite effective in moving the change process along. The EBP team can help maintain momentum with commitment and a positive attitude. Problems must be regarded as opportunities for learning. When designing a strategy to address challenges, be creative and always look for simple solutions first. EBP can take persistence, so keep moving forward.

## TIPS: Forming a Team

- Keep the team to a workable size.

- Have a clear purpose for the project and objectives for the meetings.

- Provide agendas.

- Consider identifying a facilitator to function as a knowledge translator/"sense-maker" to run the meetings.

- Regularly review or evaluate effectiveness of the team.

- Keep moving forward despite challenges.

- Choose a standing meeting time.

- Use the action plan as a working tool to help the team track work accomplished and focus on next steps.

- Regard problems as opportunities for team learning.

- When addressing challenges and designing the practice change, look for easy solutions first.

- Keep unit colleagues, leaders, and stakeholders informed of team activities and provide regular reports to quality improvement (QI).

- Report progress to QI and other committees as needed.

**EXAMPLES**

**TOOLS**

## Example 4.1    Team Representation and Communication Wheel

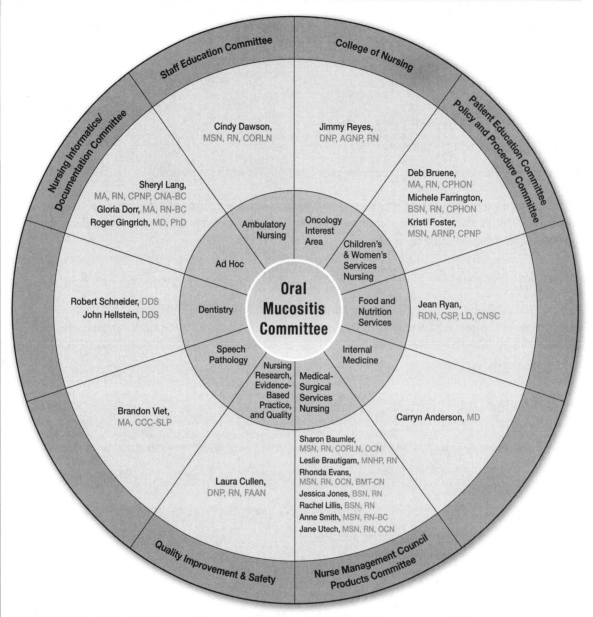

NOTE: At the UI Hospitals and Clinics, mucositis was a problem in several nursing divisions (adult, pediatric, and ambulatory services) and involved multiple departments (nursing, medicine, speech pathology, dentistry, and food services). Hospital-based committees that provided key support in developing, implementing, and tracking the protocol included patient education, quality improvement, and patient health records. A representative from the College of Nursing oncology interest group was included to expand the expertise of the team. With many team members based in different parts of the institution and university, having the communication wheel helped to ensure that no one was left out and that all viewpoints were considered.

This team communication wheel demonstrates how members of the Oral Mucositis Committee represented clinical areas and committees within the infrastructure. Team members are listed with bi-directional communication to clinical areas and essential committees.

Created: 8/11/11; Revised: 1/17/12
© Used with permission
(Cullen, Hanrahan, Tucker, Rempel, & Jordan, 2012)

## Example 4.2   EBP Project Timeline

**INSTRUCTIONS:** Insert the month as a header for each numbered column. Review the steps in the process and add any additional steps that would be helpful. Shade boxes for each step that correspond to the anticipated month it will be completed.

MONTH

| Activity | 1 | 2 | 3 | 4 | 5 | 6 | 7 | 8 | 9 | 10 | 11 | 12 | 13 | 14 | 15 | 16 | 17 |
|---|---|---|---|---|---|---|---|---|---|---|---|---|---|---|---|---|---|
| Define EBP purpose and team | ■ | ■ |  |  |  |  |  |  |  |  |  |  |  |  |  |  |  |
| Assemble, appraise, and synthesize evidence |  |  | ■ | ■ |  |  |  |  |  |  |  |  |  |  |  |  |  |
| Design practice change |  |  |  |  | ■ |  |  |  |  |  |  |  |  |  |  |  |  |
| Plan pilot and create resource materials |  |  |  |  |  | ■ |  |  |  |  |  |  |  |  |  |  |  |
| Collect baseline data |  |  |  |  |  | ■ |  |  |  |  |  |  |  |  |  |  |  |
| Prepare change agents |  |  |  |  |  |  | ■ |  |  |  |  |  |  |  |  |  |  |
| Prepare clinicians |  |  |  |  |  |  |  | ■ |  |  |  |  |  |  |  |  |  |
| Implement |  |  |  |  |  |  |  |  |  | ■ |  |  |  | ■ | ■ | ■ | ■ |
| Evaluate post-pilot |  |  |  |  |  |  |  |  |  |  |  | ■ | ■ |  |  |  |  |
| Begin project reporting |  |  |  |  |  |  |  |  |  |  |  |  | ■ |  |  |  |  |
| Begin project integration and continue monitoring |  |  |  |  |  |  |  |  |  |  |  |  |  | ■ | ■ | ■ | ■ |

| Strategy 1 Implement strategies to create awareness and interest. | Strategy 2 Implement strategies to build knowledge and commitment. | Strategy 3 Implement strategies to promote action and adoption. | Strategy 4 Implement strategies to pursue integration and sustainability. |
|---|---|---|---|

Go Live ↗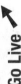

**NOTE:** EBP is not a linear process. Strategies often overlap, and time frames may need to be adjusted.

## Example 4.3    Ground Rules for Teamwork

- Create an official launch with:
  - An announcement of support from senior leaders, sponsors, and key stakeholders
  - An acknowledgment of each team member by name and credentials
  - A description of purpose
  - A description of the importance of work and how it fits organizational goals
  - Available resources described
- Schedule regular meetings (date, time, and location).
- Conflicts are identified before meeting, whenever possible.
- Agenda is sent allowing for pre-meeting preparation.
- Meetings are canceled when appropriate.
- Agenda, minutes, and action plan are posted on shared site for team members.
- Attendance is expected and meetings begin on time.
- Keep discussion focused on objective at hand and overall purpose of team.
- Limit interruptions from electronic devices.
- Listen actively.
- Establish precedent that no issue is off-limits.
- Welcome constructive criticism.
- Maintain some team discussions as confidential.
- Decision-making is done by consensus, unless deferred to a task force or otherwise noted.
- Meetings generate action steps, with written follow-up.

(*Harvard Business Review*, 2004)

## Tool 4.1 EBP Project Timeline

**INSTRUCTIONS:** Insert the month as a header for each numbered column. Review the steps in the process and add any additional steps that would be helpful. Shade boxes for each step that correspond to the anticipated month it will be completed.

| Activity | MONTH 1 | 2 | 3 | 4 | 5 | 6 | 7 | 8 | 9 | 10 | 11 | 12 | 13 | 14 | 15 | 16 | 17 |
|---|---|---|---|---|---|---|---|---|---|---|---|---|---|---|---|---|---|
| Define EBP purpose and team | | | | | | | | | | | | | | | | | |
| Assemble, appraise, and synthesize evidence | | | | | | | | | | | | | | | | | |
| Design practice change | | | | | | | | | | | | | | | | | |
| Plan pilot and create resource materials | | | | | | | | | | | | | | | | | |
| Collect baseline data | | | | | | | | | | | | | | | | | |
| Prepare change agents | | | | | | | | | | | | | | | | | |
| Prepare clinicians | | | | | | | | | | | | | | | | | |
| Implement | | | | | | | | | | | | | | | | | |
| Evaluate post-pilot | | | | | | | | | | | | | | | | | |
| Begin project reporting | | | | | | | | | | | | | | | | | |
| Begin project integration and continue monitoring | | | | | | | | | | | | | | | | | |

Go Live ➤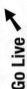

**Strategy 1** Implement strategies to create awareness and interest.

**Strategy 2** Implement strategies to build knowledge and commitment.

**Strategy 3** Implement strategies to promote action and adoption.

**Strategy 4** Implement strategies to pursue integration and sustainability.

**NOTE:** EBP is not a linear process. Strategies often overlap, and time frames may need to be adjusted.

## Tool 4.2    General Action Plan

**INSTRUCTIONS:** Identify key steps or objectives from the EBP process model. For each key step, add multiple activities that will be needed to complete that step. For each activity, list a specific person responsible, materials or resources needed, an anticipated timeline for completion, and an evaluative metric indicating successful completion (see Strategy 2-22).

**Project director name:**          **Team:**

**Project purpose:**

| Key Step or Objective | Specific Activities to Meet Objective | Person Responsible | Materials or Resources Needed | Timeline | Evaluation |
|---|---|---|---|---|---|
| | | | | | |
| | | | | | |
| | | | | | |
| | | | | | |
| | | | | | |

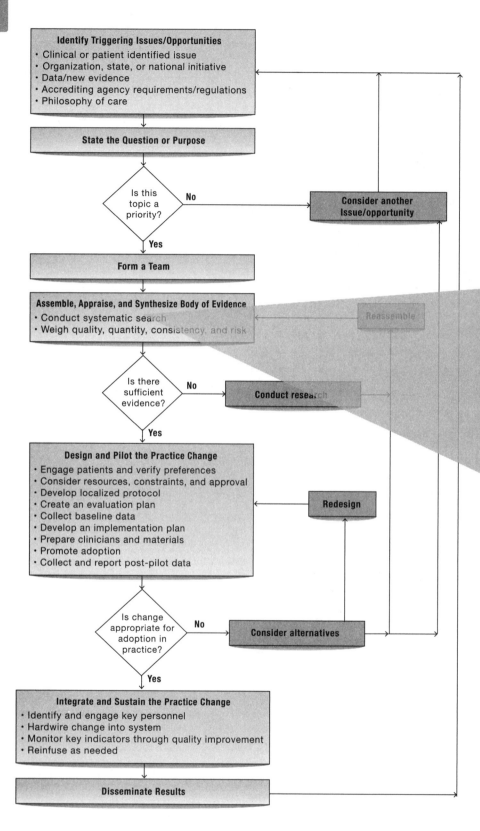

**Identify Triggering Issues/Opportunities**
- Clinical or patient identified issue
- Organization, state, or national initiative
- Data/new evidence
- Accrediting agency requirements/regulations
- Philosophy of care

**State the Question or Purpose**

Is this topic a priority?

No → **Consider another Issue/opportunity**

Yes

**Form a Team**

**Assemble, Appraise, and Synthesize Body of Evidence**
- Conduct systematic search
- Weigh quality, quantity, consistency, and risk

Reassemble

Is there sufficient evidence?

No → **Conduct research**

Yes

**Design and Pilot the Practice Change**
- Engage patients and verify preferences
- Consider resources, constraints, and approval
- Develop localized protocol
- Create an evaluation plan
- Collect baseline data
- Develop an implementation plan
- Prepare clinicians and materials
- Promote adoption
- Collect and report post-pilot data

**Redesign**

Is change appropriate for adoption in practice?

No → **Consider alternatives**

Yes

**Integrate and Sustain the Practice Change**
- Identify and engage key personnel
- Hardwire change into system
- Monitor key indicators through quality improvement
- Reinfuse as needed

**Disseminate Results**

# ASSEMBLE, APPRAISE, AND SYNTHESIZE BODY OF EVIDENCE

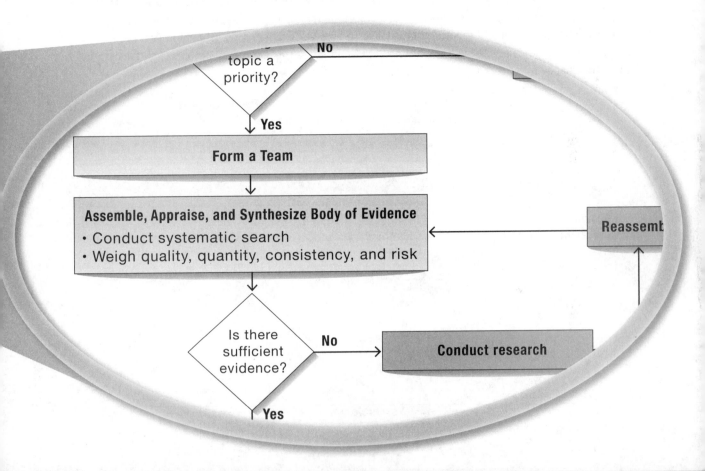

"The search for truth is in one way hard and in another way easy, for it is evident that no one can master it fully or miss it wholly. But each adds a little to our knowledge of nature, and from all the facts assembled there arises a certain grandeur."

–Aristotle

**A**fter you select your priority topic (Chapters 1–3) and form a team (Chapter 4), you will begin to search and assemble the literature, appraise articles, and synthesize the body of evidence. This step in the evidence-based practice (EBP) process can seem daunting. Follow an organized process and use tools provided in this chapter to keep the work organized and the tasks manageable. The project direction may evolve during evidence synthesis, as the interventions and outcomes in the literature inform the project purpose. Therefore, literature assembly, appraisal, and synthesis may not be linear, but rather a series of loops (see Figure 5.1). Stay focused to advance through the process. Project leaders need advanced leadership, project management, and delegation skills to manage tasks and distribute the workload. Appraisal and synthesis of evidence is a shared responsibility of the EBP team. Involving the EBP team creates a learning environment and also helps team members understand the science supporting practice change. A group approach also shares the work, helps to balance intellectual biases, and capitalizes on individual expertise. The goal is to create practice recommendations supported by the body of evidence, using a transparent and reproducible process. The evidence will arm the team with citations and research sound bites (see Strategy 1-3) to use in implementing the practice change with peers and across disciplines.

**Figure 5.1**    Assemble, Appraise, and Synthesize Process
for Identifying the Body of Evidence

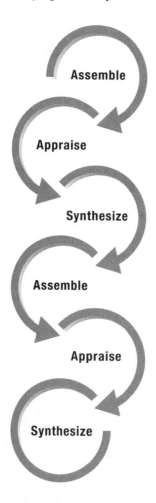

# Assemble

In conducting a search for evidence, follow a prescribed systematic process, such as a checklist, to stay organized and promote efficient use of time (see Tool 5.1). The assistance of a skilled health science librarian to design the search will increase the efficiency and yield the most relevant evidence (Deberg & Egeland, 2014; Flynn & McGuinness, 2011; Krom, Batten, & Bautista, 2010). Alternatively, user-friendly tutorials are available for developing your own search skills.

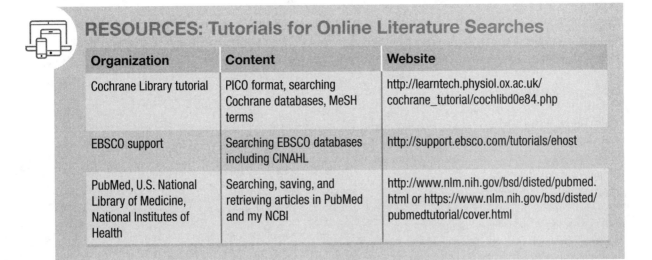

**RESOURCES: Tutorials for Online Literature Searches**

| Organization | Content | Website |
|---|---|---|
| Cochrane Library tutorial | PICO format, searching Cochrane databases, MeSH terms | http://learntech.physiol.ox.ac.uk/cochrane_tutorial/cochlibd0e84.php |
| EBSCO support | Searching EBSCO databases including CINAHL | http://support.ebsco.com/tutorials/ehost |
| PubMed, U.S. National Library of Medicine, National Institutes of Health | Searching, saving, and retrieving articles in PubMed and my NCBI | http://www.nlm.nih.gov/bsd/disted/pubmed.html or https://www.nlm.nih.gov/bsd/disted/pubmedtutorial/cover.html |

The PICO components (Patient population/problem/pilot area, Intervention, Comparison, and Outcome) from the purpose statement provide a guide to identify the most relevant literature search terms (see Chapter 2). The PICO statement will also guide the development of the basic inclusion and exclusion criteria for the search. Advanced search mechanisms are useful for combining terms. Medical Subject Headings (or MeSH terms) comprise the U.S. National Library of Medicine's standardized vocabulary (U. S. National Library of Medicine, 2008). Subject terms are useful for the searcher who is interested in searching by concept, which can enhance the relevance of search results and ensure that the search is comprehensive. Subject terms are assigned by indexers, who read entire articles and tag them from a predetermined list of headings. The MeSH browser (https://www.nlm.nih.gov/mesh/meshhome.html) is one example of a subject vocabulary and is freely available. It may be used to find descriptors, qualifiers, or concepts of interest and to see those terms in a hierarchical classification system structure (see Example 5.1). This example for pressure injury highlights the value of understanding and using established terms as these evolve and may not match local language. Other databases have different subject heading structures to organize the content, dependent on the journals and subjects included.

The scope for a search strategy will also be directed by the volume of literature available on the topic (see Table 5.1). Setting limits will affect the literature identified. Caution is advised to avoid premature elimination of articles.

## Table 5.1   Managing a Literature Search With Varying Amounts of Evidence

| Many Articles, High Quality | Few Articles, Low Quality |
|---|---|
| Inclusion criteria help to focus the topic or population: for example, peripheral IV catheters in children. | Perform the search using each concept separately. |
| Exclusion criteria further limit the population and research included, such as limiting the search to only meta-analysis, synthesis reports, or reports of guideline adherence. | Think outside the box for search terms because current terminology may have evolved over the years. |
| Narrow the search by strategically adding terms and combining with AND; consider reducing the number of terms combined with OR. | Use the "scope note" function within CINAHL to search for terms. |
| Consider narrowing the topic. | If a relevant article is found, identify the MeSH terms used for that article and search for them. |
| Limit lower levels of evidence such as expert opinions and case reports. | Do not set limits. Cast a wide net, and then refine the search as needed. |
| Organize the literature based on design of the studies included. | Be particularly careful to not set limits for only a few "most recent" years, because some literature will be missed. |
| Use subject terms and consider designating as a "major subject," which will restrict results to records that have been determined to be chiefly about the concept. | Use reference lists and "related article" searches to identify additional literature (i.e., the snowball method). |
| Consider narrowing to more recent studies with caution (e.g., those published after a high quality clinical practice guideline). | Popular consumer search engines (e.g., Google and Bing) may help to identify terms to use in scholarly bibliographic databases. |

Begin by searching the National Guideline Clearinghouse (NGC) for existing evidence-based guidelines (AHRQ, 2013a; NGC, 2011). The NGC is a federally funded resource for guidelines from around the world and is available from the Agency for Healthcare Research and Quality (AHRQ). Other international agencies offer quality clinical practice guidelines (CPGs), synthesis reports, or provide recommendations. However, online sources are rapidly emerging and frequently change content; therefore, a search for new evidence-based online resources is generally recommended. Large electronic databases such as CINAHL, Medline Plus, and PubMed are generally searched next. Systematic reviews may be located at Cochrane Library (http://www.cochranelibrary.com), the Joanna Briggs Institute Database of Systematic Reviews and Implementation Reports (http://journals.lww.com/jbisrir/pages/default.aspx), and the Campbell Collaboration Library (http://www.campbellcollaboration.org/library.html) or by setting search limits in certain bibliographic databases (e.g., PubMed has meta-analyses and scientific integrative reviews, and CINAHL has systematic reviews). Query professional organization websites for position statements with practice recommendations and/or CPGs (e.g., Oncology Nursing Society, American Association of Critical-Care Nurses). Revisiting the search is often helpful when the team is synthesizing the evidence to verify completeness of the evidence review. Consider grouping retrieved literature by type: a) CPGs, b) systematic reviews and other synthesis reports (by study design), c) research reports (by study design), d) theory articles, and e) clinical reviews.

## RESOURCES: Literature Search Engines

### EBP Guidelines

| Resource | Description | Source |
|---|---|---|
| Institute for Clinical Systems Improvement | The nonprofit ICSI organization supports and promotes the use of evidence-based healthcare in all of its scientific documents and advances improvement in patient safety and efficiency. | http://www.icsi.org<br>https://www.icsi.org/guidelines__more |
| Joanna Briggs Institute | JBI is an international, not-for-profit, membership-based, research-and-development organization based within the Faculty of Health Sciences at the University of Adelaide, Australia. | http://joannabriggs.org<br>http://journals.lww.com/jbisrir/Pages/default.aspx |
| National Guideline Clearinghouse | NGC is a public resource for summaries of evidence-based clinical practice guidelines, funded by AHRQ. | https://www.guideline.gov/ |
| National Institute for Health and Care Excellence | NICE is an independent organization responsible for providing national guidance on promoting good health and preventing and treating ill health. | http://www.nice.org.uk<br>https://www.nice.org.uk/guidance |
| University of Iowa College of Nursing | EBP guidelines are produced by and distributed through the University of Iowa College of Nursing. | http://www.iowanursingguidelines.com |
| Guidelines International Network | G-I-N is a global network whose library contains more than 6,400 guidelines, evidence reports, and related documents that have been developed or endorsed by organizational members of G-I-N. | http://www.g-i-n.net/library/international-guidelines-library |
| Registered Nurses' Association of Ontario | RNAO evidence-based practice guidelines are sponsored by the government of Ontario. | http://rnao.ca/bpg |
| U.S. Department of Veterans Affairs and the Department of Defense Clinical Practice Guidelines | VA/DoD develops government-sponsored guidelines on topics for implementation of evidence-based indicators based on high-cost, high-volume, high-risk, and problem conditions. | http://www.healthquality.va.gov |
| U.S. Preventive Services Task Force | USPSTF is an independent panel of experts in primary care and prevention who systematically review the evidence of effectiveness and develop recommendations for clinical preventive services. | http://www.uspreventiveservicestaskforce.org |

*continues*

## RESOURCES: Literature Search Engines (Continued)

| Systematic Reviews | | |
|---|---|---|
| **Resource** | **Description** | **Source** |
| Campbell Library | This international research network produces systematic reviews of the effects of social interventions. | https://www.campbellcollaboration. org/library.html |
| Cochrane | Cochrane provides systematic reviews of primary research in human healthcare and healthcare policy. | http://www.cochrane.org/evidence |
| **Large Database Search Engines** | | |
| Cumulative Index to Nursing and Allied Health Literature | CINAHL Plus with full text; indexes over 5,000 journals from the fields of nursing and allied health, with indexing back to 1937. | https://health.ebsco.com/products/ cinahl-plus-with-full-text |
| MedlinePlus National Library of Medicine National Institutes of Health | MedlinePlus provides information about diseases, conditions, and wellness issues. | http://www.nlm.nih.gov/medlineplus |
| PubMed, U.S. National Library of Medicine, National Institutes of Health | PubMed provides more than 26 million citations for biomedical literature from MEDLINE, life science journals, and online books. | http://www.ncbi.nlm.nih.gov/ pubmed |

Assembling evidence is about creating order. Keep good records of how search terms and strategies are combined with operators (AND, OR, NOT) and limits, inclusions, and exclusions for each database or website, as well as the date of searches and yield. Some databases will track and save searches for you. A tracking record for multiple searches is important for duplicating and reporting the search strategies and yields (see Tool 5.2). Develop initial criteria for inclusion or exclusion of studies before you begin appraising. Consider having two reviewers from the team screen each abstract for relevance according to inclusion/exclusion criteria and to determine the general type of evidence. Most research abstracts are incomplete (Assadi, Zarghi, Shamloo, & Nikooiyan, 2012); if in doubt about inclusion, read the full article before deciding. Continue to track articles included and excluded in your search, and maintain a complete reference list as well as full articles for those you decide to include or read. Create a standard method for labeling articles to make retrieval easier (e.g., name of first author, subject, study design, year).

## TIPS: Assembling Evidence

- Find a medical librarian to help you.

- Use PICO components to identify potential terms (keywords or subject headings) to use in the search.

- Find a relevant article, identify the MeSH terms used for that article, and then use those terms to find other articles.

- Narrow or broaden the scope of your search strategy based on the volume and quality of literature available on the topic (see Table 5.1).

- Use a combination of subject terms and keywords for the most comprehensive approach to searching. Be aware that the terms used may have a significant impact on the evidence captured.

- Partner with a medical librarian to get the best yield.

- Use subject terms and consider designating key terms as a "major subject," which will restrict results to records that have been determined to be chiefly about the concept.

- Look for CPGs first.

- Consider the credibility of the source or bibliographic database before using it.

- Consumer search engines (such as Google and Bing) indicate what is in the popular media, but sources often lack credibility, and therefore are not usually the best ways to begin a search.

- Advanced search strategies within consumer search engines may be helpful in identifying and eliminating poor-quality or market-driven websites.

- Consider using software (such as EndNote or RefWorks) for reference management. Your institution may provide this software for free or at reduced cost.

- Use a consistent process for naming reference files (e.g., first author, subject, and year), and save in folders by topic-related concepts.

- Maintain a separate file for background articles.

- Create a list of citations you have reviewed in order to avoid duplicate searches for the same articles.

- Start your synthesis tables early, even if you simply copy the citation and a link to the article.

- Use search engine tools, such as email alerts, to receive notifications of new articles.

- Provide electronic files or a direct link to articles for the EBP team to access.

- Provide a glossary of research/EBP terms, because some terms used in these reports may be unfamiliar to team members (see Appendix E).

## Appraise

Identify a systematic process for reviewing articles. A checklist for appraisal and synthesis will help to keep the process flowing (see Tool 5.3). A comprehensive, structured critique increases the scientific rigor of the review. However, this has to be balanced with the purpose, the practicality of resources and expertise available, and the intent of the critique. Though a detailed critique of methods and statistical analyses increases rigor, it is likely to be beyond the expertise and comfort of most practicing nurses (Facchiano & Hoffman Snyder, 2012). Focus attention on identifying fatal flaws in the literature, such as biased results, inappropriate methods or analyses, and conclusions that are not valid or supported by the data. Three overarching questions relate to the validity of reports:

- Can it be trusted, or is there bias?

- Does it answer the clinical question?

- Can the results be applied to the clinical setting of interest?

Catalogue articles in a way that helps to organize the evidence, such as by type, research design, subtopic, or topic-related concepts. Read articles once to screen the literature, and arrange hard copies or electronic versions in folders. Then read again, for the purpose of appraising.

1. Read CPGs to gauge recommendations for practice.

2. Review synthesis reports (e.g., meta-analyses, meta-syntheses, literature reviews) and clinical research articles, to understand the science on the topic.

3. Read clinical and theoretical articles to gain understanding of theoretical principles and concepts.

Each type of article is reviewed according to criteria specific to the methods and purpose for development. As you appraise the evidence, note the type, design, and quality, and identify any major biases, limitations, or fatal flaws. This information is used to determine whether individual articles should be included or excluded in the body of evidence. While reading the literature, complete individual article appraisals and use synthesis tables (see Tool 5.4) for summarizing and organizing evidence, and recognize any limitations or flaws in the studies. A goal is to screen for up to 10 key articles for the entire team to read while maintaining a running file of background articles to support the topic (Ogier, 1998).

## Clinical Practice Guidelines

The purpose of CPGs is to transform a large body of evidence into specific recommendations for practice in a user-friendly format. According to the current AHRQ and Institute of Medicine (IOM)—now the National Academy of Medicine—definition, "Clinical practice guidelines are statements that include recommendations intended to optimize patient care that are informed by a systematic review of evidence and assessment of benefits and harms of alternative care options" (IOM, 2010a, p. 3). The definition and methodologies for developing CPGs have evolved dramatically over the past 20 years, resulting in variability in scientific merit. Though standards are emerging, few CPGs meet them (IOM, 2011a). Therefore, it is critical to appraise the methods and the validity of practice recommendations. Poor documentation of methods used to ensure unbiased results further complicates the ability to accurately evaluate guidelines for use in clinical practice. In addition to validity, practice recommendations should be evaluated, asking the following questions:

- Is it credible? Given the evidence, would others make the same conclusions?

- Is it clinically significant? Are the guidelines interpreted consistently in similar clinical situations?

- Is it applicable? Are the recommendations applicable to the population, and are they clearly stated?

Tools for appraising CPGs evaluate the quality of development, reporting, and recommendations. Conflicts of interest, norms and values of developers, and patient involvement are important components of trustworthiness but often are not included in tools (Siering, Eikermann, Hausner, Hoffman-Eßer, & Neugebauer, 2013). The widely used and well-validated tool AGREE II (Appraisal of Guidelines, Research, and Evaluation) provides a framework for assessing the quality and reporting of CPGs (AGREE Collaboration, 2010; Brouwers et al., 2010). The electronic version, My AGREE PLUS, is a free platform that allows sharing and comparing of appraisals with team members (see Tool 5.5). Alternative tools for evaluating CPGs and other evidence are also available (see Tool 5.6).

## Systematic Reviews

The state of the science is summarized in systematic reviews such as meta-analyses (quantitative data) and meta-syntheses (qualitative data), or it might also be in the form of literature reviews, health technology assessments, integrative reviews, or consensus statements. A well-developed systematic review that includes a meta-analysis is among the best evidence. By definition, systematic reviews use explicit predetermined, transparent, and reproducible scientific methods to summarize the findings from individual studies (IOM, 2011b). However, the quality of published systematic reviews is highly variable (Pearson, 2014). Many fail to assess the quality of the included studies, use poorly defined or inappropriate methods, and do not identify potential or evident biases. To address these shortcomings, the IOM developed standards for systematic reviews. Although few systematic reviews meet these standards, expectations for methods and transparency are now clear (IOM, 2011b; Preferred Reporting Items for Systematic Reviews and Meta-Analyses [PRISMA], 2015). Poor documentation of methods makes application questionable, rendering the appraisal of systematic reviews imperative. The focus of the review should be on the processes for identifying and screening studies to include methods used, transparency, and reproducibility. Using a guide to critique each systematic review simplifies the process and ensures that important points are not missed (see Tool 5.7). Other tools and resources for appraising systematic reviews are also available (see Tool 5.6).

## Research

Systematic appraisal of a research report is needed, but a lengthy, highly detailed critique is not warranted here and would likely impede the EBP process (Facchiano & Hoffman Snyder, 2012). The purpose of this appraisal is to evaluate the quality and strength of evidence and identify limitations in order to determine whether the findings can be used in practice. Each study should be appraised in terms of the extent to which systematic bias is minimized and confounding variables are controlled. The specific criteria for appraisal are often based on the research methods used, either quantitative or qualitative. Critique of quantitative research focuses on the study design and statistical, mathematical, or computational techniques used to test hypotheses. It follows the research process, which involves identifying a clinical problem, a purpose, hypotheses, variables, methods (design, sampling, measures, and instruments), data collection procedures, analysis techniques, findings, limitations, and implications (see Tool 5.8). Quantitative research approaches include but are not limited to: randomized trial, cohort, non-randomized trial, case-control, cross-sectional, and case studies.

Qualitative research focuses on observational or investigative techniques that seek to understand and/or build theory. Because qualitative methods seek to discover and better understand at a basic level of discovery, reports include a narrative intended to build meaning and depth and a rich understanding of the topic from an insider's view. Rigor for qualitative studies is determined by trustworthiness, applicability, credibility, and auditability, so the criteria for critique are quite different (see Tool 5.9). More comprehensive tools encompass criteria for both quantitative and qualitative research and may be best for mixed methods research.

## Other Literature

Literature that is not research or a systematic synthesis of evidence (e.g., a case report, an expert opinion, theory, or a clinical report) may be included to formulate the basis for practice, particularly when other evidence is lacking. Caution is warranted because these reports are often population-specific and have the potential to be highly subjective. The review should include clear identification of the purpose, key findings, and comments or concerns (see Tool 5.10).

### TIPS: Appraising Evidence

- Use a structured review process with detailed evaluation criteria and questions for novice reviewers to build appraisal skills.

- Before starting, decide how to resolve disagreements about inclusion and exclusion: 1) Include all evidence where there is disagreement, 2) discuss until consensus is formed, or 3) have a third reviewer decide.

- Supplement systematic reviews or CPGs with newer research that was not available during development of the recommendations.

- If more than one CPG exists, use the "compare" function on the National Guideline Clearinghouse website and share with the team.

- Pay particular attention to appendixes, attachments, and other supplemental materials when critiquing CPGs. These materials may have more detailed descriptions of the methods or tools for implementation or evaluation. Because CPGs are intended to be user-friendly, often reports of detailed methods are not published or are available separately.

- Avoid the assumption that because articles appear in a nursing or other type of healthcare journal that they constitute high-quality evidence. Journals vary in their review process and standards for publication, and even with a robust review process, flaws can slip by unnoticed.

# Synthesize

Until this point, evidence has been viewed predominantly piece by piece and processed for the significance to practice. Emerging themes, similarities, and differences in the literature are apparent by using a synthesis table (see Example 5.2). Synthesis is an ongoing process of combining information in new ways to increase understanding. After the articles have been critiqued, synthesis begins in earnest. First ask the question "What must we know about this topic and why?" Then compare and contrast findings, draw together themes, and pull together ideas in writing, as described in this list:

- Begin with a topic, concept theme, or recommendation.

- Include information and citations from all sources.

- Show similarities and differences.

- Represent the evidence objectively.

Strength of the body of evidence is determined by quality, quantity, consistency, and risk. Quality of evidence is the extent to which the study design and analyses minimize systematic bias and confounding (Jones, 2010). Quantity is the magnitude of treatment effect, number of studies, and overall sample size across studies (Jones, 2010). The degree to which studies report similar results is consistency. Risk is the balance between desirable and undesirable effects and costs, comparing the current practice with the proposed change. Patient values and preferences should also be considered when weighing risks. Chapter 6 further describes grading evidence and making recommendations for practice.

## TIPS: Synthesis of the Body of Evidence

■ Use a summary table as a working document and tailor it to meet your needs. Creating a table is the beginning of the synthesis process. Add to it as the synthesis process proceeds.

■ Cut and paste the study abstract from the search site directly into the summary table, and then modify it to fit your needs. Not only does this method save time, but the links also remain intact for future retrieval and related searches, and avoids typographical errors.

■ Keep the summary table orderly and flexible so it can be used to sort literature. You may begin entering articles by author or type of evidence and sort them later by themes or concepts or according to the recommendations for practice.

■ Summarize and process data from within the article as you go. Consider what is useful and relevant.

■ Develop thesis statements based on your clinical questions. Weigh the quality, quantity, consistency, and risk of evidence supporting or refuting each thesis statement.

■ Recognize that some inconsistency in research findings is to be expected. Weigh the extent the inconsistency is critical to the quality, quantity, and risk in the body of evidence.

■ Use concepts or subject terms consistently to make searching and combining easier later. Research on the same topic may use different terms (e.g., pressure injury and pressure ulcer).

■ Bring clinical expertise into the appraisal and synthesis process for considerations in designing a practice change.

**Example 5.1    MeSH Tree Structure for Pressure Injury**

Skin and Connective Tissue Diseases [C17]

    Skin Diseases [C17.800]

        Skin Ulcer [C17.800.893]

            Buruli Ulcer [C17.800.893.295]

            Leg Ulcer [C17.800.893.592]

                Foot Ulcer [C17.800.893.592.450]  **+**

                Varicose Ulcer [C17.800.893.592.730]

            Pressure Ulcer [C17.800.893.665]

            Pyoderma Gangrenosum [C17.800.893.675]

(U.S. National Library of Medicine, 2016)

EXAMPLES

TOOLS

## Example 5.2 Synthesis Tables

### Example 1: Research studies for EBP projects

**Topic:** Probiotic use to prevent antibiotic-associated diarrhea and *Clostridium difficile* diarrhea in the medical intensive care unit (MICU)

**Team:** S. Jackson, A. Bowman, C. Bombei, K. Stenger, L. Cullen

| Author | Design /Methods | Limitations |
|---|---|---|
| Klarin, B., Wullt, M., Palmquist, I., Molin, G., Larsson, A., & Jeppsson, B. (2008). *Lactobacillus plantarum* 299v reduces colonisation of *Clostridium difficile* in critically ill patients treated with antibiotics. *Acta Anaesthesioilogica Scandinavica, 52*(8), 1096–1102. doi:10.1111/j.1399-6576.2008.01748.x | RCT in five Swedish ICUs, blinded to investigator, ward staff, and sponsor.<br>N = 44, 22 each arm.<br>Patients within 24 hours of admission to ICU. Inclusion criteria: > 18; presumed need for ICU for 3 days or longer; no known positive *C. diff* the week before enrollment; able to start enteral feeds within 24 hours of admit; not moribund. Exclusion: No feeds in 24 hours, *C. diff* on inclusion sample. | ■ Study concluded early due to low inclusion rate and decreased funding.<br><br>■ Control group had longer ICU days and days on ventilator—not statistically significant but may have contributed to findings.<br><br>■ Two of the six blinded authors had shares in Probi AB that provided the study product and performed bacterial analysis. |
| Anukam, K. C., Osazuwa, E. O., Osadolor, H. B., Bruce, A. W., & Reid, G. (2008). Yogurt containing probiotic *Lactobacillus rhamnosus* GR–1 and *L. reuteri* RC–14 helps resolve moderate diarrhea and increases CD4 count in HIV/AIDS patients. *Journal of Clinical Gastroenterology, 42*(3), 239–243. doi:10.1097/MCG.0b013e31802c7465 | Convenience sample of 24 HIV-positive women attending voluntary counseling test center in Benin City. Inclusion criteria: No history of antiretroviral therapy and CD4 count greater than 200. Given 100 ml of probiotic-supplemented yogurt versus unsupplemented yogurt for 15 days. Measures: hematologic profiles, CD4 cell counts, and quality of life at baseline, 15 and 30 days post feedings. | ■ Small size, convenience sample |

(Jackson, Bowman, Bombei, Stenger, & Cullen, n.d.)

| Finding/Safety Key Points | Product Information |
|---|---|
| *Lactobacillus plantarum* 299v reduces colonization of *C. diff* in critically ill patients treated with antibiotic.<br><br>■ No significant differences noted in stooling; significant decreased gut permeability in Lp299v group; significant difference; no cases of *C.diff* conversion in probiotic group versus four in control (p = .0485).<br><br>■ Cultures per unit protocol on patients showed more infections in control groups for blood, catheter, tracheal secretions. Urine cultures the only area more positive in probiotic group. | Lp299v containing 8 x 10 to the tenth power of *Lactobacillus plantarum* in gruel form given via enteral feeding tube dose of 100 ml every 12 hour x 3 days, and then 50cc bid daily during ICU stay. |
| ■ No bacteremia noted. Significant difference in CD4 cell counts with probiotics (P < .02); quality of life rapid resolution of GI discomfort in probiotic group versus control. Remained beyond treatment days.<br><br>■ No episodes of bacteremia!<br><br>■ Improved immune function via CD4. | ■ Conventional yogurt fermented with starter cultures of *Lactobacillus delbruekii* subsp. *Bulgaricus* and *streptococcus thermohilus* were supplemented with *L. rhmnosus*, GR–1 and *L. reuteri* RC–14 (2.5 x 10 to the 9th CFU/ml added to 990 ml of fermented yogurt). |

*continues*

## Example 5.2    Synthesis Tables (Continued)

**Example 2:** Supplemental evidence for EBP project
**Topic:** Urinary catheters for laboring patients with epidurals
**Team:** A. Hiller, J. Andrew, M. Farrington, A. Sanborn, L. Cullen

| Citation | Type/Evidence | Scope |
|---|---|---|
| Srinivas, S. (2009). Intermittent versus continuous bladder catheterization during labor: Does it matter? *Journal of Clinical Anesthesia, 20*(8), 565–566. doi:10.1016/j.jclinane.2008.11.001 | Editorial | Epidural potential complications |
| Kirton, C. A. (1997). Assessing for bladder distension. *Nursing, 27*(4), 64. | Teaching | Assessment |
| Schneiderman, E. (2012). Epidural and urinary catheters: You can have one without the other. *Journal of Obstetric, Gynecologic, & Neonatal Nursing, 41*(s1), S13. doi:10.1111/j.1552-6909.2012.01359_11.x | Innovative poster presentation | Nursing catheter care |
| McShane, F. J. (1992). Epidural narcotics: Mechanism of action and nursing implications. *Journal of Post Anesthesia Nursing, 7*(3), 155–162. | Expert teaching/review | Anesthesia/nursing |

(Hiller, Farrington, Forman, McNulty, & Cullen, in press)

| Supplemental Information | Other |
|---|---|
| Not all women need catheterization, and there is an increased risk of infection with indwelling catheters.<br><br>Epidurals appear to be associated with an increased duration of the second stage. | Intrapartum urinary retention is a known complication of epidural anesthesia and should be managed to minimize postpartum UTIs. Minimize catheter use to reduce infections. |
| Anesthesia, surgery, pregnancy, or an obstruction in the urinary tract can cause a distended bladder.<br><br>Palpate deeply with your fingertips toward the symphysis pubis.<br><br>A patient with a distended bladder must be catheterized. | |
| Proposed change:<br><br>■ Use indwelling catheter if clinically appropriate.<br><br>■ Void prior to epidural and every 2–4 hours after.<br><br>■ Assess the bladder and perform peri-care every 2 hours.<br><br>■ If unable to void, place straight catheter using sterile technique. | Indications for urinary catheter: Category III fetal heart rate or arrest of labor, closer monitoring of I & Os, receiving magnesium sulfate, or obese patients where bladder assessment is unobtainable. |
| Urinary retention rate 1–22%.<br><br>Increased bladder capacity, relaxation of detrusor muscle.<br><br>Catheterization provides relief until narcotic effect subsides. | |

*continues*

## Example 5.2    Synthesis Tables (Continued)

**Example 3:** Non-research literature from EBP project
**Topic:** Hyaluronidase for IV extravasations
**Team:** K. Hanrahan

| Citation | Type/Evidence | Scope |
|---|---|---|
| Bertelli, G., Garrone, O., Bighin, C., & Dini, D. (2001). Correspondence re: Cicchetti S, Jemec B, Gault DT: Two case reports of vinorelbine extravasation: Management and review of the literature. *Tumori, 87*(2), 112–113. | D: expert opinion | Letter discussing appropriate treatment of vinorelbine extravasations using hyaluronidase and saline flush-out. |
| European Oncology Nursing Society. (2008). Introducing the extravasation guidelines: EONS toolkit, post symposium report. Brussels, Belgium: EONS. Retrieved from http://www.cancernurse.eu/documents/EONSClinicalGuidelinesSection6-en.pdf | B2: evidence-based guideline 150–1500 units | A toolkit for implementing the European Oncology Nursing Society extravasation guidelines. |
| U.S. Food and Drug Administration, Center for Drug Evaluation and Research. (2009). FDA-approved drug products. Retrieved from http://www.accessdata.fda.gov/Scripts/cder/DrugsatFDA/index.cfm | A1: evidence-based review by regulating body; for dispersion of drugs, 50–300 units, most typically 150 units to injected solution | FDA evidence reviews and approves product labels; provides extensive information about product safety and efficacy. |

(Hanrahan, 2013)

| Conclusions RE: Hyaluronidase | Other |
|---|---|
| Suggests that simply administering hyaluronidase may have been equally or more effective than hyaluronidase and saline flush-out. Saline flush-out should be viewed as an option for treatment and not standard therapy. | ▪ Reply letter states any treatment that allows the extravasate to stay in the tissue is less than ideal. |
| Hyaluronidase is suggested as an antidote, and instructions for administration are provided; however, because of a lack of evidence, further study is recommended. | ▪ Algorithm for extravasation management<br><br>▪ Table of options for antidotes<br><br>▪ Instructions for using antidotes<br><br>▪ Table of drugs: e.g., vesicants documentation tools |
| Hyaluronidase is approved for use to increase the absorption and dispersion of other injected drugs. | ▪ Extensive information about FDA approval process for hyaluronidase product now on the market<br><br>▪ Current approved labels with extensive information about each product |

*continues*

## Example 5.2    Synthesis Tables (Continued)

**Example 4:** Research studies for evidence-based design
**Topic:** Single-family room redesign in pediatrics
**Team:** K. Hanrahan, S. Stewart, C. Kleiber, J. Kurtt, A. Gaarde

| Citation | Setting/Population | Methods |
|---|---|---|
| Domanico, R., Davis, D. K., Coleman, F., & Davis, B. O. Jr. (2010). Documenting the NICU design dilemma: Parent and staff perceptions of open ward versus single-family room units. *Journal of Perinatology, 30*(5), 343–351. doi:10.1038/jp.2009.195 | NICU<br>Parents: three groups<br>▪ Old open bay<br><br>▪ Transitioning<br><br>▪ New single-family room (SFR) | Research: Prospective study to test the efficacy of SFR NICU designs and to explore questions regarding patient clinical progress and relative patient safety |
| Smith, T. J. (2012). A comparative study of occupancy and patient care quality in four different types of intensive care units in a children's hospital. *Work, 41*(Suppl. 1), 1961–1968. doi:10.3233/WOR-2012-0415-1961 | Four intensive care units in a children's hospital: an infant care center (ICC), a medical/surgical (Med/Surg) unit, a neonatal intensive care unit (NICU), and a pediatric intensive care unit (PICU), each featuring a mix of multibed and private room (PR) patient care environments<br>HCP: nursing and house staff | Research: Comparative study of occupancy and patient care quality, before the units are upgraded to exclusive PR designs |

(Hanrahan, n.d.)

| Measures/Outcomes | Results |
|---|---|
| 1. Nurse parent support tool (NPST) and perceptions of physical facility; psychometric tested<br>2. Noise levels, illumination, and air quality measurements<br>3. LOS<br>4. Physicians estimated mortality (PERM) | Infants in the SFR unit had fewer apneic events, reduced nosocomial sepsis and mortality, and earlier transitions to enteral nutrition. More mothers sustained Stage III lactation, and more infants were discharged breastfeeding in the SFR. This study showed the SFR to be more conducive to family-centered care and to enhance infant clinical progress and breastfeeding success over that of an open ward. |
| 1. Observations of ergonomic design features<br>2. Task activity analyses of job performance of selected staff<br>3. Survey of perceptions by unit nursing and house staff (HS) of indicators of occupancy and patient care quality | The five most common task activities are interacting with patients, charting, and interacting with equipment, co-workers, and family members. Job satisfaction, patient care, work environment, patient care team interaction, and general occupancy quality rankings by ICC and/or NICU respondents are significantly higher than those by other staff respondents. Ergonomic design shortcomings noted are excess noise, problems with equipment, and work environment, job-related health, and patient care quality issues. |

## Tool 5.1   Assembling Evidence

**INSTRUCTIONS:** Review the steps outlined for planning how to assemble the best evidence. Identify dates and times for relevant steps, such as meeting with a health science librarian. Check when steps are completed. Proceed to the next step until each step has been completed.

| Date Scheduled | Activity | Done |
|---|---|---|
| | Set up meeting with healthcare librarian or use tutorial (such as PubMed) for completing your own database searches. | ☐ |
| | Identify MeSH terms, keywords, and search strategies (e.g., limits) for literature searches based on PICO (Patient population/problem/pilot area, Intervention, Comparison, Outcome) components and purpose statement. | ☐ |
| | Complete literature search; save search history and article abstracts; continue updating and recording the searches. | ☐ |
| | Locate clinical practice guidelines (if available) first, searching the National Guideline Clearinghouse and other professional organizations. | ☐ |
| | Search PubMed, CINAHL, and other large search engines appropriate to the subject or discipline. | ☐ |
| | Search the Cochrane Library. | ☐ |
| | Search professional organizations' online resources. | ☐ |
| | Search other related websites. | ☐ |
| | Have at least two reviewers read abstracts to screen articles for relevance and inclusion/ exclusion criteria. Where there is a lack of consensus, full articles may be retrieved for further review. | ☐ |
| | Retrieve full articles for review. Keep an electronic copy in a reference manager or shared file. Save references in electronic folders by topic, using a standardized format (i.e., first author, subject, year), or provide direct links for easy access by the team. | ☐ |
| | Start a reference list using RefWorks, EndNote, or another reference manager, and enter articles as they are retrieved. | ☐ |
| | Sort articles according to a) clinical practice guidelines, b) systematic reviews and other synthesis reports, c) research reports, d) theory articles, and e) clinical reviews. | ☐ |
| | Read clinical practice guidelines and systematic review articles first to gain understanding of state of practice and science, respectively. | ☐ |
| | Read research reports to gain understanding of study design and methods, intervention, variables and measures, relevance to population, and results. | ☐ |
| | Read clinical and theoretical articles to gain understanding of theoretical principles and concepts. | ☐ |
| | Identify up to 10 key clinical, research, theory, or review articles for the entire team to read. | ☐ |

## Tool 5.2    Record of Search History and Yield by Source

**INSTRUCTIONS:** When using bibliographic databases, save the search history. Include the terms used, how terms were combined, and the yield from each search.

| Database | Search or MeSH Term (List) | Approaches for Combining Terms (Boolean Operators AND/OR/NOT) | Limits Used | Yield (Combined Keywords and Numbers of Articles Identified) |
|---|---|---|---|---|
| National Guideline Clearinghouse (NGC): A public resource for summaries of evidence-based clinical practice guidelines. https://guideline.gov | | | | |
| The Cochrane Library: The leading resource for systematic reviews in healthcare. http://onlinelibrary.wiley.com/cochranelibrary/search | | | | |
| PubMed: PubMed is composed of more than 26 million citations for biomedical literature from MEDLINE, life science journals, and online books. www.ncbi.nlm.nih.gov/pubmed | | | | |
| CINAHL: CINAHL Plus with full text indexes over 5,000 journals from the fields of nursing and allied health, with indexing back to 1937. https://health.ebsco.com/products/cinahl-plus-with-full-text | | | | |
| Source:<br><br>Link: | | | | |
| Source:<br><br>Link: | | | | |
| Source:<br><br>Link: | | | | |
| Source:<br><br>Link: | | | | |

## Tool 5.3    Appraisal and Synthesis of Evidence

**INSTRUCTIONS:** Review the steps outlined for planning how to appraise and synthesize the available evidence. Identify dates and times for relevant steps, such as meetings to resolve disagreements about inclusion or exclusion. Check when steps are completed. Proceed to the next step until each step has been completed.

| Date Scheduled | Activity | Done |
|---|---|---|
| | Read articles once while searching and screening the literature. | ☐ |
| | Label each article by design (e.g., systematic review, randomized clinical trial). | ☐ |
| | Outline a systematic critique process for thoroughly reviewing evidence once. | ☐ |
| | Identify criteria for inclusion/exclusion of evidence based on the quality and relevance to practice. | ☐ |
| | Determine how to resolve disagreements. | ☐ |
| | Create a resource binder and/or electronic folders to organize materials (i.e., articles, guidelines, synthesis tables, practice recommendations, executive summaries, reference lists). | ☐ |
| | Create a summary and synthesis table for articles and guidelines and update as materials are read. | ☐ |
| | For a large number of articles, arrange literature within the synthesis table by key concepts that will relate directly to practice recommendations. | ☐ |
| | Appraise individual evidence-based guidelines and systematic reviews. | ☐ |
| | Appraise research articles. | ☐ |
| | Appraise theoretical, clinical, and other types of literature. | ☐ |
| | Determine inclusion/exclusion for each piece of evidence based on the quality and relevance to established practice criteria. | ☐ |
| | Determine the quality, relevance to practice, risks, and key findings for each article or guideline. | ☐ |
| | Resolve disagreements about inclusion/exclusion of evidence. | ☐ |
| | Compare, contrast, and synthesize information from articles on the synthesis tables. | ☐ |

## Tool 5.4 Summary and Synthesis Table

**INSTRUCTIONS:** Add a brief description for each article into a row. Include enough citation information to locate the article again later, or use APA format to save time doing this later. Briefly include the key elements found while reading that are relevant to the topic. Include only what is helpful and not a comprehensive list of findings. Include key findings and comment on strengths or weaknesses for each article.

| Guidelines, Reviews, and Other Literature | | | | |
|---|---|---|---|---|
| Citation | Critique: Type of Evidence/Limitations | Scope | Relevant Findings | Other |
| | | | | |
| | | | | |
| | | | | |
| | | | | |
| | | | | |

| Research | | | | | |
|---|---|---|---|---|---|
| Citation | Subjects | Design/ Methods | Outcomes | Relevant Results and Findings | Limitations/ Comments |
| | | | | | |
| | | | | | |
| | | | | | |
| | | | | | |
| | | | | | |

| Supplemental Evidence (not meeting inclusion criteria but supplementing guideline content and literature review) | | | | |
|---|---|---|---|---|
| Citation | Type/Evidence | Scope | Supplemental Information | Comments/Other |
| | | | | |
| | | | | |

EXAMPLES

TOOLS

## Tool 5.5  AGREE II Instrument

The Appraisal of Guidelines for Research and Evaluation (AGREE©) Instrument evaluates the process of practice guideline development and the quality of reporting. The original AGREE Instrument has been up-dated and methodologically refined. The AGREE II is now the international tool for the assessment of practice guidelines. The AGREE II, which is both valid and reliable, is composed of 23 items organized into the original six quality domains. Appraisals can be completed in hard copy (paper) form or using the MY AGREE PLUS platform for electronic appraisal, which allows individual appraisals, group appraisals, and group compari-sons.

Instructions are provided on the first pages of the instrument. Review and critique can be done individually and compared as a group for team decision-making.

AGREE Enterprise website:

http://www.agreetrust.org/agree-ii

AGREE II online training tools:

http://www.agreetrust.org/resource-centre/agree-ii-training-tools

AGREE publications about the instrument:

http://www.agreetrust.org/resource-centre/key-articles-agree-instrument

AGREE II user manual and instrument:

http://www.agreetrust.org/wp-content/uploads/2013/10/AGREE-II-Users-Manual-and-23-item-Instrument_2009_UPDATE_2013.pdf

MY AGREE PLUS platform for electronic appraisal:

Video: http://www.agreetrust.org/2013/06/important-website-upgrade

Platform:

http://www.agreetrust.org/login/?redirect_to=http%3A%2F%2Fwww.agreetrust.org%2Fmy-agree%2F

(AGREE Collaboration, 2010)

## Tool 5.6    Appraise Evidence

**INSTRUCTIONS:** Determine the kind of evidence being reviewed and associated resources. Link into each and select a resource that best meets the needs of the team.

| Organization | Content or Purpose | Website |
|---|---|---|
| **Multiple Tools** | | |
| Critical Appraisal Skills Programme | Critical appraisal skills training, workshops, and tools | http://www.casp-uk.net |
| Centre for Evidence-Based Medicine, University of Oxford | CEBM tools, examples, and downloads for the critical appraisal of medical evidence | http://www.cebm.net/index.aspx?o=1157 |
| International Centre for Allied Health Evidence | A list of critical appraisal tools, linked to the websites where they were developed | http://www.unisa.edu.au/Research/ Sansom-Institute-for-Health-Research/ Research/Allied-Health-Evidence/ Resources/CAT |
| Institute of Medicine | Book available online or as paperback. Describes standards for scholarly systematic reviews to help developers and reviewers | http://nationalacademies.org/hmd/ reports/2011/finding-what-works-in-health-care-standards-for-systematic-reviews.aspx *or* http://nationalacademies.org/hmd/ reports/2015/decreasing-the-risk-of-developing-alzheimers-type-dementia. aspx |
| **Systematic Reviews** | | |
| Assessment of Multiple Systematic Reviews, EMGO Institute, The Netherlands | AMSTAR tool for assessing the methodological quality of systematic reviews | https://amstar.ca/Amstar_Checklist.php |
| British Medical Journal Clinical Evidence | BMJ framework for assessing systematic reviews | http://clinicalevidence.bmj.com/x/set/ static/ebm/toolbox/665052.html |
| Ottawa Hospital Research Institute | Framework and tools for creating systematic reviews | http://www.prisma-statement.org/ |
| Institute of Medicine | Book available online or as paperback. Describes standards for scholarly systematic reviews to help developers and reviewers | http://nationalacademies.org/hmd/ reports/2011/finding-what-works-in-health-care-standards-for-systematic-reviews.aspx *or* http://nationalacademies.org/hmd/ reports/2015/decreasing-the-risk-of-developing-alzheimers-type-dementia. aspx |

*continues*

## Tool 5.6    Appraise Evidence (Continued)

| Clinical Practice Guidelines | | |
|---|---|---|
| The Appraisal of Guidelines for Research and Evaluation Enterprise | A generic tool (AGREE II) for evaluating the quality of reporting and quality of recommendations | http://www.agreetrust.org/agree-ii |
| Institute of Medicine | Book available online or as paperback. Describes standards for scholarly clinical practice guidelines to help developers and reviewers | http://www.nationalacademies.org/ hmd/Reports/2011/Clinical-Practice-Guidelines-We-Can-Trust.aspx |
| Institute for Quality and Efficiency in Health Care (IQWiG), Cologne, Germany | A systematic review to identify and compare appraisal tools | http://journals.plos.org/plosone/ article?id=10.1371/journal.pone.0082915 |
| Tools for Rating Evidence | | |
| U.S. Preventive Services Task Force | USPSTF grades three things: quality of the overall body of evidence, strength of evidence and magnitude of benefit for recommendations, and certainty of outcomes | http://www. uspreventiveservicestaskforce. org/Page/Name/methods-and-processes#recommendation-process |
| Grading of Recommendations Assessment, Development, and Evaluation | An informal working group whose members have developed a common, sensible, and transparent approach to grading quality of evidence and strength of recommendations | http://www.gradeworkinggroup.org |

## Tool 5.7  Systematic Review Appraisal

**INSTRUCTIONS:** Write in enough citation information to locate the article again later. Skip to "critique" section in the middle of page one. Answer each question. Return to the "overall evaluation" section for final consideration of the whole document. Answer the questions in the "overall evaluation" section and determine if the document will be used as part of the body of evidence or discarded.

### Citation

### Overall Evaluation (provide answers after completing the critique)

| | |
|---|---|
| Internal validity: Does it provide a precise and unbiased answer to the research question? | ☐ Totally adequate ☐ Moderately adequate ☐ Not adequate ☐ Can't tell |
| External validity: Can findings be applied to the population and setting of the EBP initiative? | ☐ Totally adequate ☐ Moderately adequate ☐ Not adequate ☐ Can't tell |
| Are limitations and biases reported and controlled adequately to include this study in the body of evidence for the EBP initiative? | ☐ Yes ☐ No |
| Are inclusion (and no exclusion) criteria met for EBP initiative? | ☐ Yes ☐ No |

### Critique

**Background**

| | |
|---|---|
| Is the need for a systematic review clear? | ☐ Yes ☐ No |
| Does the need for a systematic review stem from a clinical problem? | ☐ Yes ☐ No |
| Is the background literature relevant to the problem? | ☐ Yes ☐ No |

**Aim or Objective of the Report**

| | |
|---|---|
| Are elements of PICO (Patient population/problem/pilot area, Intervention, Comparison, and Outcome) discernible? | ☐ Yes ☐ No |
| Is a question about practice clearly written with a focused direction for designing the analysis? | ☐ Yes ☐ No |
| Will the answer to the question provide direction for the clinical problem? | ☐ Yes ☐ No |

**Search Strategies**

| | |
|---|---|
| Are the databases searched appropriate for the aim or objective? | ☐ Yes ☐ No |
| Are the search strategies logical and inclusive? | ☐ Yes ☐ No |

*continues*

## Tool 5.7    Systematic Review Appraisal (Continued)

### Search Strategies (Continued)

| | |
|---|---|
| Is the search process transparent and reproducible? | ☐ Yes ☐ No |
| Is the search yield sufficient for informing clinical practice? | ☐ Yes ☐ No |
| Are inclusion and exclusion criteria clear? | ☐ Yes ☐ No |
| Is the approach to addressing discrepancies clear? | ☐ Yes ☐ No |

### Methods

| | |
|---|---|
| Do at least two independent reviewers determine inclusion or exclusion of studies? | ☐ Yes ☐ No |
| Are characteristics of the included studies provided? | ☐ Yes ☐ No |
| Is the quality of the studies assessed and used appropriately in forming conclusions? | ☐ Yes ☐ No |
| Are statistical methods for combining results appropriate for the data? | ☐ Yes ☐ No |
| Are qualitative methods used to supplement quantitative methods? | ☐ Yes ☐ No |

### Results/Implications

| | |
|---|---|
| Are limitations and biases identified? | ☐ Yes ☐ No |
| Are conflicts of interest identified? | ☐ Yes ☐ No |
| Do the results provide direction for the clinical problem? | ☐ Yes ☐ No |
| Are conclusions appropriate based on the design, analysis, and results presented? | ☐ Yes ☐ No |
| Are recommendations for practice supported by evidence? | ☐ Yes ☐ No |
| Are the recommendations for practice relevant to the EBP initiative? | ☐ Yes ☐ No |

### Notes

Complete the "Overall Evaluation" section at the beginning of this tool.

## Tool 5.8   Quantitative Research Appraisal

**INSTRUCTIONS:** Write in enough citation information to locate the article again later. Skip to "critique" section in the middle of page one. Answer each question. Return to the "overall evaluation" section for final consideration of the whole article. Answer the questions in the "overall evaluation" section and determine if the study will be used as part of the body of evidence or discarded.

| Citation |
|---|
| |

| Overall Evaluation (provide answers after completing the critique) | |
|---|---|
| Internal validity: Does it provide a precise and unbiased answer to the research question? | ☐ Totally adequate<br>☐ Moderately adequate<br>☐ Not adequate<br>☐ Can't tell |
| External validity: Can findings be applied to the population and setting of the EBP initiative? | ☐ Totally adequate<br>☐ Moderately adequate<br>☐ Not adequate<br>☐ Can't tell |
| Are limitations and biases reported and controlled adequately to include this study in the body of evidence for the EBP initiative? | ☐ Yes<br>☐ No |
| Are inclusion (and no exclusion) criteria met for EBP initiative? | ☐ Yes<br>☐ No |

| Critique | |
|---|---|

### Research Question

| | |
|---|---|
| Are the research questions and/or the study aims clearly stated? | ☐ Yes<br>☐ No |
| Are the research questions relevant to the EBP initiative? | ☐ Yes<br>☐ No |
| Do the questions provide direction for the study design? | ☐ Yes<br>☐ No |

### Literature Review

| | |
|---|---|
| Are the search strategies clear, logical, and inclusive? | ☐ Yes<br>☐ No |
| Is current literature related to the research question reported? | ☐ Yes<br>☐ No |
| Is a gap in knowledge, the need for research, clear? | ☐ Yes<br>☐ No |

### Method/Design

| | | |
|---|---|---|
| ☐ Randomized controlled trial<br>☐ Experimental | ☐ Quasi-experimental<br>☐ Descriptive or observational | ☐ Mixed methods<br>☐ Other (specify) |

| | |
|---|---|
| Are the setting and population appropriate for the study question? | ☐ Yes<br>☐ No |

*continues*

## Tool 5.8    Quantitative Research Appraisal (Continued)

### Method/Design (Continued)

| | |
|---|---|
| Are the setting and sample similar to the EBP initiative setting and population? | ☐ Yes ☐ No |
| Were statistical methods used to determine a sufficient sample size? | ☐ Yes ☐ No |
| Is group randomization and assignment clear and appropriate for the study question? | ☐ Yes ☐ No |
| Is the rigor of the design sufficient for the study question and existing body of research? | ☐ Yes ☐ No |
| Are the instruments valid and reliable? | ☐ Yes ☐ No |
| Do the instruments used match the study constructs and question? | ☐ Yes ☐ No |

### Data Analysis/Results

| | |
|---|---|
| Are methods used to prevent, recognize, and control bias? | ☐ Yes ☐ No |
| Is the probability of sampling error identified? | ☐ Yes ☐ No |
| Are the numbers of participants enrolled clearly tracked from the starting sample to analyses? | ☐ Yes ☐ No |
| Are the statistical analyses appropriate for the data and study question? | ☐ Yes ☐ No |
| Are the results clear and understandable? | ☐ Yes ☐ No |
| Do the results reported and interpretation of data match? | ☐ Yes ☐ No |

### Discussion/Implications

| | |
|---|---|
| Does the discussion match the results? | ☐ Yes ☐ No |
| Is the discussion supported by other relevant research? | ☐ Yes ☐ No |
| Are limitations and threats of bias discussed? | ☐ Yes ☐ No |
| Are implications for application in practice clear and appropriate based on the results? | ☐ Yes ☐ No |
| Are the recommendations for practice relevant to the EBP initiative? | ☐ Yes ☐ No |

### Notes

Complete the "Overall Evaluation" section at the beginning of this tool.

## Tool 5.9   Qualitative Research Appraisal

**INSTRUCTIONS:** Write in enough citation information to locate the article again later. Skip to "critique" section in the middle of page one. Answer each question. Return to the "overall evaluation" section for final consideration of the whole article. Answer the questions in the "overall evaluation" section and determine if the study will be used as part of the body of evidence or discarded.

| Citation |
| --- |
|  |

| Overall Evaluation (provide answers after completing the critique) | |
| --- | --- |
| Trustworthiness: Are credibility and confidence in the true value established? Are the results an accurate reflection of the participants' experience? | ☐ Totally adequate<br>☐ Moderately adequate<br>☐ Not adequate<br>☐ Can't tell |
| Applicability: Can findings be applied to the population and setting of the EBP initiative? | ☐ Totally adequate<br>☐ Moderately adequate<br>☐ Not adequate<br>☐ Can't tell |
| Are the methods consistent (dependable) and neutral (confirmable) so as to include this study in the evidence for this EBP initiative? | ☐ Yes<br>☐ No |
| Are inclusion (and no exclusion) criteria met for the EBP initiative? | ☐ Yes<br>☐ No |

| Critique | |
| --- | --- |

**Topic/Purpose**

| | |
| --- | --- |
| Is the phenomenon of interest (topic) clear? | ☐ Yes<br>☐ No |
| Is the purpose of the study clear? | ☐ Yes<br>☐ No |
| Do the research questions provide direction for a qualitative design? | ☐ Yes<br>☐ No |
| Is the topic relevant to the EBP initiative? | ☐ Yes<br>☐ No |

**Method/Design**

| | | |
| --- | --- | --- |
| ☐ Observation<br>☐ Comparative | ☐ Triangulation<br>☐ Mixed methods | ☐ Other (specify) |

| | |
| --- | --- |
| Is sampling appropriate for the method? | ☐ Yes<br>☐ No |
| Do participants have an insider's view of the topic? | ☐ Yes<br>☐ No |
| Do the design and methods fit the study purpose? | ☐ Yes<br>☐ No |

*continues*

EXAMPLES

TOOLS

EXAMPLES

TOOLS

## Tool 5.9   Qualitative Research Appraisal (Continued)

### Method/Design (Continued)

| | |
|---|---|
| Are methods well described and replicable? | ☐ Yes ☐ No |
| Is data collection focused on the participants' experience? | ☐ Yes ☐ No |

### Data Analysis/Results

| | |
|---|---|
| Are the numbers of participants enrolled clearly tracked from the starting sample to analyses? | ☐ Yes ☐ No |
| Are analyses appropriate for the study question and data? | ☐ Yes ☐ No |
| Are data collection and methods dependable (i.e., executed consistently)? | ☐ Yes ☐ No |
| Are analysis methods and results confirmable (i.e., tracked and documented)? | ☐ Yes ☐ No |
| Do methods and results accurately reflect the participants' experience? | ☐ Yes ☐ No |
| Are analyses adequately validated (e.g., triangulation)? | ☐ Yes ☐ No |
| Are the methods and results credible? | ☐ Yes ☐ No |
| Do results add meaning or understanding to the EBP initiative? | ☐ Yes ☐ No |
| Are findings applicable to the patients in the EBP initiative? | ☐ Yes ☐ No |

### Discussion/Implications

| | |
|---|---|
| Does the report read like a narrative (i.e., telling a story)? | ☐ Yes ☐ No |
| Are the findings reported in context? | ☐ Yes ☐ No |
| Are findings supported by other relevant research? | ☐ Yes ☐ No |
| Are the implications for practice clear? | ☐ Yes ☐ No |
| Are the implications for practice relevant to the EBP initiative? | ☐ Yes ☐ No |

### Notes

Complete the "Overall Evaluation" section at the beginning of this tool.

## Tool 5.10   Other Evidence Appraisal

**INSTRUCTIONS:** Write in enough citation information to locate the document again later. Skip to "critique" section in the middle of page one. Answer each question. Return to the "overall evaluation" section for final consideration of the whole document. Answer the questions in the "overall evaluation" section and determine if the report will be used as part of the body of evidence or discarded.

| Citation |
| --- |

### Overall Evaluation (provide answers after completing the critique)

| | |
| --- | --- |
| Internal validity: Does it provide a precise and unbiased answer to the clinical question? | ☐ Totally adequate<br>☐ Moderately adequate<br>☐ Not adequate<br>☐ Can't tell |
| External validity: Can findings be applied to the population and setting of the EBP initiative? | ☐ Totally adequate<br>☐ Moderately adequate<br>☐ Not adequate<br>☐ Can't tell |
| Are limitations and biases reported and controlled adequately to include this in the body of evidence for the EBP initiative? | ☐ Yes<br>☐ No |
| Are inclusion (and no exclusion) criteria met for the EBP initiative? | ☐ Yes<br>☐ No |

| Critique |
| --- |

**Type of Evidence**

| | |
| --- | --- |
| Is other evidence limited, indicating a need to expand the pool of evidence, or does this evidence provide a unique perspective? | ☐ Yes<br>☐ No |
| Is the need for more information clear? | ☐ Yes<br>☐ No |
| Is this evidence relevant to the problem? | ☐ Yes<br>☐ No |
| Are scientific principles used? | ☐ Yes<br>☐ No |
| Are limitations and biases subjectively identified? | ☐ Yes<br>☐ No |

*continues*

## Tool 5.10   Other Evidence Appraisal (Continued)

**Type of Evidence (Continued)**

| | |
|---|---|
| Are conflicts of interest identified? | ☐ Yes ☐ No |
| Is the evidence current (the most recent update has a clear date)? | ☐ Yes ☐ No |
| Do the results provide direction for the clinical problem? | ☐ Yes ☐ No |
| Are conclusions appropriate for the methods and findings presented? | ☐ Yes ☐ No |
| Are recommendations for practice supported by evidence? | ☐ Yes ☐ No |
| Are recommendations for practice relevant to the EBP initiative? | ☐ Yes ☐ No |

**Notes**

Complete the "Overall Evaluation" section at the beginning of this tool.

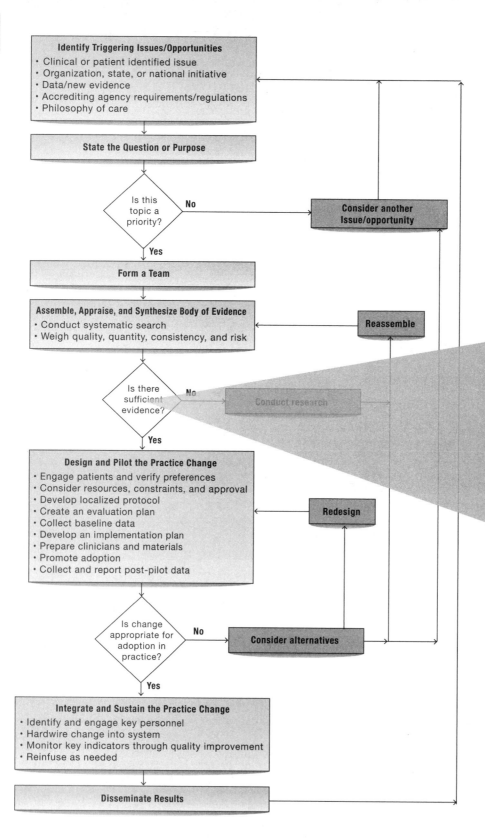

# IS THERE SUFFICIENT EVIDENCE?

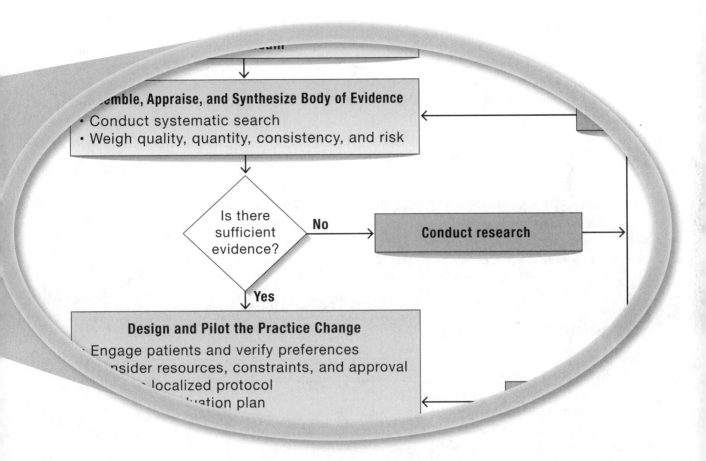

**...mble, Appraise, and Synthesize Body of Evidence**
- Conduct systematic search
- Weigh quality, quantity, consistency, and risk

Is there sufficient evidence?

**No** → **Conduct research**

**Yes**

**Design and Pilot the Practice Change**
- Engage patients and verify preferences
- ...nsider resources, constraints, and approval
- ...localized protocol
- ...ation plan

*"It is often necessary to make a decision on the basis of information sufficient for action but insufficient to satisfy the intellect."*

–Immanuel Kant

Clinical practice guidelines (CPGs) are foundational to improving healthcare (Woolf, Schünemann, Eccles, Grimshaw, & Shekelle, 2012). The goal of landmark Institute of Medicine (IOM) reports (IOM, 2010a, 2011a, 2011b) is to improve the quality and consistency of both CPGs and systematic reviews in order to promote application of evidence in practice. Likewise, the goal of assembling, appraising, and synthesizing evidence is to improve the quality of healthcare delivered to patients. Yet the jump from critiquing research and other reports to making decisions or applying research findings in practice is not always straightforward, easy, or clear-cut (Aveyard & Bauld, 2011).

Evidence-based practice (EBP) teams must move beyond synthesis to application and not get stuck reading and evaluating the literature. Instead, move forward and make a decision about using available evidence for developing practice recommendations. Team members experienced in methods for weighing evidence can help to mentor novice members and increase the reliability of recommendations (Berkman, Lohr, Morgan, Tzy-Mey, & Morton, 2013; Murad et al., 2014; Stevens, 2009). Clinicians with content expertise are key participants in weighing the evidence because they have unique perspectives and knowledge about risks, benefits, and cost of interventions, in addition to an understanding of patient values (Vaccaro et al., 2010).

Follow a well-developed analytical process for working through the literature; consider relevant sources of evidence (i.e., looking at lower levels of evidence may be indicated when other evidence is lacking), and develop an EBP protocol for local use. Use a simple checklist to keep work on track (see Tool 6.1). At the outset, make explicit decisions about the specific questions to be answered and key outcomes. As a group, determine the questions to be answered, the types of evidence that are relevant, and the criteria that will be used for making decisions (Woolf et al., 2012). While synthesizing information, begin to evaluate the quality of the evidence and strength of the recommendations for practice. This provides an efficient summary for guiding practice decisions.

## Strength of Evidence

Rarely does the answer to a clinical question come from a single study (Aslam, Georgiev, Mehta, & Kumar, 2012). Clinical decisions should be based on the body of evidence and not on individual studies (Berkman et al., 2013; Murad et al., 2014). The quality of individual studies should be determined first, based on the study design, and not the level of evidence (i.e., you can have a high-quality observational study or a poor-quality meta-analysis). Then separately, the overall strength of the evidence base can be determined (Jones, 2010). The research question should drive study design (see Table 6.1).

| Table 6.1 | Research Designs Used to Answer Clinical Questions | | | |
|---|---|---|---|---|
| **Type** | **Design** | **Description** | **Types of Questions** | **+ Strengths/ − Weaknesses** |
| Analytical experimental | Randomized controlled trial (RCT) | Efficacy of one intervention tested versus another under ideal circumstances, controlling for other influencing factors | Which intervention or therapy is most efficacious? <br><br> What are the risk factors? <br><br> What is the effect of a test on outcomes? | + High internal validity; reduced effect of confounding variables, reduced bias <br><br> − Low external validity; not generalizable to other populations |
| | Quasi-experimental | Effectiveness of one intervention, therapy, or test compared to another in real-world settings | Which intervention is most effective? <br><br> What are the risk factors? <br><br> What is the effect of a test on outcomes? | + More external validity; more generalizable to clinical practice <br><br> − Less internal validity; variables less controlled, may increase bias |
| Observational | Cohort | Prospective subjects grouped by exposure and followed over time to determine outcomes | What is the etiology/risk for rare exposures with a common outcome? <br><br> What is the prognosis? <br><br> What is the accuracy of the test? | + Time sequence best for establishing association between exposure and outcome <br><br> − Requires large sample and long-term follow-up |
| | Case-control | Retrospective subjects with a certain outcome or disease grouped and then exposures/risks compared to matched controls | What is the etiology/risk for rare outcomes with common exposures? <br><br> What are the odds for an outcome based on exposures? | + Provides rapid useful information with small sample size or diseases with a long latency period <br><br> − Recall and selection bias |
| | Cross-sectional | Prospective health status, behavior, and other risk factors of a subpopulation measured at a given time | What is the diagnostic accuracy of the test? <br><br> What is the frequency or distribution of a disease? | + No follow-up required, so relatively inexpensive to conduct <br><br> − Does not differentiate cause and effect or the sequence of events |

*continues*

**Table 6.1    Research Designs Used to Answer Clinical Questions (Continued)**

| Type | Design | Description | Types of Questions | + Strengths/ − Weaknesses |
|---|---|---|---|---|
| Descriptive | Case reports or case series | Retrospective accounts of individuals with unusual disease, intervention, or therapy documented | Which interventions or treatments have worked in practice? | + Help to generate hypotheses  − Not generalizable |
| | Ideas, opinions, editorials, anecdotal evidence | Qualitative evidence supported by theory or scientific principles | Which intervention or treatment is thought to work best in practice? | + May be useful when other evidence is lacking  − Prone to bias |

(Aslam et al., 2012; Harris & Turner, 2011

Randomized controlled trials (RCTs) are often considered the gold standard of evidence. When available, they decrease uncertainty about addressing the clinical topic but do not eliminate it (Abbott & Bakris, 2004; Aveyard & Bauld, 2011; Smith & Pell, 2003). RCTs, often used to test clinical interventions, are not practical or appropriate for certain questions and may be misleading (Smith & Pell, 2003; Vaccaro et al., 2010). Many nursing questions don't lend themselves to an RCT design. Often, nursing interventions cannot be blinded, and research findings may not be generalizable or feasible in practice settings. Also, RCTs may lack clear direction for adaptation to a specific setting or population. Other research designs may be more appropriate for certain questions (e.g., a cross-sectional design for a diagnostic study or prospective validation for a prognostic study) (Baker, Young, Potter, & Madan, 2010; Costantino, Montano, & Casazza, 2015; Woolf et al., 2012).

The overall strength of the body of evidence is determined by evidence that is consistent and best answers the clinical question. Generally, when evidence is inconsistent, the lowest level of evidence determines the overall quality. For example, if two high-quality studies show benefit and one lower-level study does not, the overall level of evidence is not automatically elevated, but remains low. In contrast, when evidence is consistent, the overall quality is that of the better evidence; for example, if two studies of high quality and one of low quality all demonstrate the same outcomes, the overall evidence is considered high quality and not lowered (Woolf et al., 2012).

# Evidence Grade and Recommendations for Practice

Decisions about evidence and recommendations require thoughtful review and consideration. There are multiple and variable scales for rating evidence (Baker et al., 2010; Berkman et al., 2015; Gugiu & Gugiu, 2010; Jones, 2010) sponsored by independent groups, government agencies, and specialty organizations. In choosing a method for rating recommendations, consider the system adapted by your institution or specialty organization (Baker et al., 2010). Using an explicit and systematic approach to rating the evidence will help the team prevent errors, critically appraise the body of evidence, and communicate when making complex judgments about recommendations for practice (GRADE Working Group, 2016). However, users should also know that, particularly for more complex topics, grading systems have poor inter-rater reliability (Berkman et al., 2015; Berkman et al., 2012) and have not been validated (Halawa, 2014).

The Grading of Recommendations Assessment, Development and Evaluation (GRADE) Working Group is a widely adopted method created by an independent group and intended for guideline users and developers (Guyatt et al., 2011). The GRADE approach rates certainty of the body of evidence (quality, including study design, risk of bias, precision, consistency, generalizability, and effect size) as high, moderate, low, or very low across studies and clinical outcomes (Balshem et al., 2011). Strength of recommendations for practice and the extent to which you can be confident about the results are characterized as strong or weak, according to the quality of evidence, balance between desirable and undesirable outcomes, values and preferences, and costs. Weak recommendations are often conditional, discretionary, or qualified (Andrews et al., 2013; Guyatt et al., 2008). For more complex problems on a broader scope, more sophisticated systems such as that of the U.S. Preventive Services Task Force (USPSTF) resources and grading schema are available (see Table 6.2) (USPSTF, 2016a, 2016b).

**Table 6.2    U.S. Preventive Services Task Force (USPSTF) Grading Schema**

**USPSTF Strength of Recommendation Definitions***

| Grade | Definition | Suggestions for Practice |
|---|---|---|
| A | The USPSTF recommends the service. There is high certainty that the net benefit is substantial. | Offer or provide this service. |
| B | The USPSTF recommends the service. There is high certainty that the net benefit is moderate or there is moderate certainty that the net benefit is moderate to substantial. | Offer or provide this service. |
| C | The USPSTF recommends selectively offering or providing this service to individual patients based on professional judgment and patient preferences. There is at least moderate certainty that the net benefit is small. | Offer or provide this service for selected patients depending on individual circumstances. |
| D | The USPSTF recommends against the service. There is moderate or high certainty that the service has no net benefit or that the harms outweigh the benefits. | Discourage the use of this service. |
| I Statement | The USPSTF concludes that the current evidence is insufficient to assess the balance of benefits and harms of the service. Evidence is lacking, of poor quality, or conflicting, and the balance of benefits and harms cannot be determined. | Read the "Clinical Considerations" section of the USPSTF recommendation statement. If the service is offered, patients should understand the uncertainty about the balance of benefits and harms. |

*\* The USPSTF changed its grade definitions based on a change in methods in May 2007 and again in July 2012, when it updated the definition of and suggestions for practice for the grade C recommendation.*

*continues*

## Table 6.2   U.S. Preventive Services Task Force (USPSTF) Grading Schema (Continued)

| USPSTF Levels of Certainty Regarding Net Benefit | |
|---|---|
| Level of Certainty* | Description |
| High | The available evidence usually includes consistent results from well-designed, well-conducted studies in representative primary care populations. These studies assess the effects of the preventive service on health outcomes. This conclusion is therefore unlikely to be strongly affected by the results of future studies. |
| Moderate | The available evidence is sufficient to determine the effects of the preventive service on health outcomes, but confidence in the estimate is constrained by such factors as:<br><br>■ The number, size, or quality of individual studies.<br>■ Inconsistency of findings across individual studies.<br>■ Limited generalizability of findings to routine primary care practice.<br>■ Lack of coherence in the chain of evidence.<br><br>As more information becomes available, the magnitude or direction of the observed effect could change, and this change may be large enough to alter the conclusion. |
| Low | The available evidence is insufficient to assess effects on health outcomes. Evidence is insufficient because of:<br><br>■ The limited number or size of studies.<br>■ Important flaws in study design or methods.<br>■ Inconsistency of findings across individual studies.<br>■ Gaps in the chain of evidence.<br>■ Findings not generalizable to routine primary care practice.<br>■ Lack of information on important health outcomes.<br><br>More information may allow estimation of effects on health outcomes. |

* The USPSTF defines certainty as "likelihood that the USPSTF assessment of the net benefit of a preventive service is correct." The net benefit is defined as benefit minus harm of the preventive service as implemented in a general, primary care population. The USPSTF assigns a certainty level based on the nature of the overall evidence available to assess the net benefit of a preventive service.

(USPSTF, 2016b)

If no system is in place, choose one based on the project focus and clinical needs with consideration of the purpose and scope. For direct application to a clinical problem, select a simple system. For example, at University of Iowa Hospitals and Clinics, standards cite evidence that is simply noted to be based on research (R), non-research literature (L), national guidelines (N), or expert opinion (E) (see Example 6.1).

# The Decision Point

At this juncture, the team must decide whether the evidence is sufficient for pilot testing or if further research is needed (see Figure 6.1). The decision for recommending a practice change based on evidence cannot be derived from a formula but must rely on an understanding and consideration of the strength of the body of evidence, risk and benefits, the clinical need and setting, and expert clinical judgment. Practice recommendations must be made to meet the needs of current and future patients and be adapted to the local setting. These recommendations are designed to optimize benefits and minimize risk (e.g., by ensuring ready access to appropriate equipment). A priority factor is always safety, weighing the benefits and the risks/harm to patients (e.g., early ambulation to reduce pneumonia versus risk of fall).

**Figure 6.1**     Indications for Deciding: Is There Sufficient Evidence?

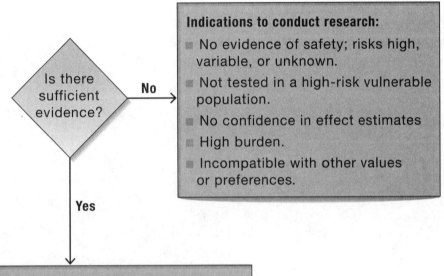

**Indications to conduct research:**

- No evidence of safety; risks high, variable, or unknown.
- Not tested in a high-risk vulnerable population.
- No confidence in effect estimates
- High burden.
- Incompatible with other values or preferences.

**Indications to move forward with pilot:**

- Themes are repeated in several articles.
- The same citations and conclusions repeat among references.
- There is sufficient research to organize the articles by study design (e.g., grouping citations with similar themes on the synthesis table can provide a sense of the extent of the evidence), and there are a number of articles, including those with high-quality study design (e.g., randomized control trials or multisite experiments).
- At least one relevant clinical practice guideline is available.

Overall, confidence in clinical practices having more benefit than harm can be achieved when high-quality systematic reviews with high-quality studies designed to answer the specific question in a variety of populations are evident (Costantino et al., 2015). Unfortunately, clear, consistent, high-quality evidence is rarely the case. Finding one absolute and consistent recommendation for practice reported in the literature is unlikely. Making practice decisions based on imperfect evidence may feel premature, yet there is a need to move forward with making clinical decisions. Practice recommendations (i.e., nursing assessments or interventions) can be developed even when evidence is of a lower level; examples of this are abundant in the literature (see Example 6.2) (Heneghan, 2011). Four additional domains the USPSTF considers for making clinical decisions when evidence is insufficient are: 1) potential for preventable burden, 2) potential harm, 3) costs, and 4) current practice. The GRADE Working Group and USPSTF acknowledge that clinicians don't have the luxury or time to wait for certain evidence; therefore, whenever possible, it is best to use the evidence available and, if necessary, use judgment to guide practice recommendations (Andrews et al., 2013; Petitti et al., 2009).

## Evidence Is Sufficient

Creating practice recommendations based on evidence is complex and requires skill. Recommendations for practice should include clear rationale statements that summarize the risks, benefits, and outcomes considered and link to the supporting evidence (see Example 6.3). Recommendations should not reach beyond the supporting evidence. Regardless of conclusion, transparency about the process is best—explaining what evidence, values, or preferences went into decision-making. Recommendations should be worded carefully, concisely, and precisely in behavioral terms that favorably influence integration in practice (Woolf et al., 2012). An *executive summary* is a concise way (one or two pages maximum) to summarize the work completed. It can be updated through the project to communicate progress to the team and other stakeholders (see Example 6.4). In the next steps, the team needs to consider other contextual factors (e.g., patient preferences, values, and local resources) and determine whether change is indicated. An evidence-based practice change should always be pilot tested so that a systematic evaluation can be used to make decisions about integration and widespread implementation or rollout.

## Evidence Is Not Sufficient

In some cases, clinicians cannot be confident that the desired effects of an intervention outweigh the undesired effects. In other cases, critical aspects of an intervention may be unknown (e.g., frequency or dose of flushes for peripheral IV catheters in neonates). Particularly when confidence in effect is low, risk is high, and values are not known, there may be insufficient evidence to change practice. New knowledge can be generated when existing evidence is insufficient. Research is a systematic investigation—including development, testing, and evaluation—designed to develop or contribute to generalizable knowledge (U.S. Department of Health & Human Services [USDHHS], n.d.-b). Be clear when differentiating research from EBP and quality processes (see Tool 6.2). When evidence is insufficient, conduct of research to generate or expand knowledge available for making practice decisions is indicated (Anderson, Kleiber, Greiner, Comried, & Zimmerman, 2016). The difficulty is that the time required to conduct research is often not conducive to patient care decisions. When new knowledge is generated by research and other sources (including pilot testing), evidence should be reassembled, appraised, and synthesized as the body of evidence has changed.

## RESOURCES: The GRADE Working Group Resources

The Grading of Recommendations Assessment, Development and Evaluation (GRADE) Working Group began in the year 2000 as an informal collaboration of people with an interest in addressing the shortcomings of grading systems in healthcare. The working group has developed a common, sensible, and transparent approach to grading certainty/quality of evidence and strength of recommendations. Many international organizations have provided input into the development of the GRADE approach, which has created a standard for evidence grading.

| Page Description | Link |
|---|---|
| Home page | http://www.gradeworkinggroup.org |
| Online learning modules to help guideline developers and authors of systematic reviews use the GRADE approach to grade the evidence in systematic reviews, create summary of findings tables and GRADE evidence profiles, and move from collecting evidence to making recommendations | https://cebgrade.mcmaster.ca |
| Suggested criteria for stating that the GRADE system was used | http://www.gradeworkinggroup.org/docs/Criteria_for_using_GRADE_2016-04-05.pdf |
| A selected list of GRADE publications | http://www.gradeworkinggroup.org/#pub |
| GRADEpro Guideline Development Tool, an all-in-one web solution for summarizing and presenting information for healthcare decision-making; also includes the GRADE handbook | https://gradepro.org |

(GRADE Working Group, 2016)

## TIPS: Determine if There Is Sufficient Evidence

- Look for existing systematic reviews and evidence-based guidelines that address the clinical questions. Update older reviews with current evidence. Don't reinvent.

- Determine the analytical process before you begin.

- Recommend that your institution or organization adopts a practical, consistent system for rating strength of evidence and clinical recommendations.

- Supplement the team with members who have expertise in literature review and synthesis. Mentor clinicians who have no experience in the process.

- Consider the strength of the total body of evidence; when high-quality evidence is lacking, look to lower levels of evidence.

- Further develop synthesis tables with the strength of evidence and strength of recommendation.

- Develop recommendations for practice from clinical questions and thesis statements. Weigh the evidence supporting or refuting, identify the cumulative strength of evidence, and then make recommendations for practice accordingly.

- Use informed clinical judgment and patient perspectives to determine best course when faced with insufficient evidence.

- Keep notes about how decisions are made, and demonstrate transparency in your process.

- Begin to create an executive summary to concisely communicate progress to the team and other stakeholders.

- Reassemble evidence when new knowledge from research or pilot testing emerges.

## RESOURCES: U.S. Preventive Services Task Force

The USPSTF is an independent, volunteer panel of national experts in prevention- and evidence-based medicine. The task force works to improve the health of all Americans by making evidence-based recommendations about clinical preventive services such as screenings, counseling services, and preventive medications.

| Description of Resource | Link |
|---|---|
| Home page | http://www.uspreventiveservicestaskforce.org |
| Searchable, evidence-based recommendations for primary care practice | http://www.uspreventiveservicestaskforce.org/Page/Name/recommendations |
| Task Force 101 Resources fact sheet and videos | http://www.uspreventiveservicestaskforce.org/Page/Name/task-force-101-resources |
| Understanding How the USPSTF Works: USPSTF 101 | http://www.uspreventiveservicestaskforce.org/Page/Name/understanding-how-the-uspstf-works |
| Grade definitions (2012)<br><br>A, B, C, D, or I | http://www.uspreventiveservicestaskforce.org/Page/Name/grade-definitions |
| USPSTF procedures manual, methods, commentaries, and resources for practice | http://www.uspreventiveservicestaskforce.org/Page/Name/methods-and-processes |

(USPSTF, 2016a)

**Example 6.1    Policy on Referencing Within Policies and Procedures**

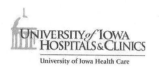 Policy and Procedure Manual

University of Iowa Health Care

| References: Guidelines for Documenting | N-A-13.003 |
| --- | --- |

A.    <u>Research References</u>:

Research references should be footnoted as $R_1$, $R_2$, $R_3$, etc. in the body of the policy, procedure or document where the citation takes place.  Specific footnote information should then be listed at the end of the document.

*Example*:

<u>Research References</u>:

$R_1$      Goode, C.J., Titler, M., Rakel, B., Ones, K.S., Kleiber, C., Small, S., & Triolo, P.K. (1991).  A meta-analysis of effects of heparin flush and saline flush:  Quality and cost implications.  *Nursing Research*, 40, 423-430, 423-430. doi:xx.xxxxxxxxxx or Retrieved from http://www.xxxxxxxx.

If there are more than seven authors, reference should be listed as:

$R_1$      Goode, C.J., Titler, M., Rakel, B., Ones, K.S., Kleiber, C., Small, S.,…Triolo, P.K. (1991).  A meta-analysis of effects of heparin flush and saline flush:  Quality and cost implications.  *Nursing Research*, 40, 423-430, 423-430. doi:xx.xxxxxxxxxx or Retrieved from http://www.xxxxxxxx.

B.    <u>Literature References</u>:

Literature references can be cited in two ways:

1.    If an entire document is based on an article(s), the literature reference may be noted as such at the end of the document.

2.    If a specific statement or section is based on information in the literature, that section should be <u>footnoted</u> as $L_1$, $L_2$, etc. with the specific footnote information noted at the end of the document.

*Example*:

<u>Literature References</u>:

$L_1$      Danek, G.D. & Norris, E.M. (1992). Pediatric IV catheters:  Efficacy of saline flush. *Pediatric Nursing, 18*(2), 111-113.  doi:xx.xxxxxxxxxx or Retrieved from http://www.xxxxxxxx

C.    <u>National Guideline References</u>:

1.  If an entire document is based on published guidelines, the National Guideline Reference may be noted as such at the end of the document.

**Example 6.1    Policy on Referencing Within Policies and Procedures (Continued)**

2.  If a specific statement or section is based on information in the guideline, that section should be footnoted as N1, N2, etc. with the specific footnote information noted at the end of the document.

    Example:

    N1    Herr, K. et al. (2000). *Evidence-Based Guideline: Acute Pain Management in the Elderly.* AHRQ #1R01 HS10482-01. Bethesda, MD: Agency for Healthcare Research and Quality.

D.    Expert Opinion/Consultation/Collaboration:

1.  Consultants may be individual or departments.

    *Example:*

    Expert Opinion References:

    E1    Beverly Folkedahl, RN, BSN, CWOCN, APN/Clinical Nurse Specialist, University of Iowa Health Care (personal communication, <date>).

    E2    Department of Respiratory Care, University of Iowa Health Care (personal communication, <date>).

E.    General Form for Electronic References (from the 6th Edition of the APA Publication Manual).

Electronic sources include aggregated databases, online journals, Web sites or Web pages, newsgroups, Web- or e-mail-based discussion groups, and Web- or e-mail-based newsletters.  Electronic references should be integrated into one of the above 4 categories (e.g., R; L; N; E).

*Examples*

1.  Online periodical:

    Author, A. A., Author, B. B., & Author, C. C. (2000).  Title of article. *Title of Periodical, xx,* xxxxxx.  doi:xx.xxxxxxxxxx or retrieved from http://www.xxxx.xxx.

2.  Online document:

    Author, A. A. (2000). *Title of work.*  Retrieved from http:/www.xxxx.xx..

Written:        4/95
Last Reviewed: 2/98, 10/08, 11/11, 6/13
Last Revised:   6/01, 8/05, 11/14

References: Guidelines for Documenting
NA 13.003

## Example 6.2    Practice Recommendations Using Low-Level Evidence

### Classic Examples

**Parachutes** to prevent death and injury from jumping out of airplanes have not been tested by RCT studies. This report demonstrates why low-level evidence is sometimes needed to guide practice (Smith & Pell, 2003).

**Hand hygiene** efficacy tested through RCTs is limited (Ejemot-Nwadiaro, Ehiri, Arikpo, Meremikwu, & Critchley, 2015) and complicated by risk factors and other intervention strategies (McLaws, 2015), yet there is sufficient evidence from other observational studies to be a well-established, evidence-based practice (Blouin, 2010; CDC, 2002; World Health Organization, 2009).

### Other Examples

**Fall prevention guidelines** in hospitals have not been demonstrated to prevent falls (Clyburn & Heydemann, 2011), even though fall prevention literature includes randomized trials (Dykes et al., 2010). Research evaluating the effectiveness of individual fall prevention interventions is difficult to complete because of issues with control, feasibility, measurement, and patient safety. Nonetheless, using a multi-faceted fall prevention program can reduce fall rates (Choi & Hector, 2011; Michael et al., 2010; Spoelstra, Given, & Given, 2011; Titler et al., 2016; The Joint Commission, 2015).

**Nurse rounding** has been widely adopted as a common-sense intervention. Evidence is limited by non-randomized samples, small samples, and short durations (Hicks, 2015) with mixed findings on sustained fall reduction rates (Tucker, Bieber, Attlesey-Pries, Olson, & Dierkhising, 2011). It is difficult to develop a randomized controlled trial to evaluate the effectiveness of rounding, because rounding is a patient care routine. In addition, the risk of rounding is minimal, the gains are multiple, and rounding is an independent nursing intervention that may be relatively easy to use. Research may still provide direction about the best procedure and frequency for rounding, but nurses are moving forward with adoption.

**Bedside handoff report** was identified as a National Patient Safety Goal in 2009 and an important determinant of quality and safety. Limited but low-level qualitative studies (Sherman, Sand-Jecklin, & Johnson, 2013) are beginning to provide direction about how to implement bedside handoff report while addressing the challenges of maintaining privacy (Ferguson & Howell, 2015) and the needs of special populations (Clarke & Persaud, 2011; Foronda, VanGraafeiland, Quon, & Davidson, 2016; Kamath et al., 2016).

**Flush solutions** for maintaining patency of peripheral arterial lines for adults have conflicting recommendations reported from research (AACN Thunder Project Task Force, 1993; Caixeta et al., 2011; Classen, Jaser, & Budnitz, 2010; Del Cotillo, Grané, Llavoré, & Quintana, 2008; Fanikos et al., 2004; Infusion Nurses Society, 2011). Evidence is of poor quality due to risk of bias, and there is insufficient, not definitive, information to support adding heparin (1–2U/ml) to saline for maintaining arterial catheter patency (Robertson-Malt, Malt, Farquhar, & Greer, 2014). Nurses and interprofessional teams must weigh the evidence and make practice decisions for patient care.

## CITATIONS

AACN, 1993; Blouin, 2010; Caixeta et al., 2011; CDC, 2002; Choi & Hector, 2011; Clarke & Persaud, 2011; Classen, Jaser, & Budnitz, 2010; Clyburn & Heydemann, 2011; Del Cotillo, Grané, Llavoré, & Quintana, 2008; Dykes et al., 2010; Ejemot-Nwadiaro, Ehiri, Arikpo, Meremikwu, & Critchley, 2015; Fanikos et al., 2004; Ferguson & Howell, 2015; Foronda, VanGraafeiland, Quon, & Davidson, 2016; Hicks, 2015; Infusion Nurses Society, 2011; The Joint Commission, 2015; Kamath et al., 2016; McLaws, 2015; Michael et al., 2010; Robertson-Malt, Malt, Farquhar, & Greer, 2014; Sherman, Sand-Jecklin, & Johnson, 2013; Smith & Pell, 2003; Spoelstra, Given, & Given, 2011; Titler et al., 2016; Tucker, Bieber, Attlesey-Pries, Olson, & Dierkhising, 2011; World Health Organization (WHO), 2009.

**Example 6.3    Practice Recommendations: Vancomycin**

## Prophylactic Use of Vancomycin Prior to Removal of Peripherally Inserted Central Catheter (PICC) in the Neonatal Intensive Care Unit (NICU)

Gail Reynolds, DNP, ARNP, CPNP

### Practice Recommendation

■ Prophylactic vancomycin x 1 prior to peripherally inserted central catheters (PICC) removal with the goal to decrease the incidence of post catheter removal sepsis (PCRS, defined as requiring a sepsis evaluation and antibiotics) in low birth weight infants admitted to the neonatal intensive care unit (Reynolds, Tierney, & Klein, 2015).

### Recommended Implementation

Create standard-of-care protocol and standing order-set to support clinician decision-making:

■ Vancomycin 15 mg/kg once prior to PICC line removal in neonates $\leq$ 2500 grams at birth, with a PICC line >/= to 10 days and the last dose of antibiotics >12 hours prior to the PICC removal (Reynolds et al., 2015).

■ Administration of vancomycin prior to the PICC removal outside these guidelines may be ordered based on prescriber assessment (Reynolds et al., 2015).

### Rationale

■ When a PICC is placed, bacteria can colonize at the tip of the catheter. Upon removal of the catheter, there is a risk of bacteria being released into the bloodstream from the biofilm becoming dislodged and the neonate may become septic (de Silva et al., 2002).

■ Coagulase negative staphylococci (CoNS) are the most common pathogen identified in late-onset sepsis in neonates admitted to the NICU and the use of indwelling central lines increases the risk of hospital-acquired infections (Baier, Bocchini, & Brown, 1998; Borghesi & Stronati, 2008; Cooke et al., 1997; Garland, Alex, Henrickson, McAulife, & Maki, 2005; Hemels, van den Hoogen, Verboon-Maciolek, Fleer, & Krediet, 2011; Lee, 2011; Lodha, Furlan, Whyte, & Moore, 2008; Powers & Wirtschafter, 2010; Stoll et al., 2002; van den Hoogen, Brouwer, Gerards, Fleer, & Krediet, 2008) with gram positive pathogens accounting for as much as 80% of CLABSIs (Garland & Uhing, 2009).

■ CoNS are particularly adept at adhering to catheters and forming biofilms (Marchant, Boyce, Sadarangani, & Lavoie, 2013) leading to this organism being responsible for the majority of catheter-associated sepsis; other organisms associated with sepsis in the presence of central venous catheters include: Staphylococcus aureus, Enterobacter, Klebsiella, and Escherichia coli (van den Hoogen et al., 2008).

■ Other factors that may increase a neonate's risk for CLABSI, including length of time the catheter is in place (Sengupta, Lehmann, Diener-West, Peri, & Milstone, 2010; Njere, Islam, Parish, Kuna, & Keshtgar, 2011) and placement in the upper versus lower extremity (Hoang et al., 2008).

■ A retrospective study (van den Hoogen et al., 2008) and a prospective randomized study (Hemels et al., 2011) both determined that the use of prophylactic cefazolin at the time of removal of a central line decreased the incidence of neonatal sepsis.

- Vancomycin is the drug of choice when treating hospital-acquired gram positive or CoNS sepsis (Cooke et al., 1997; Craft, Finer, & Barrington, 2000; Spafford, Sinkin, Cox, Reuens, & Powell, 1994).

- No reports found vancomycin as harmful or ineffective in the treatment of CLABSI in the neonatal population.

- The key to minimizing the development of vancomycin resistance is to achieve optimal drug exposure. It is possible to select for vancomycin-resistant mutants by using low doses along with prolonged exposure to vancomycin (Rybak, 2006).

- Retrospective chart audits showed that when antibiotics were given within 12 hours before PICC line removal, only 2% of the line removal episodes (1/48) resulted in a neonate developing clinical sepsis versus 13% (21/165) when no antibiotics were given prior to removal ($p = 0.03$, Fisher's exact test). There was an 11% absolute decrease and a six-fold relative decrease in post-catheter removal clinical sepsis events in premature neonates who received antibiotics prior to PICC line removal (Reynolds et al., 2015).

- Despite the increased use of elective antibiotics with line removal, there was no increase in total antibiotic usage due to the overall decrease in episodes of clinical sepsis or changes in antibiogram susceptibility patterns (Reynolds et al., 2015).

## Revisiting This Recommendation

Ongoing surveillance and quality monitoring is warranted. Review literature annually for new citations for updating the practice. Re-evaluate prior to policy review in 2 or 3 years.

For more information: The complete Prophylactic Use of Vancomycin Prior to Removal of Peripherally Inserted Central Catheter (PICC) in the Neonatal Intensive Care Unit (NICU) report and references can be obtained by contacting Gail Reynolds at gail-reynolds@uiowa.edu.

## CITATIONS

Baier, Bocchini Jr, & Brown, 1998; Borghesi & Stronati, 2008; Cooke et al, 1997; Craft, Finer, & Barrington, 2000; de Silva et al., 2002; Garland, Alex, Henrickson, McAuliffe, & Maki, 2005; Garland & Uhing, 2009; Hemels, van den Hoogen, Verboon-Maciolek, Fleer, & Krediet, 2011; Hoang et al., 2008; Lee, 2011; Lodha, Furlan, Whyte, & Moore, 2008; Marchant, Boyce, Sadarangani, & Lavoie, 2013; Njere, Islam, Parish, Kuna, & Keshtgar, 2011; Powers & Wirtschafter, 2010; Reynolds, Tierney, & Klein, 2015; Rybak, 2006; Sengupta, Lehmann, Diener-West, Peri, & Milstone, 2010; Spafford, Sinkin, Cox, Reuens, & Powell, 1994; Stoll et al., 2002; van den Hoogen, Brouwer, Gerards, Fleer, & Krediet, 2008.

EXAMPLES

TOOLS

## Example 6.4   Executive Summary

### Critical Congenital Heart Disease Screening in the Newborn Nursery

Danielle Wendel, DNP, ARNP, CPNP

### Introduction of Problem

Congenital heart disease is the most common congenital disorder in newborns and is also the leading cause of death in infants. In the United States, about 7,200 (18 per 10,000) infants are born every year with a critical congenital heart disease (CCHD). Approximately 30% of infants with CCHD are diagnosed after leaving the hospital as a newborn. Pulse oximetry screening in the newborn unit can help detect CCHD early so that evaluation and treatment can be promptly initiated, thereby reducing morbidity and/or mortality. The purpose of this capstone project was to develop, implement, and evaluate a pulse oximetry screening protocol to be used in the newborn nursery at The University of Iowa Hospitals and Clinics (UIHC).

### Literature Review

Several studies have shown that the risk of morbidity and mortality increases when there is a delay in diagnosis of CCHD. Pulse oximetry screening has been shown to be an effective screening measure of CCHD. Pulse oximetry, when used in detection of critical congenital heart disease, has high specificity and moderate sensitivity. Although there is some cost associated with the screening, it is significantly off set by the avoided costs of care in newborns with undiagnosed CCHD. When we diagnose infants earlier before they become acutely ill, we will avoid costs caused by prolonged hospitalization and decrease long-term morbidity. The cost of screening per case diagnosed is approximately $5,198, and the cost of an infant readmitted in circulatory collapse is approximately $5,233. This does not account for the costs of long-term morbidity that is averted with a timely diagnosis. The theoretical model employed was Rogers Diffusion of Innovations Theory. This model leads to advances in health promotion and disease prevention by the diffusion or spread of new ideas such as evidence-based practices.

### Methodology

At UIHC, an interprofessional group including nurse managers, nurse educators, cardiologists, physicians, neonatologists, advanced registered nurse practitioners, and respiratory therapists was formed to address the need of a pulse oximetry screening protocol. The project leader (DNP student) was a pediatric nurse practitioner, practice expert, and nurse educator. A variety of implementation strategies were used. The group developed an evidence-based pulse oximetry protocol, algorithm, and parent education. Nurses were provided training on the screening protocol using a presentation and mentored hands-on experience. How to correctly apply the pulse oximetry probe and correctly read the pulse oximeter was emphasized. The pulse oximetry screening policy was implemented in the newborn nursery at UIHC. The resources needed to implement the protocol (pulse oximeter, probes, echocardiography, and pediatric cardiology specialist) were already in place at the facility. Data were collected from chart reviews on the number of positive screenings, echocardiogram results, and the number of infants diagnosed with CCHD over a 12-month period. The project was determined as not being human subjects research by the IRB.

## Evaluation

The CCHD screening protocol was developed and implemented at UIHC in the newborn nursery. All infants are screened for CCHD prior to being discharged. In the first 12 months, 1,325 patients were screened. There were three positive screenings. All three newborns had an echocardiogram showing a patent foramen ovale. No CCHD was found in the first year of implementation. Unexpected outcomes would be to identify newborns with other causes of low-oxygen saturations, such as pneumonia. We did not have any unexpected outcomes in the first year of implementation. One challenge with the implementation of the protocol was timing of the screening. We changed the timing of the screen to 0400 to decrease the amount of time parents and clinicians would have to wait for a diagnosis via echocardiogram if there was a positive screen.

## Impact on Practice

Pulse oximetry screening of newborns has been endorsed by the American Academy of Pediatrics, the American Heart Association, and the American College of Cardiology Foundation. In 2011, the U.S. Department of Health and Human Services recommended adopting pulse oximetry screening for CCHD in the uniform screening panel for all newborns. Many states have already mandated screening for CCHD. Iowa passed legislation in the Senate, and it is under consideration in the House. The number of newborns who are diagnosed earlier with CCHD will increase through uniform screening.

## Conclusions

Pulse oximetry screening for CCHD is easy to use, quick to administer and get values, inexpensive with a good cost-benefit ratio, safe, non-invasive, and acceptable to use as a screening tool in our specific population. By developing and implementing a pulse oximetry protocol to screen for CCHD in the newborn, we will aid in diagnosing infants with previously undiagnosed CCHD prior to discharge. Earlier detection of CCHD may decrease morbidity and mortality.

## For More Information

The complete *Critical Congenital Heart Disease Screening in the Newborn Nursery* reports and references can be obtained by contacting Danielle Wendel at danielle-wendel@uiowa.edu.

## CITATION

Wendel, n.d.

## Tool 6.1   Determine if There Is Sufficient Evidence

**INSTRUCTIONS:** Review the steps outlined for determining if evidence is sufficient for an EBP change. Identify dates and times for relevant steps, such as meetings to make a list of practice recommendations. Check when steps are completed. Proceed to the next step until each step has been completed.

| Date Scheduled | Activity | Done |
|---|---|---|
| | Determine the process for analyzing evidence. | ☐ |
| | Determine the criteria for making clinical decisions (e.g., strength of evidence, risk, benefit, outcomes). | ☐ |
| | Define the key clinical questions and outcomes of interest. | ☐ |
| | Review the synthesis table for themes or concepts related to the questions and outcomes of interest. | ☐ |
| | Determine the quality and strength of the body of evidence for each question and each outcome. | ☐ |
| | Create a list of potential risks for patients associated with the question (e.g., pharmacologic interventions for post-operative pain and slowed return of motility). | ☐ |
| | Create a list of potential benefits for patients associated with the question (e.g., pharmacologic interventions for post-operative pain and increased mobility; increased mobility reducing the risk of DVT and pneumonia). | ☐ |
| | Draft a list of recommendations for practice, including citations. | ☐ |
| | Determine the strength of each recommendation. | ☐ |
| | Determine the clinical roles (e.g., nursing, pharmacy) responsible for the recommended practice to ensure that each one is represented in decision-making. | ☐ |
| | Convene a team meeting; include additional stakeholders. | ☐ |
| | Discuss each potential practice recommendation, the body of evidence supporting the recommendation, and potential risks and benefits. | ☐ |
| | Create a project executive summary to concisely update the team and stakeholders; update as project work progresses. | ☐ |

## Tool 6.2 Determining Quality Improvement, EBP, or Research

**INSTRUCTIONS:** Answer each question in the column on the left by checking which box most closely reflects the intent of the work to be accomplished. Review responses as a team. Recognize that all three methods are systematic evaluative methods that include living individuals as part of the evaluation. Discuss and select as a team the method most closely matching the intent. Proceed with relevant notifications and approvals.

| | Quality Improvement | Evidence-Based Practice | Research |
|---|---|---|---|
| Which definition fits? | ☐ QI is an organizational strategy that formally involves the analysis of process and outcomes data and the application of systematic efforts to improve performance (AHRQ, 2011a).<br><br>☐ The degree to which healthcare services for individuals and populations increases the likelihood of desired health outcomes and are consistent with current professional knowledge (IOM, 2004, para. 3). | ☐ Evidence-based practice is the process of shared decision-making between practitioner, patient, and others significant to them based on research evidence, the patient's experiences and preferences, clinical expertise or know-how, and other available robust sources of information (STTI, 2008).<br><br>☐ Healthcare delivery based on the integration of the best research evidence available combined with clinical expertise, in accordance with the preferences of the patient and family (Sackett et al., 1996; Sackett, Straus, Richardson, Rosenberg, & Haynes, 2000). | ☐ Systematic investigation, including research development, testing, and evaluation, designed to develop or contribute to generalizable knowledge; (USDHHS, n.d.-b).<br><br>☐ Systematic investigation designed to contribute to generalizable knowledge (USDHHS, n.d.-b). |
| | Intent | | |
| Who benefits? | ☐ Current patients/families<br>☐ Current clinicians<br>☐ Organization | ☐ Future patients/families<br>☐ Future clinicians<br>☐ Organization | ☐ Clinicians<br>☐ Scientific community<br>☐ Subjects (on occasion) |
| What is the purpose? | ☐ Improve quality or safety of processes or patient experience within the local clinical setting.<br>☐ Evaluate changes in efficiency or flow. | ☐ Improve quality and safety within the local clinical setting by applying evidence in healthcare decisions. | ☐ Contribute to and/or generate new knowledge that can be generalized. |
| What is the scope of interest? | ☐ Specific unit or patient population within an organization | ☐ Specific unit or patient population within an organization | ☐ Generalize to populations beyond organization |

*continues*

**Tool 6.2    Determining Quality Improvement, EBP, or Research (Continued)**

| | Quality Improvement | Evidence-Based Practice | Research |
|---|---|---|---|
| | **Methodology** | | |
| Which process or outcome measurements are used? | ☐ Measures are simple, easy to use, and administer.<br><br>☐ Measures are for key indicators only. | ☐ Measures for key indicators using tools with face validity and may be without established validity or reliability.<br><br>☐ Measures include knowledge, attitude, behavior/practices, outcomes, and balancing measures (Bick & Graham, 2010; Institute for Healthcare Improvement [IHI], 2017). | ☐ Measures are complex.<br><br>☐ Increased time is required to fill out the measure.<br><br>☐ Measures require a detailed administration plan.<br><br>☐ Estimates of reliability, validity, specificity, and/ or sensitivity are required. |
| Which design fits? | ☐ Examples include:<br>  ☐ Six Sigma<br>  ☐ Plan Do Study Act (PDSA)<br>  ☐ LEAN<br>  ☐ Continuous Quality Improvement (CQI) | ☐ Iowa Model or another EBP process model | ☐ Randomized control<br><br>☐ Quantitative<br><br>☐ Qualitative |
| What is the timing? | ☐ Rapid cycle (for example, PDSA) | ☐ Planned<br><br>☐ Variable timeline based on available clinical practice guidelines or other synthesis reports | ☐ Planned and longer |
| Are there extraneous variables? | ☐ Acknowledged but not measured | ☐ Acknowledged but not measured | ☐ Controlled and/or measured<br><br>☐ Tight protocol control |
| What is the sample? | ☐ Convenience sample | ☐ Convenience sample | ☐ Varied sampling based on study question; may include an established process to improve generalizability of results |

**CHAPTER 6:** IS THERE SUFFICIENT EVIDENCE?     99

| | Quality Improvement | Evidence-Based Practice | Research |
|---|---|---|---|
| What is the sample size? | ☐ Small, but large enough to observe changes<br><br>☐ Feasible for data collection | ☐ Small, but large enough to observe changes<br><br>☐ Feasible for data collection | ☐ Size based on estimates of adequate power or saturation |
| Which data collection is used? | ☐ Minimal time, resources, cost | ☐ Minimal time, resources, cost | ☐ Complex, tightly controlled plan for resources constructed |
| Which data analysis is used? | ☐ Descriptive statistics, run chart, or statistical process control charts for trended data | ☐ Descriptive statistics, run chart, or statistical process control charts for trended data; may use inferential statistics | ☐ Complex with inferential statistics to promote generalizability of results |
| Are there relevant regulating bodies? | ☐ Organization<br><br>☐ Influenced by:<br>  ☐ The Joint Commission<br>  ☐ Centers for Medicare & Medicaid Services | ☐ Organization | ☐ Organization, Office of Human Research Protections, FDA, state and local laws |
| Are there additional burdens or risks? | ☐ Patient and/or population is expected to benefit directly from improved flow or process.<br><br>☐ Risk of participation is the same as receiving usual clinical care.<br><br>☐ If risk or burden is higher than with usual care, consider research and IRB. | ☐ Patient and/or population is expected to benefit directly from observations.<br><br>☐ Risk of participation is the same as receiving usual clinical care.<br><br>☐ If risk or burden is higher than with usual care, consider research and IRB. | ☐ Participant is aware of risks.<br><br>☐ Informed consent is required.<br><br>☐ IRB is required.<br><br>☐ Subject may or may not benefit from participation in study. |
| Is IRB approval needed? | ☐ Generally not required unless per organizational policy; recommend checking policy and/or with an organizational leader. | ☐ Generally not required when evaluation is limited to QI unless per organizational policy. Recommend a human subject's research determination if there are questions or organization policy/requirements. | ☐ Required |

*continues*

EXAMPLES

TOOLS

## Tool 6.2   Determining Quality Improvement, EBP, or Research (Continued)

| | Quality Improvement | Evidence-Based Practice | Research |
|---|---|---|---|
| Is dissemination possible? | ☐ Expected to disseminate within the organization; may be expected for public accountability and transparency based on CMS regulations; may be published.<br><br>☐ "The intent to publish is an insufficient criterion for determining whether a quality improvement activity involves research. Planning to publish an account of a quality improvement project does not necessarily mean that the project fits the definition of research; people seek to publish descriptions of nonresearch activities for a variety of reasons, if they believe others may be interested in learning about those activities." (USDHHS, n.d.-b, para. 6) | ☐ Expected to disseminate within the organization; publication is increasingly becoming an expectation.<br><br>☐ Does not indicate generalizability of findings or research (see disseminating quality improvement data).<br><br>☐ Adopt SQUIRE 2.0 criteria (Standards for Quality Improvement Reporting Excellence [SQUIRE], 2015) | ☐ Expected |

## CITATIONS

AHRQ, 2011a; Bick & Graham, 2010; IHI, 2017; IOM, 2004; OHRP, 2009; Sackett et al., 1996; Sackett et al., 2000; Sigma Theta Tau International 2005–2007 Research and Scholarship Advisory Committee, 2008; SQUIRE, 2015; USDHHS, n.d.-b.

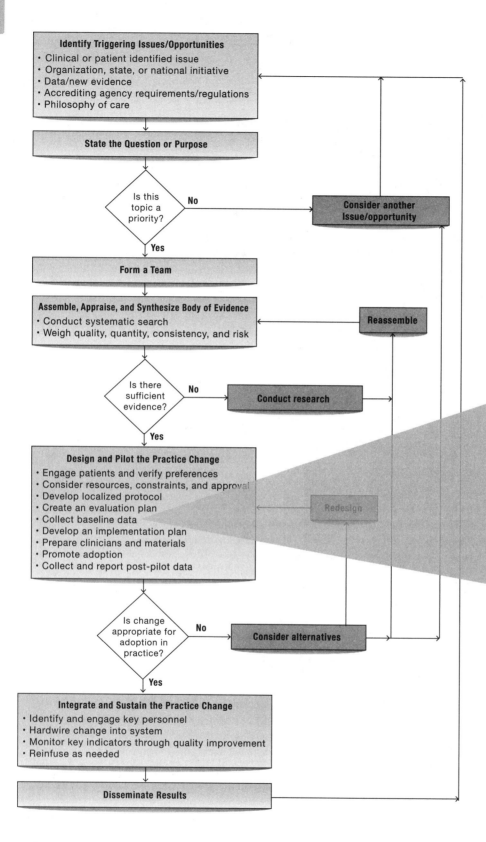

**Identify Triggering Issues/Opportunities**
- Clinical or patient identified issue
- Organization, state, or national initiative
- Data/new evidence
- Accrediting agency requirements/regulations
- Philosophy of care

**State the Question or Purpose**

Is this topic a priority?

**No** → **Consider another Issue/opportunity**

**Yes**

**Form a Team**

**Assemble, Appraise, and Synthesize Body of Evidence**
- Conduct systematic search
- Weigh quality, quantity, consistency, and risk

← **Reassemble**

Is there sufficient evidence?

**No** → **Conduct research**

**Yes**

**Design and Pilot the Practice Change**
- Engage patients and verify preferences
- Consider resources, constraints, and approval
- Develop localized protocol
- Create an evaluation plan
- Collect baseline data
- Develop an implementation plan
- Prepare clinicians and materials
- Promote adoption
- Collect and report post-pilot data

← **Redesign**

Is change appropriate for adoption in practice?

**No** → **Consider alternatives**

**Yes**

**Integrate and Sustain the Practice Change**
- Identify and engage key personnel
- Hardwire change into system
- Monitor key indicators through quality improvement
- Reinfuse as needed

**Disseminate Results**

# DESIGN AND PILOT THE PRACTICE CHANGE

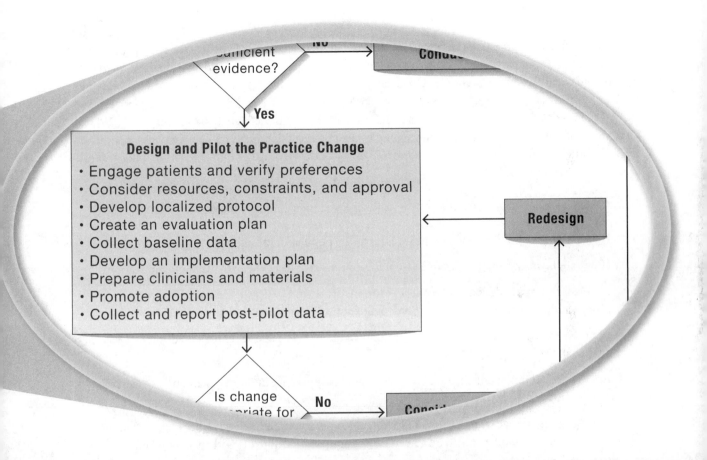

"*What would life be if we had no courage to attempt anything?*"

–Vincent van Gogh

When the evidence-based practice (EBP) team decides to move forward, the next step is to design a pilot test of the change. Pilot testing the practice change is a critically important step in implementing EBP (Shapiro & Donaldson, 2008). In the Iowa Model, this step was expanded to provide more specific guidance on the process. The purpose of the pilot is to determine whether the practice change works as intended, whether the implementation plan results in adoption of the change, and whether other patient care areas would benefit from a rollout. Failing to plan a systematic and thorough pilot test can lead to confusion among the EBP users and may make it difficult to interpret the post-change data. Without credible data to show that the EBP had the intended effect, it may be difficult to convince users and stakeholders to maintain the change.

Pilot testing often requires more time and effort than assembling, appraising, and synthesizing the evidence, so adjust the timeline for the project accordingly. Shapiro and Donaldson (2008) provide a useful example of a timeline for making triage changes in emergency departments. Involve the right people in the planning. At this point in the process, new team members may need to be added. If the EBP might incorporate patient or family preferences (e.g., family presence during resuscitation), engage patients and families in the discussion. Select a pilot area that has an enthusiastic manager, known opinion leaders, and change champions. Supportive leadership is vital for the success of the initiative (Sandström et al., 2011). Be mindful of other initiatives that are happening in the pilot area that may compete for resources and time. The strategies described in Chapter 8 provide ideas for developing the implementation plan and promoting adoption of the EBP.

Questions to consider when using the body of evidence to design and pilot the practice change are:

- How is the evidence relevant and meaningful to the population of interest?

- How can the intervention be adapted to fit the cultural norms of the patients and organization?

- How can recommendations be adapted to be consistent with patient preferences (e.g., promoting independence vs. limiting independent mobility to prevent falling)?

- What are the risks and how can they be minimized to benefit patients, clinicians, or the organization?

- Are the costs (human and material) associated with the practice and implementation of the practice change outweighed by the benefits?

- Is the practice change complex? Are there threats to intervention fidelity (ability to carry out intervention as intended)? Is there a need for training and monitoring anticipated outcomes?

- What are the consequences for ineffective use or failure of the practice change? How can these consequences be addressed or minimized?

- Is the practice recommendation consistent with existing institutional policies? How can policy updates be approved and adopted after a pilot?

- Does the practice fit within nursing's scope of practice, or are the relevant providers participating in developing the practice recommendation?

# Engage Patients and Verify Preferences

Early EBP approaches focused largely on determining the best research evidence related to a clinical problem or decision and applying that evidence to resolve the issue (Haynes, Devereaux, & Guyatt, 2002). Contemporary models go beyond the evidence and recognize that success of a practice or an intervention is influenced by a host of other factors, including patient preferences and values, which may differ from clinician advice or recommendations (Burman, Robinson, & Hart, 2013). "Patient preferences refer to patient perspectives, beliefs, expectations and goals for health and life, and to the processes that individuals use in considering potential benefits, harms, costs and inconveniences of the management options in relation to one another" (Montori, Brito, & Murad, 2013, p. 2503). Integrating preferences supports the movement toward patient-centered healthcare, which emphasizes their experience rather than diseases and increases patient involvement in decision-making (Krahn & Naglie, 2008). Practicing patient-centered healthcare means finding out what patients want, helping them find relevant information, and supporting their decision-making processes (Krahn & Naglie, 2008). Engaging patients and families in the implementation of the best evidence for a patient's situation, disease, and care is imperative to providing safe, patient-centered, efficient, equitable, timely, and effective care systems (Kemper, Blackburn, Doyle, & Hyman, 2013).

# Consider Resources, Constraints, and Approval

EBP is a complex, multifactorial process that requires the art and science of nursing as well as consideration of resources from the time the purpose statement is developed and the initiative is deemed an institutional priority (Hauck et al., 2013). After it is determined a priority, important next steps are to ensure that adequate resources (human and material) exist to formulate the team, organize and synthesize the relevant literature (which requires basic searching and article-reviewing skills as well as time [Majid et al., 2011]), develop a plan, collect pre-implementation data, implement the practice changes with the host of implementation strategies, collect and evaluate the post-implementation data, move forward with a larger rollout, and disseminate the initiative outcomes. Constraints to be considered are the necessary human and material resources to execute the project, including, but not limited to, equipment, information technology and design, and statistical expertise (Majid et al., 2011). Moreover, leadership is needed that understands change and innovation theory (Hauck et al., 2013), articulates the value of evidence, and appreciates the engagement of nurses in EBP. Organizational readiness (Hauck et al., 2013) and organizational approval bodies (e.g., quality and safety oversight committees, institutional review boards; Hockenberry, 2014) must also be understood within each organization to ensure successful EBP initiatives.

**TIPS: Engaging Patients and Families**

■ Seek qualitative research to understand the patient/family experience.

■ Involve patient/family representatives on teams and councils.

■ Interview patient/family about their questions and experiences in care.

■ Seek patient/family suggestions for priorities and EBP care.

■ Request patient/family review and edits for teaching tools, decision aids, and reminders.

■ Seek patient/family input in healthcare decisions.

■ Adapt tools and interactions to meet the needs of vulnerable patients/families.

■ Encourage patient advocacy by family or a caregiver.

A process should also be in place to assist students from any discipline to obtain approval to develop and implement EBP within the nursing department (see Example 7.1) (Basol, Larsen, Simones, & Wilson, 2017; Foote, Conley, Williams, McCarthy, & Countryman, 2015; Selker et al., 2011). Student work will need to follow all organizational policies, including confidentiality, data security, and protection of patient information. Faculty members can be an important bridge between students and agencies (Moch, Quinn-Lee, Gallegos, & Sortedahl, 2015). Supporting student projects can promote learning for current and future employees, provide student time as a resource addressing an important topic, and support collaboration across academia and practice settings (Barnsteiner, Reeder, Palma, Preston, & Walton, 2010; Moch et al., 2015). Developing skills in the EBP process and leadership for application of EBP in practice addresses an important national agenda for nursing and nursing education (IOM, 2010b). Developing EBP skills, including implementation skills, remains a priority for healthcare organizations because of the impact on quality, safety, and cost (Braithwaite, Marks, & Taylor, 2014; Stevens, 2009). In addition, EBP improvements can also provide a beneficial edge in a competitive market.

# Develop Localized Protocol

Most published evidence-based guidelines provide recommendations for practice but lack the specific instructions necessary to implement the practice in the real world. For example, one small part of a comprehensive evidence-based guideline for the prevention of chemotherapy-induced mucositis suggests using cryotherapy (Keefe et al., 2007). The guideline recommends that people receiving certain kinds of chemotherapy hold ice or cold liquids in their mouths during the medication infusion in order to prevent or minimize mucositis. Exactly how cryotherapy should be administered is not discussed in the guideline. It is up to the various professionals who want to implement cryotherapy to develop a local protocol that is specific to the setting. An example of a localized protocol is in Example 7.2. The protocol is made up of a policy (a statement of what the expected practice should be, who should receive it, and who should not receive it) and a procedure (a series of detailed steps describing exactly how the practice is accomplished). The policy helps the practitioner decide whether the patient should receive cryotherapy; the procedure tells the practitioner how to do it. Some EBPs don't require a formal protocol (e.g., providing opportunities for clinicians to take exercise breaks during their shifts). The checklist provided in Tool 7.1 will help to determine the need for a policy or procedure.

**TIPS: Developing a Localized EBP Protocol to Pilot**

- Make appropriate equipment and information easily accessible.
- Make the procedure repeatable by multiple clinicians.
- Design the protocol to be feasible for the majority of patients and in the majority of clinical scenarios.
- Listen to clinician questions and incorporate solutions.

## Create an Evaluation Plan

Evaluation is an important part of the pilot. Standard components for EBP evaluation include process and outcome indicators. A comprehensive process evaluation includes knowledge, perceptions/attitudes, and practice behaviors (Bick & Graham, 2010; Parry, Carson-Stevens, Luff, McPherson, & Goldmann, 2013). Outcomes that are evaluated may address patient, family, clinicians, and/or organizational perspectives. Outcome measures should also include relevant balancing measures (Institute for Healthcare Improvement, 2015). A parallel evaluation is used to seek patient or family feedback. Topic-specific indicators and evaluation tools can be identified by reviewing relevant clinical practice guidelines, research, or other reports. Chapter 9 has additional information related to creating an evaluation plan.

## Collect Baseline Data

Evaluation of project-specific process and outcome indicators is completed before implementation of the practice change. Baseline process indicators may be obtained through clinician and patient or family questionnaires that capture knowledge, perceptions, and practice behaviors. Baseline clinician and patient or family perceptions can help guide implementation planning. Further information regarding collecting baseline data is shared in Chapter 9.

## Develop an Implementation Plan

Implementation is one of the most challenging steps in the EBP process. Use baseline data to guide selecting implementation strategies. Implementation plans should be detailed and thorough. A phased approach is recommended (Cullen & Adams, 2012; Rogers, 2003). Tools and tips for planning implementation are described in Chapter 8. As part of a phased approach to implementing the EBP, prepare clinicians and materials for the practice change and use interactive implementation strategies to promote adoption among clinicians and patients or families.

## Prepare Clinicians and Materials

A variety of educational methods and opportunities for learning can be used. In addition to the usual in-service and one-to-one communication, consider reminders (see Strategy 3-1), pocket guides (see Strategy 2-2), and concise targeted messages (Ruhe et al., 2005). An effective leader will address the individual concerns of users who will be affected by the change (Sandström et al., 2011). Build buy-in by cultivating change champions (see Strategy 2-4) and engaging users and stakeholders in discussions (Powell et al., 2012).

Link the change to institutional and unit values and needs (see Strategy 1-2). These can be financial, as in reducing or avoiding cost, or regulatory, as in meeting government or agency standards. Also ensure easy access to the necessary equipment and resources, to make it easy for clinicians to get it right.

## Promote Adoption

Enthusiastic, hands-on involvement of leaders is essential to successful implementation of EBP (Stetler, Ritchie, Rycroft-Malone, & Charns, 2014). Ruhe et al. (2005) write about "malleable moments" to influence the acceptance of change, by being in the right place at the right time. Consider having change champions available on all shifts while the change in practice is being piloted, especially early in the process. Unexpected issues will arise in even the best-planned implementation. Leaders must ensure that implementation issues are listened to honestly, addressed, and quickly resolved (Schifalacqua, Costello, & Denman, 2009). For late adopters, continue to motivate acceptance of the change by building the case. Tactics include asking users to self-reflect on why the practice change is important and finding incentives for adoption. Additional strategies to consider are outlined in detail in Chapter 8.

## Collect and Report Post-Pilot Data

Evaluation of the process and outcome indicators is also completed after implementation of the practice change. A comparison of pre- and post-pilot data demonstrates whether the desired outcome was achieved as anticipated (success of the pilot), effectiveness of the evidence-based protocol, and need for modification of either the implementation plan or the practice protocol. After the post-pilot data collection, the pilot area (or areas) should receive actionable and timely data feedback (see Strategies 3-12, 3-13, and 4-6) regarding the results and next steps. Additional reporting should follow the institution's shared governance process (see Chapter 12). Chapter 9 includes a more comprehensive description of collecting and reporting post-pilot data.

**Example 7.1   Policy for Student Projects**

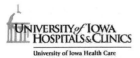

## Policy and Procedure Manual

| Approval for Students to do Course Projects | N-A-12.004 |
|---|---|

**PURPOSE:**      To promote coordination, communication and provision of safe quality care.
To document the presence of and provide approval for students' project work within the Department of Nursing.

**POLICY:**

I.   Placement approval

    A.   UI students work with their faculty for placement; approvals from University of Iowa Hospitals and Clinics are already established.

    B.   An affiliation agreement and request for placement with follow-up screening is required for all non-University of Iowa (UI) undergraduate and graduate students. Work with your faculty advisor to contact the Director – Nursing Education for assistance. (See attached table of Approvals Needed for Student Projects)

II.   For all student EBP, quality and research projects, approval is required from the Director – Office of Nursing Research, Evidence-Based Practice (EBP) and Quality.

III.   No project activities, including data collection, should be initiated within the Department of Nursing until the appropriate approvals are obtained.

IV.   Each student must work with a UI Hospitals and Clinics (UIHC) sponsor.

V.   Use of UIHC data must be discussed with the UIHC sponsor. If the sponsor has questions about data or any other aspects of the project, she/he may contact the Director – Nursing Education or Director – Office of Nursing Research, EBP and Quality for assistance and clarification of policies.

VI.   UI IRB (institutional review board) or HSRD (human subjects research determination) review is required for all student projects completed at UIHC, regardless if the project has already been reviewed and approved by the student's non-UI college or university.

**PROCEDURE:**

I.   Collaborative Agreement and Concept Approval

    A.   The student and faculty member will agree on a scholarly student project. For project ideas, a list of UIHC and nursing priorities is available at this <link>.

*continues*

**Example 7.1    Policy for Student Projects (Continued)**

   B.   Non-UI faculty/students will contact the Director – Nursing Education to discuss the general plans for the student project, determine the procedure to be followed for approval, and initiate an agreement regarding the project.

   1.   The Director – Nursing Education initiates or verifies that a current Cooperating Agency Agreement is in place and necessary screening, paperwork, orientation and accesses are completed  prior to signing Form 3.

   2.   UI students are exempt from this step.

   C.   Following the placement approval, students doing EBP, quality and research work are responsible for forwarding their requests to the Director – Office of Nursing Research, EBP and Quality and/or the Nursing Research and EBP Committee (NREC).

I.   Student Research

   A.   The student must complete Form I, "Request for Approval of Research" and file a proposal as outlined for research approval in policy N-A-12.001 "Approval to do Research Within the Department of Nursing Services and Patient Care", if the project is research.

II.   Other Student Projects, (i.e. non-research) including EBP, quality improvement (QI), education, etc.

   A.   The student must complete Form 3, "Student Projects within UIHC Department of Nursing Services and Patient Care".

   1.   Complete student information (Form 3 – Step 1, see procedure I. C. above).

      a.   Non-UI students must obtain signature from Director of Nursing Education, to verify a cooperative agency agreement and clear it for placement.

      b.   UI students are exempt from this signature.

   2.   Outline project scope with UIHC sponsor (Form 3 – Step 2, policy statements III & IV and procedure I. A. & I. B.  above).

      a.   Obtain Nursing Information Technology Team Lead signature if applicable (only when a change in the electronic health record [EHR] is planned).

      b.   Prepare a Human Subjects Research Determination (HSRD) through HawkIRB to determine the work is not research. Draft content, but <u>do not submit</u> to IRB yet, see steps 6 and 8 below.

         1)   Students should discuss the processes and methods used (e.g., EBP, QI) and refer to the "project," "project director," etc.

**Example 7.1   Policy for Student Projects (Continued)**

        2)    Students are cautioned to avoid use of terminology, such as "study", "sample size", "primary investigator", etc. which may be confused with research.

        3)    If the student is not a UIHC employee or UI student, the student will need to work with their UIHC sponsor to enter the HSRD.

3.    Obtain Nurse Manager and Clinical Nursing Director signatures for each area involved in the project (Form 3 – Step 3).

4.    Complete internal reporting and integration agreement (Form 3 – Step 4).

5.    Complete confidentiality and external sharing agreement (Form 3 – Step 5).

6.    Review HSRD with UIHC Sponsor and Faculty Advisor and obtain required signatures (Form 3 – Step 6). See step 8 below before submitting to IRB.

7.    Obtain NREC approval (Form 3 – Step 7).

    a.    Submit Form 3 and the HSRD application as an e-mail attachment for NREC approval. See instructions on Form 3.

    b.    When NREC approves your project or makes recommendations for changes, you will be notified by an e-mail.

    c.    Most approvals will be returned in 2 weeks.

    d.    Approvals will include an attachment with Form 3 signed by the Director – Office of Nursing Research, EBP and Quality and/or an NREC Chairperson.

8.    Upload the signed Form 3 as an attachment to the HSRD application and submit to IRB through the UI HawkIRB system (Form 3 – Step 8).

    a.    Additional questions about the project may come to the student from the IRB through the UI HawkIRB system.

    b.    The student will be notified via e-mail when the HSRD is completed/approved (usually in less than a week).

    c.    Go to the UI HawkIRB system to obtain the HSRD memo.

        1)    If the project is determined NOT to be human subjects research, save the memo from the IRB for a personal record and for step 9 below.

*continues*

**Example 7.1    Policy for Student Projects (Continued)**

> 2) If the project is determined to be Human Subjects Research, the student should consult the Faculty Advisor and follow the directions and steps outlined in procedure II above, and policy N-A-12.001 "Approval to do Research Within the Department of Nursing Services and Patient Care".

> 9. Submit completed Form 3 and HSRD memo to your college and the NREC (Form 3 – Step 9).

IV. Dissemination of student research or other student projects.

   A. Any reporting beyond UIHC or the class requires additional written approval.

   B. Use of data or the project for publication or presentation will be discussed with the Director of Nursing Research, Evidence-Based Practice and Quality prior to dissemination.

**RELATED STANDARDS LINK:**

■ Policies and Guidelines for the Nursing Student and Nursing Instructor Experiences at UIHC

■ N-A-12.001 "Approval to do Research Within the Department of Nursing Services and Patient Care"

**APPENDICES:**

■ Appendix A – Approvals needed for student projects

■ Appendix B – Contacts for approvals and workflow

■ Appendix C – Form 3

■ Appendix D – Instructions for creating 'printer friendly' version and PDF file of HSRD application

**Written:**    2/74

**Revised:**    4/79, 5/81, 11/82, 9/84, 1/86, 2/92, 8/94, 6/98, 6/01, 8/05, 10/08; 4/09, 2/12, 7/13, 2/14, 2/16; 6/16; 8/16, 12/16

**Reviewed:**  11/83, 6/89, 5/04; 5/08, 2/16

**Example 7.2    EBP Protocol as a Procedure: Cryotherapy**

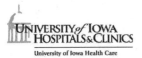

# Policy and Procedure Manual

| Department of Nursing Services and Patient Care Standards of Practice | N-02.036 |
| --- | --- |

**SUBJECT/TITLE:**    Cryotherapy (ice or cold therapy) for Chemotherapy Patients Receiving Bolus Doses or Short Infusions (<30 minutes) of Fluorouracil, Edatrexate, and/or Melphalan

**PURPOSE:**    Nursing intervention to assist in preventing or decreasing the severity of oral mucositis.

**POLICY:**

1.  Cryotherapy is used for adult and pediatric patients receiving bolus doses or short infusions (<30 minutes) of Fluorouracil [L1, L3, N1, R3, R7], Edatrexate [L1, L3], and/or Melphalan [L1, L3, N1, R1, R4, R5] who are able to tolerate oral intake.

2.  Cryotherapy is contraindicated for patients receiving Oxaliplatin or other patients for whom sucking on ice chips or popsicles is contraindicated.

**PROCEDURE:**

1.  Patients will be offered ice chips, popsicles, or an alternative material 30 minutes prior to infusion of the indicated chemotherapeutic agent, throughout the infusion, and for 30 minutes after the infusion or to the extent they can tolerate the ice chips, popsicles, or alternative material before, during, and after infusion of the chemotherapeutic agent. [L1, L2, L3, N1, R1, R4, R5, R6]

    A.    Alternatives to ice chips that may be used are slush drinks, sherbet, or ice cream. [R5, R6]

2.  Patients should be instructed to move the cold material (e.g., at least one ounce of ice chips, popsicles, or sherbet) around in the mouth to make contact with all mucosal surfaces. [L3, R4, R5, R6]

    A.    Cryotherapy material should be replenished as soon as it melts. [R2, R4, R5, R6]

    B.    Patients should avoid eating or drinking hot or warm items while performing cryotherapy. [R4]

3.  Documentation of the use of cryotherapy will be in the electronic patient record (e.g., Oral Care Row).

*continues*

EXAMPLES

TOOLS

## Example 7.2   EBP Protocol as a Procedure: Cryotherapy (Continued)

**REFERENCES:**

**Literature References:**

L1   Kwong, K. K. (2004). Prevention and treatment of oropharyngeal mucositis following cancer therapy: Are there new approaches? *Cancer Nursing, 27,* 183–205.

L2   Migliorati, C. A., Oberle-Edwards, L., & Schubert, M. (2006). The role of alternative and natural agents, cryotherapy and/or laser for management of alimentary mucositis. *Supportive Care in Cancer, 14,* 533–540.

L3   Scully, C., Sonis, S., & Diz, P. D. (2006). Oral mucositis. *Oral Diseases, 12*(3), 229–241.

L4   Worthington, H. V., Clarkson, J. E., Bryan, G., Furness, S., Glenny, A. M., Littlewood, A., … Khalid, T. (2011). Interventions for preventing oral mucositis for patients with cancer receiving treatment. *Cochrane Database of Systematic Reviews, 2011*(4). doi:10.1002/14651858.CD000978.pub5

L5   Stokman, M. A., Spijkervet, F. K. L., Boezen, H. M., Schouten, J. P., Roodenburg, J. L. N., & de Vries, E. G. E. (2006). Preventative intervention possibilities in radiotherapy- and chemotherapy-induced oral mucositis: Results of meta-analyses. *Journal of Dental Research, 85*(8), 690–700.

**National Guidelines:**

N1   Keefe, D. M., Schubert, M. M., Elting, L. S., Sonis, S. T., Epstein, J. B., Raber-Durlacher, J. E., … Peterson, D. E. (2007). Updated clinical practice guidelines for the prevention and treatment of mucositis. *Cancer, 109*(5), 820–831.

**Research References:**

R1   Aisa, Y., Mori, T., Kudo, M., Yashima, T., Kondo, S., Yokoyama, A., … Okamoto, S. (2005). Oral cryotherapy for the prevention of high-dose melphalan-induced stomatitis in allogeneic hematopoietic stem cell transplant recipients. *Supportive Care in Cancer, 13,* 266–269.

R2   Karagozoglu, S., & Ulusoy, M. F. (2005). Chemotherapy: The effect of oral cryotherapy on the development of mucositis. *Journal of Clinical Nursing, 14,* 754–765.

R3   Katranci, N., Ovayolu, N., Ovayolu, O., & Sevinc, A. (2011). Evaluation of the effect of cryotherapy in preventing oral mucositis associated with chemotherapy-A randomized controlled trial. *European Journal of Oncology Nursing, 16*(4), 339–344. doi:10.1016/j.ejon.2011.07.008

R4   Lilleby, K., Garcia, P., Gooley, T., McDonnell, P., Taber, R., Holmberg, L., … Bensinger, W. (2006). A prospective, randomized study of cryotherapy during administration of high-dose melphalan to decrease the severity and duration of oral mucositis in patients with multiple myeloma undergoing autologous peripheral blood stem cell transplantation. *Bone Marrow Transplantation, 37*(11), 1031–1035.

R5   Mori, T., Yamazaki, R., Aisa, Y., Nakazato, T., Kudo, M.,Yashima, T., … Okamoto, S. (2006). Brief oral cryotherapy for the prevention of high-dose melphalan-induced stomatitis in allogeneic hematopoietic stem cell transplant recipients. *Supportive Care in Cancer, 14*(4), 392–395.

R6   Nikoletti, S., Hyde, S., Shaw, T., Myers, H., & Kristjanson, L. J. (2005). Comparison of plain ice and flavoured ice for preventing oral mucositis associated with the use of 5-fluorouracil. *Journal of Clinical Nursing, 14*(6), 750–753.

**EXAMPLES**

**TOOLS**

**Example 7.2     EBP Protocol as a Procedure: Cryotherapy (Continued)**

R7     Papadeas, E., Naxakis, S., Riga, M., & Kalofonos, C. H. (2007). Prevention of 5-fluorouracil-related stomatitis by oral cryotherapy: A randomized controlled study. *European Journal of Oncology Nursing, 11*(1), 60–65.

R8     Svanberg, A., Öhrn, K., & Birgegård, G. (2010). Oral cryotherapy reduces mucositis and improves nutrition—A randomised controlled trial. *Journal of Clinical Nursing, 19*(15–16): 2146–2151.doi: 10.1111/j.1365-2702.2010.03255.x

| | |
|---|---|
| **Date Created:** | 9/08 |
| **Source:** | Oral Mucositis Committee |
| | Department of Nursing Services and Patient Care |
| **Initial Approval Date:** | 3/09 |
| **Initial Effective Date:** | 3/09 |
| **Date Revised:** | 3/12 |
| **Date Last Reviewed:** | 12/15 |

## Tool 7.1    Determining a Need for a Policy or Procedure

**INSTRUCTIONS:** Several considerations would determine the need for a practice policy or procedure. This tool outlines when to consider developing an evidence-based policy or procedure. If any answer is yes, consider developing a practice policy or procedure.

| | |
|---|---|
| Gap in available policy or procedure on the topic | ☐ Yes |
| | ☐ No |
| Low volume or infrequent patient care issue | ☐ Yes |
| | ☐ No |
| High-risk patient care issue | ☐ Yes |
| | ☐ No |
| Strong commitment to the traditional practice | ☐ Yes |
| | ☐ No |
| Drastic change in practice indicated by current evidence | ☐ Yes |
| | ☐ No |
| Current variation in practice or high probability of variation in practice | ☐ Yes |
| | ☐ No |
| Concern about fidelity of practice change (ability to carry out as intended) | ☐ Yes |
| | ☐ No |
| Variation in practice increases patient risk for poor outcome or increased length of stay | ☐ No |
| | ☐ No |
| Critical steps indicated by current evidence | ☐ Yes |
| | ☐ No |
| Documentation changes needed to support clinicians at the point of care | ☐ Yes |
| | ☐ No |
| New medication or equipment that changes current monitoring or treatments | ☐ Yes |
| | ☐ No |

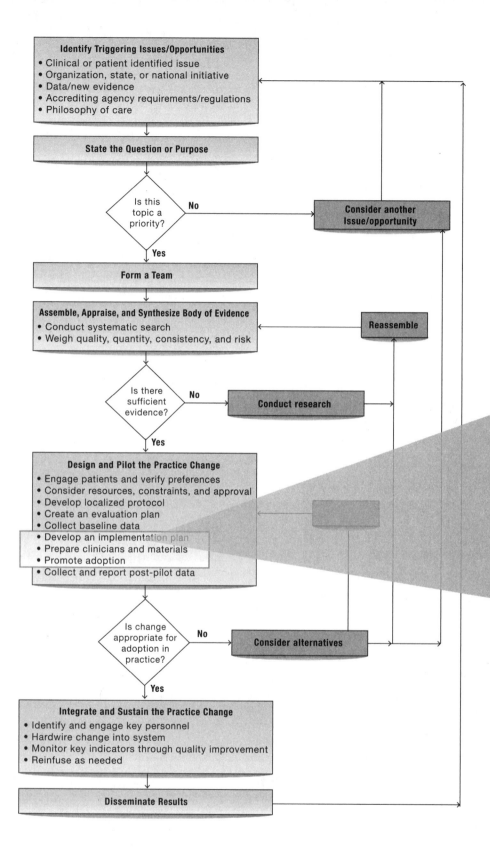

**Identify Triggering Issues/Opportunities**
• Clinical or patient identified issue
• Organization, state, or national initiative
• Data/new evidence
• Accrediting agency requirements/regulations
• Philosophy of care

**State the Question or Purpose**

Is this topic a priority?

**No** → **Consider another Issue/opportunity**

**Yes**

**Form a Team**

**Assemble, Appraise, and Synthesize Body of Evidence**
• Conduct systematic search
• Weigh quality, quantity, consistency, and risk

**Reassemble**

Is there sufficient evidence?

**No** → **Conduct research**

**Yes**

**Design and Pilot the Practice Change**
• Engage patients and verify preferences
• Consider resources, constraints, and approval
• Develop localized protocol
• Create an evaluation plan
• Collect baseline data
• Develop an implementation plan
• Prepare clinicians and materials
• Promote adoption
• Collect and report post-pilot data

Is change appropriate for adoption in practice?

**No** → **Consider alternatives**

**Yes**

**Integrate and Sustain the Practice Change**
• Identify and engage key personnel
• Hardwire change into system
• Monitor key indicators through quality improvement
• Reinfuse as needed

**Disseminate Results**

# IMPLEMENTATION

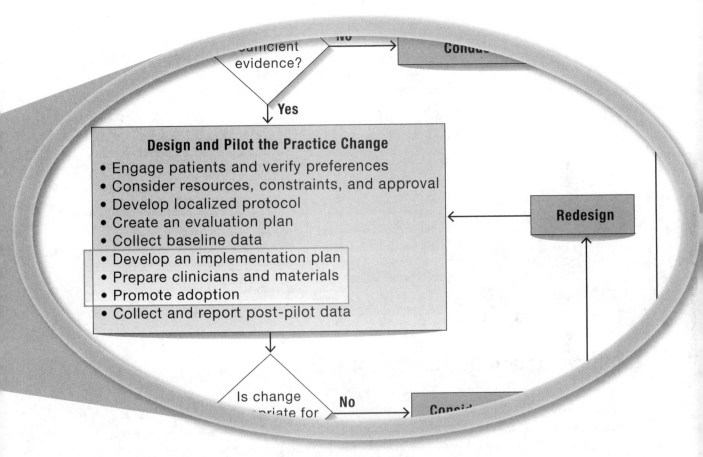

…ficient evidence? → **No** → Condu…

**Yes**

**Design and Pilot the Practice Change**
- Engage patients and verify preferences
- Consider resources, constraints, and approval
- Develop localized protocol
- Create an evaluation plan
- Collect baseline data
- Develop an implementation plan
- Prepare clinicians and materials
- Promote adoption
- Collect and report post-pilot data

**Redesign**

Is change …priate for → **No** → Consi…

*"A journey of a thousand miles begins with a single step."*

–Lao Tzu

Implementation can be a challenging step in the evidence-based practice (EBP) process (Saunders & Vehviläinen-Julkunen, 2016). The Iowa Model highlights broad considerations for implementation during the pilot. These considerations need to be expanded into a full implementation plan. A phased approach to implementation may facilitate adoption (Rogers, 2003). Four broad phases are adapted from Rogers' (2003) Diffusion of Innovation Theory for use in healthcare (see Figure 8.1). This chapter is organized using the Implementation Strategies for EBP as a guide. An overview of the process is described, and tools and examples follow. The last part of the chapter includes a description of 63 of the most complex implementation strategies (see Figure 8.2). Each strategy has a definition, identified benefit(s), a procedure for how to operationalize the strategy, an example, and select citations. Strategies are arranged by phases. Select from among the strategies to create a comprehensive implementation plan (see Tool 8.1). Strategies are organized to enhance movement through four phases of implementation: Create awareness and interest, build knowledge and commitment, promote action and adoption, and pursue integration and sustainability. Using a phased approach can help team leaders organize their implementation plans. Complete Phases 1 and 2 before the actual "go live" begins to prepare clinicians for the scheduled EBP change. In Phase 3, active adoption of the practice change begins with the pilot "go live." Each phase is essential to achieve a sustained improvement.

**Figure 8.1**   Implementation Phases

Create Awareness & Interest → Build Knowledge & Commitment → Promote Action & Adoption → Pursue Integration & Sustained Use

# Implementation Strategies for EBP

The Implementation Strategies for EBP (Figure 8.2) was designed to help EBP team leaders select effective strategies to use (Cullen & Adams, 2012). The columns in the implementation guide (see Figure 8.2) represent implementation phases progressing from awareness through sustained change. Each column includes strategies addressing the goal for that phase. Implementation strategies targeting two distinct groups are arranged in rows. The first row specifically targets the clinicians and organizational leaders, including key stakeholders. The second row of strategies builds support for the practice change within the organizational system or context. Project leaders select implementation strategies that are appropriate for the topic, their particular unit/clinic, and organization as the EBP initiative progresses. This implementation planning is an important step during the pilot step of the Iowa Model.

**Figure 8.2**    Implementation Strategies for Evidence-Based Practice

| Create Awareness & Interest | Build Knowledge & Commitment | Promote Action & Adoption | Pursue Integration & Sustained Use |
|---|---|---|---|

**Connecting With Clinicians, Organizational Leaders, and Key Stakeholders**

| Create Awareness & Interest | Build Knowledge & Commitment | Promote Action & Adoption | Pursue Integration & Sustained Use |
|---|---|---|---|
| ■ Highlight advantages* or anticipated impact*<br>■ Highlight compatibility*<br>■ Continuing education programs*<br>■ Sound bites*<br>■ Journal club*<br>■ Slogans & logos<br>■ Staff meetings<br>■ Unit newsletter<br>■ Unit inservices<br>■ Distribute key evidence<br>■ Posters and postings/fliers<br>■ Mobile 'show on the road'<br>■ Announcements & broadcasts | ■ Education (e.g., live, virtual, or computer-based)*<br>■ Pocket guides<br>■ Link practice change & power holder/stakeholder priorities*<br>■ Change agents (e.g., change champion*, core group*, opinion leader*, thought leader, etc.)<br>■ Educational outreach or academic detailing*<br>■ Integrate practice change with other EBP protocols*<br>■ Disseminate credible evidence with clear implications for practice*<br>■ Make impact observable*<br>■ Gap assessment/gap analysis*<br>■ Clinician input*<br>■ Local adaptation* & simplify*<br>■ Focus groups for planning change*<br>■ Match practice change with resources & equipment<br>■ Resource manual or materials (i.e., electronic or hard copy)<br>■ Case studies | ■ Educational outreach/academic detailing*<br>■ Reminders or practice prompts*<br>■ Demonstrate workflow or decision algorithm<br>■ Resource materials and quick reference guides<br>■ Skill competence*<br>■ Give evaluation results to colleagues*<br>■ Incentives*<br>■ Try the practice change*<br>■ Multidisciplinary discussion & troubleshooting<br>■ "Elevator speech"<br>■ Data collection by clinicians<br>■ Report progress & updates<br>■ Change agents (e.g., change champion*, core group*, opinion leader*, thought leader, etc.)<br>■ Role model*<br>■ Troubleshooting at the point of care/bedside<br>■ Provide recognition at the point of care* | ■ Celebrate local unit progress*<br>■ Individualize data feedback*<br>■ Public recognition*<br>■ Personalize the messages to staff (e.g., reduces work, reduces infection exposure, etc.) based on actual improvement data<br>■ Share protocol revisions with clinician that are based on feedback from clinicians, patient, or family<br>■ Peer influence<br>■ Update practice reminders |

**Building Organizational System Support**

| Create Awareness & Interest | Build Knowledge & Commitment | Promote Action & Adoption | Pursue Integration & Sustained Use |
|---|---|---|---|
| ■ Knowledge broker(s)<br>■ Senior executives announcements<br>■ Publicize new equipment | ■ Teamwork*<br>■ Troubleshoot use/application*<br>■ Benchmark data*<br>■ Inform organizational leaders*<br>■ Report within organizational infrastructure*<br>■ Action plan*<br>■ Report to senior leaders | ■ Audit key indicators*<br>■ Actionable and timely data feedback*<br>■ Non-punitive discussion of results*<br>■ Checklist*<br>■ Documentation*<br>■ Standing orders*<br>■ Patient reminders*<br>■ Patient decision aids*<br>■ Rounding by unit & organizational leadership*<br>■ Report into quality improvement program*<br>■ Report to senior leaders<br>■ Action plan*<br>■ Link to patient/family needs & organizational priorities<br>■ Unit orientation<br>■ Individual performance evaluation | ■ Audit and feedback*<br>■ Report to senior leaders*<br>■ Report into quality improvement program*<br>■ Revise policy, procedure, or protocol*<br>■ Competency metric for discontinuing training<br>■ Project responsibility in unit or organizational committee<br>■ Strategic plan*<br>■ Trend results*<br>■ Present in educational programs<br>■ Annual report<br>■ Financial incentives*<br>■ Individual performance evaluation |

* Implementation strategy is supported by at least some empirical evidence in healthcare.

For permission to use, go to https://uihc.org/implementation-strategies-evidence-based-practice-evidence-based-practice-implementation-guide

© Copyright of the Implementation Strategies for Evidence-Based Practice is retained by Laura Cullen, MA, RN, FAAN, and the University of Iowa Hospitals and Clinics.

Cullen, L., & Adams, S. L. (2012). Planning for implementation of evidence-based practice. *Journal of Nursing Administration, 42*(4), 222–230. doi:10.1097/NNA.0B013E31824CCD0A

# Select Implementation Strategies

Selecting strategies and knowing how to use them and how to package them together is complex (Proctor, Powell, & McMillen, 2013). Collect and use pre-data from the pilot evaluation (see Chapter 9) to guide identification of appropriate implementation strategies. The Implementation Strategies for EBP (see Figure 8.2) includes a long list of strategies from which to choose.

When choosing implementation strategies, ask these questions (Cullen & Adams, 2012):

- What EBP changes have been successfully implemented previously? How were those practice changes implemented?

- Who are stakeholders or others who might be interested in this EBP? What is the potential impact or advantage for them? What are their priorities, and how can those priorities be addressed in the EBP protocol, workflow, or implementation plan?

- How can the process be simplified and built into the system to make adoption easier?

- What are barriers and facilitators to adoption of this EBP? What creative and simple solutions can address the barriers and/or optimize the facilitators?

- What information or data are the clinicians and stakeholders accustomed to seeing? What information or data are typically shared with practice changes?

- How can we design memorable messages for clinicians and leaders describing the EBP that includes credible evidence, description of the importance of the change, description of how the EBP change will work, and description of anticipated outcomes?

An implementation planning tool (see Tool 8.1) may be helpful. Some strategies are particularly effective and will be useful in most EBP changes, including use of change agents (see Table 8.1), educational outreach or academic detailing (see Strategy 2-9), audit (see Strategy 3-12) and actionable feedback (see Strategy 3-13), and reporting to senior leaders (see Strategy 2-23). Change agents play variable but important roles as influential people who can impact implementation (see Table 8.1). Combining a number of different change agent roles is useful. Intensive strategic planning for implementation is needed to increase the speed with which evidence is put into practice (Esposito, Heeringa, Bradley, Croake, & Kimmey, 2015).

## Table 8.1  Change Agents

| Name | Perspective | Educational Role | Impact |
|------|-------------|------------------|--------|
| Change champion (Strategy 2-4) | Focus is local and is from inside the organization. | Reviews evidence, designs practice change (e.g., policy), assists with creating resources for implementation, trains peers | Assists project leader and links evidence with reality of clinical practice |
| Core group (Strategy 2-5) | Focus is local and is from the unit/clinic adopting the EBP. | Reviews key evidence, trains, role models, reinforces, and troubleshoots with colleagues | Point-of-care learning |
| EBP facilitator/ mentor (Strategy 2-8) | Broad program focus may be from inside or outside the organization. | Provides leadership throughout the EBP process | Mentors or functions as project director |
| Knowledge broker (Strategy 1-8) | Broad program focus is from outside the organization to build local capacity for EBP. | Assesses facilitators and barriers, locates best evidence, trains, networks, mentors, and reports results | Leads and connects with project directors |
| Opinion leader (Strategy 2-6) | Focus is on the program and across the continuum of care from inside the organization. | Reviews evidence and judges fit, educates peers, influences practice of others | Peer influence |
| Thought leader* (Strategy 2-7) | Focus is local and may be from inside or outside the organization. | Provides persuasive information | Some indication that the program preparation influences practice change of the thought leader serving as an educator, with little anticipated impact on audience. |

**\*NOTE:** Emerging concept yet to be tested in healthcare. Designed to change attitudes about the practice change.

### CITATIONS

Abdullah et al., 2014; Bornbaum, Kornas, Peirson, & Rosella, 2015; Dobbins et al., 2009; Dogherty, Harrison, Graham, Vandyk, & Keeping-Burke, 2013; Fleuren, van Dommelen, & Dunnink, 2015; Flodgren, Parmelli et al., 2011; Harvey & Kitson, 2016; Hauck, Winsett, & Kuric, 2013; Prince & Rogers, 2012; Rogers, 2003; Stetler et al., 2006; Titler, 2008.

# Combine Implementation Strategies

Choose and use implementation strategies cumulatively from the early phases throughout the implementation process (see Tool 8.1). Highlight potential advantages, key evidence, project logo, and results of a gap analysis throughout the implementation process to help busy clinicians stay focused. Continue to add strategies as needed, creating a proactive, comprehensive implementation plan.

Implementation is fluid, complex, highly interactive, and impacted by contextual variations. Prescriptive and rigid timing of strategies is not appropriate (Spyridonidis & Calnan, 2011; Wensing, Bosch, & Grol, 2010). Team leaders will almost certainly need to adjust or add implementation strategies as the work progresses (Esposito et al., 2015). Selecting implementation strategies has been described as an art. "Research-based evidence can provide some guidance but cannot show decisively which intervention is most appropriate," yet a structured approach to selecting implementation strategies may be helpful (Wensing et al., 2010, p. E85). EBP projects in different clinical areas addressing different topics may need different implementation strategies (Herr et al., 2012; Titler et al., 2009; Titler et al., 2016), and flexibility is the key (see Example 8.1). The need to adjust both the practice change procedure and the implementation procedures may become evident. Team members should have regular discussions about which implementation strategies are working and revise the implementation plan when needed. Keep track of the implementation process using this worksheet (see Tool 8.2). Rely on questions from users as a guide for developing creative solutions.

## TIPS: Implementation Planning

- Use Implementation Strategies for Evidence-Based Practice for planning implementation.

- Use multiple reinforcing and interactive implementation strategies.

- Have trusted change agents who provide consistent messages.

- Use simple solutions first.

- Build on the natural learning style of clinicians (i.e., seeking information from trusted colleagues).

- Build on the power of lateral (peer) influence.

- Use creative troubleshooting.

- Add humor where appropriate; make it fun.

## Example 8.1  Different Implementation Strategies by Topic and Clinical Areas

| Strategies for Energy Through Motion© for Cancer Survivors in Ambulatory Care | Strategies Used for Adult and Pediatric Oral Mucositis Assessment in Acute and Ambulatory Care |
|---|---|
| **PHASE 1: Create Awareness and Interest** | |
| ■ Highlight the advantages<br>■ Highlight compatibility<br>■ Continuing education programs<br>■ Slogans and logos<br>■ Staff meetings<br>■ Senior executive announcements<br>■ Publicize new equipment | ■ Highlight the advantages<br>■ Highlight compatibility<br>■ Report anticipated impact<br>■ Slogan and logo<br>■ Staff meetings<br>■ Unit inservices<br>■ Postings and posters<br>■ Announcements and broadcasts<br>■ Knowledge broker |
| **PHASE 2: Build Knowledge and Commitment** | |
| ■ Education<br>■ Link practice change and stakeholder priorities<br>■ Change agents (change champion, core group)<br>■ Disseminate credible evidence with clear implications for practice<br>■ Gap assessment<br>■ Clinician input<br>■ Local adaptation and simplify<br>■ Match practice change with resources and equipment<br>■ Teamwork<br>■ Troubleshoot use/application<br>■ Inform organizational leaders<br>■ Action plan | ■ Education<br>■ Pocket guide<br>■ Link practice change with stakeholders' priorities<br>■ Change agents<br>■ Educational outreach<br>■ Try the practice change<br>■ Disseminate credible evidence<br>■ Gap assessment<br>■ Clinician input<br>■ Local adaptation<br>■ Match the practice change with resources<br>■ Sound bites<br>■ Resource manual<br>■ Teamwork<br>■ Troubleshoot use of the protocol<br>■ Inform organizational leaders<br>■ Action planning<br>■ Link topics with organizational priorities |

*continues*

EXAMPLES

TOOLS

## Example 8.1    Different Implementation Strategies by Topic and Clinical Areas (Continued)

| Strategies for Energy Through Motion© for Cancer Survivors in Ambulatory Care | Strategies Used for Adult and Pediatric Oral Mucositis Assessment in Acute and Ambulatory Care |
|---|---|
| **PHASE 3: Promote Action and Adoption** | |
| <ul><li>Educational outreach/academic detailing</li><li>Reminders or practice prompts</li><li>Resource materials</li><li>Give evaluation results to colleagues</li><li>Try the practice change</li><li>Report progress and updates</li><li>Change agents (change champion, core group)</li><li>Role model</li><li>Troubleshooting at the point of care/bedside</li><li>Provide recognition at the point of care</li><li>Audit key indicators</li><li>Actionable and timely data feedback</li><li>Report into quality improvement program</li><li>Action plan</li><li>Link to patient/family needs</li></ul> | <ul><li>Educational outreach</li><li>Reminders or practice prompts</li><li>Resource materials and quick reference guide</li><li>Skill competency</li><li>Feedback evaluation results</li><li>Incentives</li><li>Try the change</li><li>Multidisciplinary discussion and troubleshooting</li><li>"Elevator speech"</li><li>Data collection by clinicians</li><li>Report progress</li><li>Role model practice change</li><li>Change agents provide troubleshooting and recognition at point of care</li><li>Audit key indicators</li><li>Feedback of actionable evaluative data</li><li>Non-punitive discussions</li><li>Documentation changes</li><li>Rounding by unit leaders</li><li>Report within the quality improvement program</li><li>Report to senior leaders</li><li>Action plan</li><li>Link to patient needs</li><li>Orientation</li></ul> |
| **PHASE 4: Pursue Integration and Sustained Use** | |
| <ul><li>Public recognition</li><li>Personalize the messages to staff, based on actual improvement data</li><li>Present in educational programs</li></ul> | <ul><li>Personalize the "What's in it for me?" messages</li><li>Share protocol revisions</li><li>Peer influence</li><li>Update practice reminders</li><li>Audit and feedback</li><li>Report to senior leaders</li><li>Report within quality improvement program</li><li>Revise policy</li><li>Trend results</li><li>Present in educational programs</li></ul> |
| **CITATIONS** | |

Cullen, Baumler et al., in press; Farrington, Cullen, & Dawson, 2010; Farrington, Cullen, & Dawson, 2013; Farrington, Cullen, & Dawson, 2014; Huether, Abbott, Cullen, Cullen, & Gaarde, 2016.

## Tool 8.1    Selecting Implementation Strategies for EBP

**INSTRUCTIONS:** Use this worksheet to select strategies and organize an EBP implementation plan. Review considerations outlined in each phase. Add the person responsible, the planned date, and notes for each strategy. Attach this worksheet outlining the implementation plan to the project action plan (see Tool 4.2).

### PHASE 1 CONSIDERATIONS: CREATE AWARENESS AND INTEREST

- What are the positive aspects of the EBP?
- Think of this as marketing the EBP.
- Be fun, eye-catching, and memorable.

|  | Strategies | Resources Needed | Whom to Involve | Date to Initiate |
|---|---|---|---|---|
| **Clinician, Organizational Leaders, and Stakeholders** | ☐ Highlight advantages or anticipated impact | | | |
| | ☐ Highlight compatibility | | | |
| | ☐ Continuing education programs | | | |
| | ☐ Sound bites | | | |
| | ☐ Journal club | | | |
| | ☐ Slogans and logos | | | |
| | ☐ Staff meetings | | | |
| | ☐ Unit newsletter | | | |
| | ☐ Unit inservices | | | |
| | ☐ Distribute key evidence | | | |
| | ☐ Posters and postings/fliers | | | |
| | ☐ Mobile "show on the road" | | | |
| | ☐ Announcements and broadcasts | | | |
| | ☐ Knowledge broker(s) | | | |
| | ☐ Senior executive announcements | | | |
| **Building Systems** | ☐ Publicize new equipment | | | |

*continues*

*EXAMPLES*

*TOOLS*

## Tool 8.1    Selecting Implementation Strategies for EBP (Continued)

**PHASE 2 CONSIDERATIONS: BUILD KNOWLEDGE AND COMMITMENT**

- How do clinicians within a discipline/setting like to learn?
- Build on the natural tendency of clinicians to learn from each other.
- Complete before "go live."

| Strategies | Resources Needed | Whom to Involve | Date to Initiate |
|---|---|---|---|
| ☐ Education (e.g., live, virtual, or computer-based) | | | |
| ☐ Pocket guides | | | |
| ☐ Link practice change and power holder/stakeholder priorities | | | |
| ☐ Change agents (e.g., change champion, core group, opinion leader, or thought leader) | | | |
| ☐ Educational outreach or academic detailing | | | |
| ☐ Integrate practice change with other EBP protocols | | | |
| ☐ Disseminate credible evidence with clear implications for practice | | | |
| ☐ Make impact observable | | | |
| ☐ Gap assessment/gap analysis | | | |
| ☐ Clinician input | | | |
| ☐ Local adaptation and simplify | | | |
| ☐ Focus groups for planning change | | | |
| ☐ Match practice change with resources and equipment | | | |
| ☐ Resource manual or materials (i.e., electronic or hard copy) | | | |
| ☐ Case studies | | | |

Clinician, Organizational Leaders, and Stakeholders

## PHASE 2 CONSIDERATIONS: BUILD KNOWLEDGE AND COMMITMENT

**Building Systems**

| | |
|---|---|
| ☐ | Teamwork |
| ☐ | Troubleshoot use/application |
| ☐ | Benchmark data |
| ☐ | Inform organizational leaders |
| ☐ | Report within organizational infrastructure |
| ☐ | Action plan |
| ☐ | Report to senior leaders |

## PHASE 3 CONSIDERATIONS: PROMOTE ACTION AND ADOPTION

- Use highly interactive and personal approaches.
- Demonstrate, encourage return demonstration, and provide reinforcement.
- Keep an eye toward building the EBP into the system and to make it easy to do it right.

**Clinician, Organizational Leaders, and Stakeholders**

| Strategies | Resources Needed | Whom to Involve | Date to Initiate |
|---|---|---|---|
| ☐ Educational outreach/academic detailing | | | |
| ☐ Reminders or practice prompts | | | |
| ☐ Demonstrate workflow or decision algorithm | | | |
| ☐ Resource materials and quick reference guides | | | |
| ☐ Skill competence | | | |
| ☐ Give evaluation results to colleagues | | | |
| ☐ Incentives | | | |
| ☐ Trying the practice change | | | |
| ☐ Multidisciplinary discussion and troubleshooting | | | |
| ☐ "Elevator speech" | | | |

*continues*

## Tool 8.1    Selecting Implementation Strategies for EBP (Continued)

### PHASE 3 CONSIDERATIONS: PROMOTE ACTION AND ADOPTION (Continued)

| | Strategies | Resources Needed | Whom to Involve | Date to Initiate |
|---|---|---|---|---|
| Building Systems | Data collection by clinicians | | | |
| | Report progress and updates | | | |
| | Change agents (e.g., change champion, core group, opinion leader, thought leader) | | | |
| | Role model | | | |
| | Troubleshooting at the point of care/bedside | | | |
| | Provide recognition at the point of care | | | |
| | Audit key indicators | | | |
| | Actionable and timely data feedback | | | |
| | Non-punitive discussion of results | | | |
| | Checklist | | | |
| | Documentation | | | |
| | Standing orders | | | |
| | Patient reminders | | | |
| | Patient decision aids | | | |
| | Rounding by unit and organizational leadership | | | |
| | Report into quality improvement program | | | |
| | Report to senior leaders | | | |
| | Action plan | | | |
| | Link to patient/family needs and organizational priorities | | | |
| | Unit orientation | | | |
| | Individual performance evaluation | | | |

## PHASE 4 CONSIDERATIONS: PURSUE INTEGRATION AND SUSTAINED USE

- Think about booster shots or periodic reinfusion.
- Build toward the EBP becoming the norm or the standard way to practice.
- Building EBP into the system is critical to help clinicians.

### Clinician, Organizational Leaders, and Stakeholders

| | Strategies | Resources Needed | Whom to Involve | Date to Initiate |
|---|---|---|---|---|
| ☐ | Celebrate local unit progress | | | |
| ☐ | Individualize data feedback | | | |
| ☐ | Public recognition | | | |
| ☐ | Personalize the messages to staff (e.g., reduces work, reduces infection exposure) based on actual improvement data | | | |
| ☐ | Share protocol revisions with clinicians that are based on feedback from clinicians, patient, or family | | | |
| ☐ | Peer influence | | | |
| ☐ | Update practice reminders | | | |

### Building Systems

| | Strategies | Whom to Involve | Date to Initiate | Notes |
|---|---|---|---|---|
| ☐ | Audit and feedback | | | |
| ☐ | Report to senior leaders | | | |
| ☐ | Report into quality improvement program | | | |
| ☐ | Revise policy, procedure, or protocol | | | |
| ☐ | Competency metric for discontinuing training | | | |
| ☐ | Project responsibility in unit or organizational committee | | | |
| ☐ | Strategic plan | | | |

*continues*

EXAMPLES

TOOLS

## Tool 8.1 Selecting Implementation Strategies for EBP (Continued)

| | Strategies | Whom to Involve | Date to Initiate | Notes |
|---|---|---|---|---|
| | **PHASE 4 CONSIDERATIONS: PURSUE INTEGRATION AND SUSTAINED USE (Continued)** | | | |
| ☐ | Trend results | | | |
| ☐ | Present in educational programs | | | |
| ☐ | Annual report | | | |
| ☐ | Financial incentives | | | |
| ☐ | Individual performance evaluation | | | |

**Building Systems**

## Tool 8.2   Collecting Pilot Process Issues

**INSTRUCTIONS:** This worksheet is to help track successes and problems during the pilot of the EBP change. Use this worksheet throughout each of the implementation phases and add comments and observations as the process unfolds. If needed, add more space to each category to maintain a complete and meaningful record. This will provide valuable information when moving into the "integrate and sustain" step of the EBP process.

### QUESTIONS TO KEEP IN MIND

What was the evidence-based change?

How different is the change from existing practice?

How were the pilot units/areas chosen? What criteria were used for selection?

What implementation strategies were used and how effective were they?

What resources were needed to implement the pilot? Were there any difficulties in obtaining those resources?

What policies and/or procedures were affected by the change?

Were there any groups that should have been included in planning the rollout?

Was there variability in the success of the pilot among pilot areas? If so, why?

Was the change adapted at any time during the pilot? If so, why?

*continues*

EXAMPLES

TOOLS

## Tool 8.2    Collecting Pilot Process Issues (Continued)

Were there any special circumstances that affected the rollout of the pilot (i.e., major changes within the institution such as new patient population, new documentation system, unforeseen leadership or workforce changes)?

How were the outcome indicators chosen?

Were there any difficulties in retrieving outcome data?

Were there any unexpected road blocks to implementing the pilot?

# Implementation Strategies for Evidence-Based Practice
## PHASE 1: CREATE AWARENESS & INTEREST

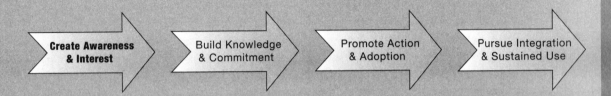

| STRATEGY NAME | PAGE |
|---|---|

The most complex implementation strategies to perform are described. The evidence on how to use the procedures is provided to improve their effectiveness. Use in combination for a comprehensive implementation plan.

## Strategy 1-1    Highlight Advantages or Anticipated Impact

| PHASE | 1: Create Awareness & Interest |
|---|---|
| FOCUS | Connecting With Clinicians, Organizational Leaders, & Key Stakeholders |

### DEFINITION

To highlight advantages or anticipated impact describes the expected benefit of the new EBP over the traditional practice or "the degree to which an innovation is perceived as being better than the idea it supersedes." The relative advantage is a characteristic of the innovative new practice that facilitates adoption (Rogers, 2003, p. 229).

### BENEFITS

- Motivates clinicians to improve adoption.
- Used to encourage buy-in or build a positive perception about the EBP by the clinical team, based on meeting patient/family, clinician, or organizational needs.
- May increase the social status of the user who is adopting the new practice.

### PROCEDURE

- Use the evidence from clinical practice guidelines or research to identify the potential patient, staff, or organizational outcomes; identify reported improvements in relevant processes or outcomes.
- Report anticipated improvement, matching the purpose of the EBP with research findings or clinical practice guidelines recommendations.
- Compare reported outcomes with current patient, clinicians, or organizational outcomes.
- Calculate estimated improvement (e.g., reduced adverse events or cost savings based on current patient volume). Include estimated or anticipated impact in early communications with clinicians and stakeholders.
- Keep the message about the advantage or impact simple and memorable.
- Repeat messages about the advantage in all information and resources about the EBP and across implementation phases.
- Compare the advantages achieved to those reported in the clinical practice guidelines or research when disseminating project results. Report comparison with actual processes or outcomes to clinicians and leaders.

## EXAMPLES

### Example 1: Thermoregulation in Adult Trauma Patients

**Purpose:**

- Decreased hypothermia for adult trauma patients while in the emergency department.

**Evidence:**

- Hypothermia is a known complication of trauma that contributes to poor patient outcomes and increased mortality, which occurs in 2–33% of trauma admissions to the emergency department.
- Some patients even experience increasing hypothermia during treatment in the emergency department.
- The goal is to maintain or rewarm a patient to achieve a temperature greater than 35°C without causing a thermal injury.
- Only 38–40% of patients have their temperature taken upon arrival in the emergency department, but our data demonstrate that 90% of trauma patients have their temperature taken upon arrival.
- Large variations in hypothermia management have been reported when a protocol is not in place.

**Statement of anticipated impact:**

- Use of a protocol for prevention and treatment has led to a 50% reduction in hypothermia, as a complication of trauma. An EBP protocol is being piloted to manage hypothermia in adult trauma patients during the time they are in the emergency department, with a similar reduction in hypothermia and related outcomes expected.

(Block, Lilienthal, Cullen, & White, 2012)

### Example 2: Low-Dose Ketamine for Orthopaedic Surgery Patients

**Purpose:**

- To improve post-operative pain for opioid-tolerant orthopaedic spine surgery patients by using low-dose ketamine infusion post-operatively.

**Evidence:**

- Benefits opioid-tolerant patients.
- May reset opioid receptors.
- Monitor for side effects.

**Relative advantage:**

- Low-dose ketamine may reduce morphine consumption.

(Farrington, Hanson, Laffoon, & Cullen, 2015)

## CITATIONS

Atkinson, 2007; Block, Lilienthal, Cullen, & White, 2012; Carlfjord, Lindberg, Bendtsen, Nilsen, & Andersson, 2010; Dogherty, Harrison, Graham, Vandyk, & Keeping-Burke, 2013; Fabry, 2015; Farrington, Hanson, Laffoon, & Cullen, 2015; Grant & Hofmann, 2011; Green & Aarons, 2011; Harris, Erwin, Smith, & Brownson, 2015; Harron & Titterington, 2016; Khong, Holroyd, & Wang, 2015; Morris & Clarkson, 2009; Rogers, 2003; ten Ham, Minnie, & van der Walt, 2016; van Bodegom-Vos, Davidoff, & Marang-van de Mheen, 2016.

## Strategy 1-2   Highlight Compatibility

| PHASE | 1: Create Awareness & Interest |
|---|---|
| FOCUS | Connecting With Clinicians, Organizational Leaders, and Key Stakeholders |

### DEFINITION

"Compatibility is the degree to which an innovation is perceived as being consistent with the existing values, past experiences, and needs of potential adopters" (Rogers, 2003, p. 240).

### BENEFITS

- Compatibility has been shown to correspond with attitudes about adoption of the EBP. EBPs are adopted more rapidly when the innovation is compatible with the values of the practitioners, needs or values of patients or practitioners, practitioners' previous experiences, and the healthcare system (e.g., resources, equipment, priorities, etc.).
- Compatibility makes the relationship between existing values and norms to the EBP changes clear.

### PROCEDURE

- Identify practitioner, group, and leader values.
- Identify patient needs (e.g., preventive healthcare services).
- Determine characteristics or outcomes of the EBP that match clinician values, patient values, or organizational mission.
- Use the clinical practice guidelines or research report to identify an impact on patient, clinician, or organizational outcomes matching these values.
- Include a statement of compatibility with early information about the EBP.
- Repeat statement of compatibility to keep clinicians focused on the value and potential impact from the EBP through later phases of implementation.

### EXAMPLE

**Topic:** Healthcare worker vaccination to prevent influenza has benefits that are compatible with a variety of value paradigms. Any of these may be selected and communicated to varying audiences.

#### Compatibility matching professional commitment

- Reduces risk of transmitting influenza to patients.
- Reduces risk of mortality for most at-risk patents.

#### Compatibility matching organizational priorities

- Reduces lost work days due to illness.
- Reduces healthcare cost associated with hospitalization for unvaccinated people.

#### Compatibility personal benefit

- Reduces risk of being infected with influenza.
- Reduces risk of HCW transmitting influenza to their family.

### CITATIONS

Abraham & Roman, 2010; Aletraris, Edmond, & Roman, 2015; Bosch, Tavender, Brennan, Knott, Gruen, & Green, 2016; Carlfjord, Lindberg, Bendtsen, Nilsen, & Andersson, 2010; Green & Aarons, 2011; Kastner et al., 2015; Khong, Holroyd, & Wang, 2015; Knudsen & Roman, 2015; Pankratz, Hallfors, & Cho, 2002; Putzer & Park, 2012; Rogers, 2003; Tandon et al., Bass, 2007.

**PHASE 1**

## Strategy 1-3   Sound Bites

| PHASE | 1: Create Awareness & Interest |
|---|---|
| FOCUS | Connecting With Clinicians, Organizational Leaders, and Key Stakeholders |

### DEFINITION

Sound bites are short and memorable phrases of three important points that are relevant to the target audience. They may include identification of the need for change, one key point about the evidence, the expected outcome from the practice change, or the behavior/practice change needed.

### BENEFITS

- Captures the attention of busy clinicians.
- Combines "chunks" of information that create awareness of an issue needing to be addressed.
- Statements are concise, catchy, and memorable.

### PROCEDURE

- Identify key messages.
- Consider messages that motivate action: perceived susceptibility, importance, severity, or risks associated with the problem, emphasis on desired outcomes or benefits, developing a plan of action, a goal one wants to achieve, or rate of goal achieved from intervention.
- Select three important points relevant to clinicians, such as:
  - The need for change (e.g., gap analysis)
  - One key fact from the evidence
  - Expected outcome or benefit from the practice change
  - Behavior/practice change needed (a required element to include)
  - When, where, or how to provide the new practice
- Create a short and memorable phrase from the important points.
- Tailor the message toward relevant intrinsic values (e.g., costs, personal goals or motivators, perceived threat, supporting a positive attitude, supportive of group norms).
- Tie or link to the project logo as a visual cue.
- Include an action step as one important part of the message.

*continues*

## Strategy 1-3  Sound Bites (Continued)

### EXAMPLES

**Oral Mucositis Prevention**

- Over 90% of head and neck cancer patients will develop oral mucositis.

- Magic mouthwash is ineffective and should be avoided.

- Oral care should include fluoride toothpaste, a soft toothbrush, and regular saline or bicarbonate oral rinses.

(American Academy of Nursing, 2014; Bonomi & Batt, 2015; DeSanctis et al., 2016; Lalla, Saunders, & Peterson, 2014)

**Pain Management After Surgery**

- Pain hurts!

- Seventy-five percent of patients experiencing post-operative pain report moderate to extreme pain.

- Combine pharmacologic and non-pharmacologic interventions as multimodal analgesia after surgery.

(Chou et al., 2016)

### CITATIONS

Albarracín et al., 2003; American Academy of Nursing, 2014; Bonomi & Batt, 2015; Chou et al., 2016; De Sanctis et al., 2016; Lalla, Saunders, & Peterson, 2014; Manika, Ball, & Stout, 2014; Morris & Clarkson, 2009; Pelletier & Sharp, 2008; Smith et al., 2009; Tessier, Sarrazin, Nicaise, & Dupont, 2015; Web Sites and Sound Bites, 2011; Whitehill King, Freimuth, Lee, & Johnson-Turbes, 2013; Wylie, 2009; Yudkin, 2011.

## Strategy 1-4    Journal Club

| PHASE | 1: Create Awareness & Interest |
|---|---|
| FOCUS | Connecting With Clinicians, Organizational Leaders, and Key Stakeholders |

### DEFINITION

Journal clubs are organized sessions for clinicians to review and discuss research articles published in scientific journals to facilitate use of research findings and to promote EBP (Kirchhoff, 1999).

### BENEFITS

- Easy-to-follow technique, using discussion for learning.
- Improves participants' familiarization with research study design.
- Improves participants' skills in reading and critiquing research.
- Positively influences attitude toward use of research findings.
- Increases confidence in applying research into practice.
- Promotes interprofessional collaboration, team building, professional growth, and empowerment.

### PROCEDURE

- Market event through email, flyers, and word-of-mouth.
- Open to voluntary participation and professional development.
- Determine a facilitator.
- Determine whether continuing education credits will be offered.
- Develop an evaluation tool to determine whether learning objectives are met.
- Choose a topic.
- Decide how to select and assign articles.
- Distribute articles with identical critique forms.
  - Provide enough time for participants to read articles and complete critique forms before discussion session.
- Schedule discussion sessions for review.
  - Determine meeting location (e.g., near work unit), time (e.g., repeat sessions, during work hours), length, and frequency (e.g., monthly, quarterly).
  - Determine available discussion formats (e.g., in-person, online, conference call).
- Capture discussion/findings.
  - Identify related policy/procedure/protocol.
  - Suggest policy/procedure/protocol revisions.
  - Follow institutional approval process for policy/procedure/protocol revisions.
  - Consider implications for an implementation plan.

*continues*

## Strategy 1-4 Journal Club (Continued)

### EXAMPLE

Presentation on critiquing and appraising evidence and the proposed structure for a new journal club series.

---

*Journal Article Review and Evidence-Based Practice: How to Begin*

**Sharon Tucker, PhD, RN, PMHCNS-BC, FAAN**
Director, Nursing Research, Evidence-Based Practice and Quality
sharon-tucker@uiowa.edu; 356-0518

BJ Wagner, Marilyn Wurth, Julie Williams, Lori Jenkins
ASC Perioperative Nurse Enrichment Series

---

### Overall Series Objective

- Increase understanding of the research process and importance of EBP.
- Enhance use of research findings to improve clinical practice.
- Identify potential research opportunities in the ASC.

---

### Structure

- Unit-based
- One article reviewed each month
- Articles to be chosen by the Journal Club Committee
  - All staff nurses will be on a rotation to assist/work with the committee during a particular month

---

### Structure (cont.)

- Committee will formulate 4-6 questions
  - Focus on the research presented
  - Evaluate the strength of the article and data
  - Encourage thought and discussion
  - How does this relate to the ASC?

---

### Structure (cont.)

- Article and questions will be ready for distribution at the beginning of the month
  - Briefly introduce each article during the first staff meeting of the month
- Review and discuss article as a group during the last staff meeting of the month
  - 15-25 minute discussion
- Summary of discussion posted for all to review

---

### Expectations for Journal Series

- Learn about reading current literature
- Raise questions and participate in discussion
- Consider leading or co-leading one session
- Stimulate further interest in building scholarship and possibly research into ASC practices
- Identify resources available for mentorship and assistance at UI Hospitals and Clinics

## Session Objectives

- Articulate the importance of reviewing research articles and the relevance to EBP in health care.
- Identify the process of evaluating the strength of evidence and relationships to practice.
- Discuss journal article review as one mechanism for the larger EBP process.

## Value of EBP for Nursing

- What is EBP?
- Why is it important?
- How have perioperative nurses applied EBP?
- What are you hoping for with this series?

## Evidence-Based Practice

- Integration of best research evidence with clinical expertise and patient values (Sackett et al., 2000; Titler, 2008)
- Evidence-based practice is the process of shared decision-making between practitioner, patient, and others significant to them based on *research evidence, the patient's experiences and preferences, clinical expertise or know-how, and other available robust sources of information* (STTI, 2008)

## Sources of Evidence

- Systematic reviews of multiple randomized controlled trials (experiments) or single experiments
- Quasi-experimental studies
- Nonexperimental research including qualitative studies
- Quality management databases
- Consensus of respected authorities
- Clinician expertise

**The Iowa Model Revised: Evidence-Based Practice to Promote Excellence in Health Care**

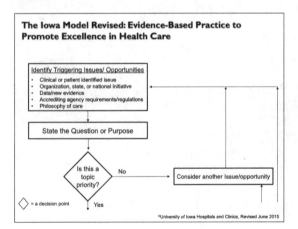

**The Iowa Model Revised: Evidence-Based Practice to Promote Excellence in Health Care (cont.)**

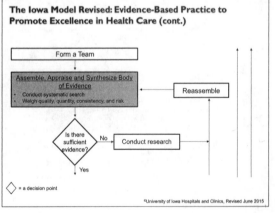

*continues*

## Strategy 1-4    Journal Club (Continued)

### EXAMPLE

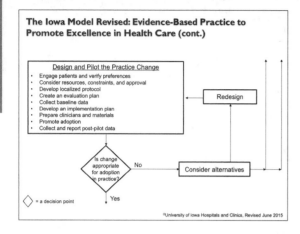

The Iowa Model Revised: Evidence-Based Practice to Promote Excellence in Health Care (cont.)

**Design and Pilot the Practice Change**
- Engage patients and verify preferences
- Consider resources, constraints, and approval
- Develop localized protocol
- Create an evaluation plan
- Collect baseline data
- Develop an implementation plan
- Prepare clinicians and materials
- Promote adoption
- Collect and report post-pilot data

Redesign

Is change appropriate for adoption in practice?    No    Consider alternatives

◇ = a decision point    Yes

©University of Iowa Hospitals and Clinics, Revised June 2015

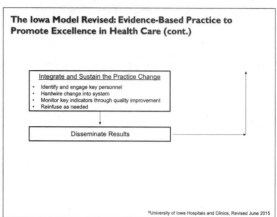

The Iowa Model Revised: Evidence-Based Practice to Promote Excellence in Health Care (cont.)

**Integrate and Sustain the Practice Change**
- Identify and engage key personnel
- Hardwire change into system
- Monitor key indicators through quality improvement
- Reinfuse as needed

Disseminate Results

©University of Iowa Hospitals and Clinics, Revised June 2015

## Value of Reading Research Articles

- Solve clinical problems
- Improve outcomes
- Find cost-effective practices
- Learn consumer perspectives
- Acquire new ideas and technologies

## General Tips for Getting Started

- Competence and confidence in reviewing articles grows with practice and experience
- Remember that all studies and clinical practice guidelines are not created equal
- Authors may not always reveal or present the data accurately and reviewers are human and have limits too
- Patient safety should never be compromised when considering a practice change
- Mentors and resources are available to help; don't hesitate to ask

## Dissecting an Article

- Identify type of article
  - Research study, conceptual paper, literature review, systematic review, integrated review, meta-analysis, opinion paper
  - Research design
    - Quantitative: experimental, quasi-experimental, predictive, correlational, descriptive, survey
    - Qualitative: phenomenology, grounded theory, ethnography
- Start with abstract, introduction and discussion
- Get a mentor
- Use resources such as textbooks and checklist
- Don't give up
- Practice, practice, practice

## Common Format to Research Reports

- Abstract
- Introduction/Background/Literature Review
- Method including Design
- Results
- Discussion
- Implications for Practice/Research
- Conclusions
- References
- Appendices

### Reading Research Articles and the Literature

- Critique and appraisal of research studies is a step in the EBP process
- Can be seen as time intensive and "over the head" of many nurses
- Rapid Critical Appraisal is one recommended approach for busy clinicians
  - User-friendly, efficient approach to critically appraising a published RCT

### Critique and Appraisal: Using Research Results

- Questions to ask
  - Is the study potentially helpful to your practice?
  - Would the application of the results be consistent with current healthcare agency policies, procedures, and standards?
  - Would it be reasonable to implement the study findings?
  - If a practice change is suggested, are the benefits for patients worth the effort of obtaining necessary resources to make any changes?
    - Any safety issues or risks; human subject issues

### Examples of Research Articles that Have Made a Difference at UI Hospitals and Clinics

- Bacteriostatic normal saline for IV starts
- IV flushes…heparin versus saline
- Intravenous therapy and interventions for IV infiltration/extravasation
- Implementing pre-operative screening for undiagnosed obstructive sleep apnea
- Listening to bowel sounds in adult abdominal surgery patients

### ASC Resources

- Journal Club
- Unit leadership
- Resource textbooks with glossary and checklists
- Librarian: Jennifer DeBerg
- Research and EBP Resources
  - Sharon Tucker, PhD, RN, PMHCNS-BC, FAAN
  - Laura Cullen, DNP, RN, FAAN
  - Kirsten Hanrahan, DNP, ARNP
  - Nursing Research and EBP Committee
- Departmental advanced practice nurses and other leaders

### References

- Burns, B., & Grove, S. (2009). *The practice of nursing research* (6th ed.). Philadelphia: Saunders/Elsevier.
- Burns, B., & Grove, S. (2011). *Understanding nursing research* (5th ed.). Philadelphia: Saunders/Elsevier.
- Davies, B., & Logan, J. (2003). *Reading research: A user friendly guide for nurses and other health professionals.* Canada: Elsevier.
- Fineout-Overholt, E., Mazurek Melnyk, B., Stillwell, S., & Williamson, K. (2010). Critical appraisal of the evidence: Part II. *American Journal of Nursing, 110*(9), 41-48.
- Lasserson, D. (2009). *Rapid critical appraisal of controlled trials.* Clinical Lecturer, Department of Primary Health Care, University of Oxford.
- Mazurek Melnyk, B., & Fineout-Overholt, E., (2005). Rapid critical appraisal of randomized controlled trials (RCTs): An essential skill for evidence-based practice (EBP). *Pediatric Nursing, 31*(1), 50-52.
- Ogier, M. (1998). *Reading research: How to make research more approachable* (2nd ed.). London: Bailliere Tindall.

(Tucker, 2011)

### CITATIONS

Berta, Ginsburg, Gilbart, Lemieux-Charles, & Davis, 2013; Duffy, Thompson, Hobbs, Niemeyer-Hackett, & Elpers, 2011; Ellen et al., 2013; Gardner Jr., 2016; Häggman-Laitila, Mattila, & Melender, 2016; Kirchhoff, 1999; Lachance, 2014; McKeever, Kinney, Lima, & Newall, 2016; Schreiner, Kudrna, & Kenney, 2015; Tucker, 2011, August; Wilson, Ice et al., 2015.

## Strategy 1-5   Distribute Key Evidence

| PHASE | 1: Create Awareness & Interest |
|---|---|
| FOCUS | Connecting With Clinicians, Organizational Leaders, and Key Stakeholders |

### DEFINITION

To distribute key evidence is to provide strategic articles to inform the intended audience about a practice.

### BENEFITS

- Reading articles provides scientific support to align beliefs about the efficacy and willingness to use interventions more closely with expert opinion.
- Brings clinicians into the project early, creating ownership.
- Gains support of early adoptors, building a critical mass.
- Begins to identify clinician feedback and barriers to practice change.
- Arms clinicians with evidence to construct a rationale for a practice change.

### PROCEDURE

- Set a limit of one to five best articles, or fewer than 20 pages total, to keep the attention of busy clinicians.
- Distribute written material in easily accessible electronic format.
- Select articles strategically; a systematic review to create awareness of current evidence, a clinical practice guideline to identify recommendations for practice, and best evidence in a similar population.
- Provide a short, 1-2 sentence synopsis of why each piece of evidence is important for determining a practice change.
- Consider position statements and clinical practice guidelines from authoritative sources respected by clinicians.
- Consider discussing articles in journal club format (see Strategy 1-4).

### EXAMPLE

Block, J., Lilienthal, M., & Cullen, L. (2015). Thermoregulation for adult trauma patients. In M. Farrington (Series Ed.) *EBP to Go®: Accelerating evidence-based practice.* Iowa City, IA: Office of Nursing Research, Evidence-Based Practice and Quality, Department of Nursing Services and Patient Care, University of Iowa Hospitals and Clinics.

Clinical Overview

Block, J., Lilienthal, M., Cullen, L., & White, A. (2012). Evidence-based thermoregulation for adult trauma patients. *Critical Care Nursing Quarterly, 35*(1), 50–63. doi:10.1097/CNQ.0b013e31823d3e9b

Detailed Literature Review

Ireland, S., Murdoch, K., Ormrod, P., Saliba, E., Endacott, R., Fitzgerald, M., & Cameron, P. (2006). Nursing and medical staff knowledge regarding the monitoring and management of accidental or exposure hypothermia in adult major trauma patients. *International Journal of Nursing Practice, 12*(6), 308–318. doi:10.1111/j.1440-172X.2006.00589.x

Research Article

Ireland, S., Endacott, R., Cameron, P., Fitzgerald M., & Paul, E. (2011). The incidence and significance of accidental hypothermia in major trauma—A prospective observational study. *Resuscitation, 82*(3), 300–306. doi:10.1016/j.resuscitation.2010.10.016

## CITATIONS

Benishek, Kirby, Dugosh, & Padovano, 2010; Block, Lilienthal, & Cullen, 2015; Breimaier, Halfens, & Lohmann, 2015; Haxton, Doering, Gingras, & Kelly, 2012; Rash, DePhillipps, McKay, Drapkin, & Petry, 2013.

PHASE 1

## Strategy 1-6    Posters and Postings/Fliers

| PHASE | 1: Create Awareness & Interest |
|---|---|
| FOCUS | Connecting With Clinicians, Organizational Leaders, and Key Stakeholders |

### DEFINITION

Posters and postings are abbreviated informational or educational materials for display in areas that will catch the attention of clinicians.

### BENEFITS

- Provides a mechanism to share standard information in an easy-to-read format.
- Easy to develop and duplicate at minimal cost.
- Mobile method to reach members of the team in various clinical areas.

### PROCEDURE

- Determine the space available for poster dimensions and how to prop or hang.
- Determine focus based on current step of project work and design targeting that focus (e.g., report need for the EBP, report evidence, report progress with adoption, or lessons learned).
- Develop content to tell the project work as a story that includes:
  - Team
  - Project title
  - Purpose statement
  - Rationale or background (optional)
  - Method (EBP process model used)
  - Synthesis of evidence
  - Practice change
  - Implementation strategies
  - Evaluation/results
  - Conclusion
  - Implications (optional)
- Design content to be visually appealing; consider colors, font, format, graphs and visual elements.
- Design to be simple and easy to read.
- Organize to read from left to right and from the top down if audience is from Western countries.
- Design content for readability at a distance and in a short amount of time.
- Update periodically to keep clinicians informed and involved.
- Add humor, when appropriate, to draw attention.
- Rotate location of the poster or make duplicates to reach clinicians in other areas.
- Include simple action steps for reader to take.

PHASE 1

## Evidence-Based Patient Preference
### for Pain Assessment Among Hospitalized Older Adults

Laura Cullen, DNP, RN, FAAN; Kara Prickett, MSN, RN-BC; Jessica Lower, BSN, RN; Kasey Ostrander, ADN, RN; Wes Pollpeter, BSN, RN; Shey Stillings, ADN, RN; Rebecca Wolf, BSN, RN; Kelsey Smith, BSN, RN-BC

Department of Nursing Services and Patient Care, University of Iowa Hospitals and Clinics, Iowa City, IA

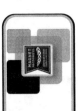

### Purpose

To provide evidence-based pain assessment matching patient preferences for older adults on a cardiac/cardiac surgery step-down unit

### Process

Iowa Model of Evidence-Based Practice to Promote Quality Care (Titler, et al., 2001)

### Synthesis of Evidence

- Hospitalized older adults often experience moderate to severe pain; their pain is under treated, and interferes with their recovery (Gianni et al., 2010; Gregory & Haigh, 2008; Haller et al., 2011; Sawyer et al., 2010).
- Practice recommendations include assessment as an important step in pain management (Gordon et al., 2005; Hadjistavropoulos et al., 2007; Herr et al., 2006; RNAO, 2007).
- Nurses often are not aware of patient preferences for even basic care such as pain management (Florin et al., 2006).
- Understanding patient preferences and actively involving patients in decisions are important for improving patient satisfaction with pain control. Patient preferences vary and must be assessed (Florin et al., 2008).
- Both cognitively intact and cognitively impaired older adults are able to self-report pain (Shega et al., 2010; Ware et al., 2006).
- Several tools have been evaluated for use with older adults: Numeric Rating Scale (NRS), Verbal Descriptor Scale (VDS), Faces Pain Scale (FPS), Faces Pain Scales-Revised (FPS-R), and the Iowa Pain Thermometer (IPT) (Flaherty, 2008; Ware et al., 2006).
- Despite valid, reliable and feasible pain scales, med-surg nurses don't consistently use them and assess pain less frequently than recommended (Coker et al., 2010; Haller et al., 2011; Michaels et al., 2007). Even when assessed, pain may not be documented consistently, making trending and treatment difficult (Haller et al., 2011).
- Nurse's pain assessment improves after EBP implementation (Abdalrahim et al., 2011; Haller et al., 2011; Zhang et al., 2008), as do other pain management practices (Haller et al., 2011; Hansson et al., 2006) and nursing knowledge (Abdalrahim et al., 2011; Mezey et al., 2009; Sawyer et al., 2010).

### Choosing a Pain Assessment Tool

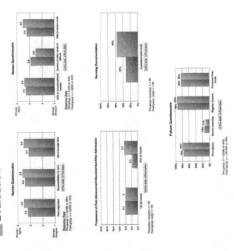

Used with permission K. Herr, PhD, RN, FAAN

### Implementation Strategies Used

Cullen, L. & Adams, S. (2012). Planning for Implementation of Evidence-Based Practice. *Journal of Nursing Administration, 42*(4), 222-230.

### Evaluation

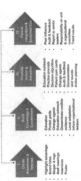

### Conclusion and Next Steps

- EBP improved nurse's pain assessment processes.
- Despite these gains, patient perceptions were largely unchanged.
- Next steps include reinfusion and expanded evidence-based pain management to improve patient satisfaction with pain control.

Williams & Cullen, 2016

*continues*

**PHASE 1**

## Strategy 1-6    Posters and Postings/Fliers (Continued)

### EXAMPLE: Posting/Flier

# Did I trace all my IV lines?
# Do I know what is infusing where?

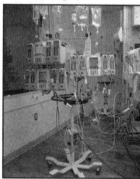

## It's a jungle out there!

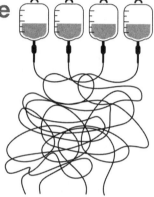

# Know where you are - at all times
# or bad things happen!

(Hannon, n.d.)        A Quality Quip from your QIS Committee

### CITATIONS

Arslan, Koca, Tastekin, Basaran, & Bozcuk, 2014; Butz, Kohr, & Jones, 2004; Cullen et al., 2013, April; Drouin, Campbell, & Kaczorowski, 2006; Ellerbee, 2009; Fineout-Overholt, Gallagher-Ford, Melnyk, & Stillwell, 2011; Forsyth, Wright, Scherb, & Gaspar, 2010; Hannon, n.d.; Turck, Silva, Tremblay, & Sachse, 2014; Williams & Cullen, 2016; Wood & Morrison, 2011.

## Strategy 1-7     Announcements & Broadcasts

| PHASE | 1: Create Awareness & Interest |
|---|---|
| FOCUS | Connecting With Clinicians, Organizational Leaders, and Key Stakeholders |

### DEFINITION

Announcements and broadcasts include information for broad dissemination in verbal or written format (often done as email from senior leaders).

### BENEFITS

- Announcements and broadcasts can be timely and reach a large audience.
- Information from the senior leader in the form of an announcement adds a sense of urgency to the work.
- Senior leadership communication about priorities is important to create awareness.

### PROCEDURE

- Identify key messages and actions to be taken.
- Determine delivery method (e.g., email).
- Be brief and focused.
- Include senior leader's endorsement or call to action with actionable activities and expectations.
- Eliminate protected health information.
- Proofread and consider the tone before sending.
- Consider the timing and when to send to increase readership (e.g., early morning).
- Distribute widely.

*continues*

**PHASE 1**

## Strategy 1-7    Announcements & Broadcasts (Continued)

### EXAMPLE

| | |
|---|---|
| **From:** | CEO; VP Nursing; CQO |
| **Sent:** | \<date\> |
| **To:** | All Clinicians |
| **Subject line:** | Quality Care Announcement |
| **Attachment:** | [W] Announcement |

This evidence-based practice announcement is sent on behalf of the VP for Patient Care Quality and Safety, \<name\>, \<credentials\>, \<organization\>.

Dear Colleagues,

In an effort to reduce hospital acquired infections for patients with a central line, we will begin daily **CHG (chlorhexidine gluconate) bathing** for all inpatients with a central line unless there is a rationale for non-use listed in the provider orders. Literature consistently shows the CHG treatment is associated with a reduction in central line infections. Please see N-02.105, a new policy which provides direction for the procedure.

**Effective date:** \<month/day/year\>
**Inventory number:** \<XXXX\>

Please note a very small sample of patients may have a **skin sensitivity or allergic reaction**, as reported to the FDA and in the literature. Reactions are to be treated per protocol (NP-08.120) and sensitivity warrants discontinuation with a rationale and use of alternative bathing cloths or skin care based on age and condition.

Please inform all clinicians within your departments and clinical areas of this practice update.

Thank you for your commitment to quality and safety,

\<signature\>
\<name and credentials\>

### CITATIONS

Al Ayubi, 2016; Alfonso, Blot, & Blot, 2016; Badran, Pluye, & Grad, 2015; De Leon, Fuentes, & Cohen, 2014; Farrell, 2016; Frost et al., 2016; Grad et al., 2008; Jamal et al., 2016; Kalman & Ravid, 2015; Kim et al., 2016; Middaugh, 2015; Summerfield & Feemster, 2015.

**PHASE 1**

## Strategy 1-8    Knowledge Broker(s)

| PHASE | 1: Create Awareness & Interest |
|---|---|
| FOCUS | Building Organizational System Support |

### DEFINITION

A knowledge broker is an external facilitator who increases knowledge sharing and use of the best evidence to address clinician-users and organizational system-context issues proactively through learning networks for adaptation to meet local needs. The broker functions as a trusted intermediary to improve understanding among researchers, clinicians, and decision-makers.

### BENEFITS

■ Provides a resource to improve clinicians' knowledge and skill about how to apply EBP.

■ Increases networking among clinicians addressing similar clinical issues during adoption of practice recommendations and interchange between researchers and end-users.

### PROCEDURE

■ Selecting a knowledge broker:
  ● Consult an agency external to the healthcare setting for expertise in the EBP process, networking, and creating learning communities.
  ● Facilitates EBP process by applying extensive EBP expertise and ability to adapt efforts to fit the local setting.
  ● Requires a diverse set of skills including strong communication and writing skills that are persuasive, consistent with a master's (or higher) degree preparation.

■ Elements of the knowledge broker role:
  ● Establishes collaborative relationships; develops rapport and credibility with clinicians, senior leaders, and other stakeholders.
  ● Creates and maintains a system for communication promoting collaboration among participants and participating organizations to promote mutual understanding and exchange of information.
  ● Addresses organizational change; garners senior leadership perceptions about priorities, strengths, and barriers for planning adoption of the EBP.
  ● Establishes need for EBP.
  ● Uses senior leader focus groups to describe strengths and barriers and identify implementation strategies to create a plan of action:
    □ Establish credibility and authority for process change.
    □ Describe value of EBP for organization.
    □ Identify practice preferences and attitudes toward the EBP.
    □ Determine decision-making style of senior leaders.
    □ Assess knowledge needs.

*continues*

## Strategy 1-8    Knowledge Broker(s) (Continued)

### PROCEDURE (Continued)

- ☐ Assess extent of EBP or conduct of research activities and skills.
- ☐ Investigate infrastructure supporting EBP.
- ☐ Determine organizational resources (e.g., human, computers, databases, electronic library).
- ☐ Determine recent restructuring, staff turnover, or other barriers.
- ☐ Establish a link with quality improvement initiatives, experts, or organizations.
- Creates networks or partnerships across clinical areas or organizations.
- Assesses clinician perceptions about strengths and barriers for adoption of the EBP.
- Uses clinician focus groups to describe strengths and barriers and to identify implementation strategies to create a plan of action:
  - ☐ Describe value of the EBP for unit/clinical area.
  - ☐ Identify practice preferences and attitudes toward the EBP.
  - ☐ Assess knowledge needs.
  - ☐ Establish a link with quality improvement initiatives, experts, and resources.
  - ☐ Identify knowledge sources accessed frequently (e.g., reading research, local experts).
  - ☐ Determine format preferences for receiving evidence summaries.
  - ☐ Determine usual implementation strategies to use that are effective.
- Develops expertise with critical review of research and evidence summaries.
- Assists with and guides project management.
- Facilitates adoption.
- Distributes key evidence or evidence summary updates.
- Reports results internally and facilitates sharing within network/learning community.
- Reports to the funding agency.

### EXAMPLES

Dobbins, M., Robeson, P., Ciliska, D., Hanna, S., Cameron, R., O'Mara, L., . . . Mercer, S. (2009). A description of a knowledge broker role implemented as part of a randomized controlled trial evaluating three knowledge translation strategies. *Implementation Science, 4*(23), 1–9. doi: 10.1186/1748-5908-4-23

Urquhart, R., Porter, G. A., & Grunfeld, E. (2011). Reflections on knowledge brokering within a multidisciplinary research team. *Journal of Continuing Education in the Health Professions, 31*(4), 283–290. doi:10.1002/chp.20128

PHASE 1

## CITATIONS

Bornbaum, Kornas, Peirson, & Rosella, 2015; Conklin, Lusk, Harris, & Stolee, 2013; Dobbins et al., 2009; Gerrish et al., 2011; Long, Cunningham, & Braithwaite, 2013; Waring, Currie, Crompton, & Bishop, 2013; Willems, Schröder, van der Weijden, Post, & Visser-Meily, 2016.

# Implementation Strategies for Evidence-Based Practice
## PHASE 2: BUILD KNOWLEDGE & COMMITMENT

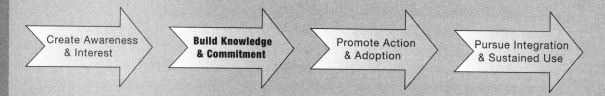

Create Awareness & Interest → **Build Knowledge & Commitment** → Promote Action & Adoption → Pursue Integration & Sustained Use

The most complex implementation strategies to perform are described. The evidence on how to use the procedures is provided to improve their effectiveness. Use in combination for a comprehensive implementation plan.

## Strategy 2-1    Education

| STRATEGY | 2: Build Knowledge & Commitment |
| --- | --- |
| FOCUS | Connecting With Clinicians, Organizational Leaders, and Key Stakeholders |

### DEFINITION

Education is the process of providing or acquiring knowledge or skills related to the EBP process and changes.

### BENEFITS

- Education is a familiar approach.
- Formats are flexible, easily accessed, and fairly inexpensive.
- Reach and availability expand when education is provided in multiple settings and through different formats.
- Face-to-face sessions allow for bidirectional communication about the practice change.
- Education targets knowledge gaps and behaviors critical to success of the practice change.

### PROCEDURE

- Perform needs assessment.
- Determine topic and content/key messages to include.
  - Consider adult learning principles.
  - Plan for brief, standardized sessions.
  - Link scope of project and relevance with organizational priorities and benefits for patients.
- Determine educational learning objectives (refer to Bloom's taxonomy learning domains and standard list).
- Determine whether continuing education credits will be provided.
- Develop an evaluation plan to determine effectiveness of the program.
  - Enhance subsequent teaching strategies based on learner feedback.
- Select delivery methods (e.g., train-the-trainer, self-learning, computer-based training, simulation, face-to-face, social media, online tools).
  - Format (offer a range of options and multifaceted strategies; consider available technology):
    - ☐ Individual or group sessions
    - ☐ In-person or remote/distance learning
    - ☐ Didactic presentation, written educational manual/materials
    - ☐ Deliberate practice, if acquisition of skills is needed
  - Frequency (is it something that can be available 24 hours per day and 7 days per week?)
  - Length (and depth of information to be covered).
  - Interactive learning should be used versus passive learning.
  - Application of content must be included.
  - Arrange face-to-face session;
    - ☐ Consider venue/facility.
    - ☐ Determine speakers to deliver content.
    - ☐ Schedule the education sessions (offer repeat or recorded sessions).

*continues*

PHASE 2

## Strategy 2-1   Education (Continued)

### PROCEDURE (Continued)

- Market education sessions through email, flyers, website, intranet, and word-of-mouth.
- Deliver presentations or educational materials.
  - Communicate using plain language.
  - Target communication to specific, relevant audience.
- Determine format and frequency for periodic reinforcement ("booster doses") of key messages.

### EXAMPLE

Lipmanowicz, H., & McCandless, K. (2014). *The surprising power of liberating structures: Simple rules to unleash a culture of innovation.* Seattle, WA: Liberating Structures Press.

*What, So What, Now What? W³* is a technique that can be used for group reflection (Lipmanowicz & McCandless, 2014).

- Collect facts about "What" happened.
- Make sense of the facts: "So What."
- Determine the next actions to take: "Now What."

An example of how the *What, So What, Now What? W³* technique could be modified to reflect W⁴, which can be used at the end of an educational session about an EBP change.

- What
  - Write down one thing that you learned/relearned.
  - Write down what you have found helpful.
- So What
  - Write down how it was meaningful.
- What Else
  - Write down what additional clarification would be helpful.
- Now What
  - Write down your next one or two steps for application.
  - Report to the group for discussion and to reinforce learning

### CITATIONS

Bloom's Taxonomy, 2016; Burke et al., 2015; Champagne, Lemieux-Charles, Duranceau, MacKean, & Reay, 2014; Clay-Williams, Nosrati, Cunningham, Hillman, & Braithwaite, 2014; Fleiszer, Semenic, Ritchie, Richer, & Denis, 2016a; Holmes, Schellenberg, Schell, & Scarrow, 2014; Jacobs et al., 2014; Kwok, Callard, & McLaws, 2015; Levin & Chang, 2014; Lipmanowicz & McCandless, 2014; Lugtenberg, Burgers, Han, & Westert, 2014; Mauger et al., 2014; Rushmer, Hunter, & Steven, 2014; Shah et al., 2014; Taylor, Clay-Williams, Hogden, Braithwaite, & Groene, 2015; van Riet Paap et al., 2015; Walker, Mwaria, Coppola, & Chen, 2014.

## Strategy 2-2   Pocket Guides

| PHASE | 2: Build Knowledge & Commitment |
|---|---|
| FOCUS | Connecting With Clinicians, Organizational Leaders, and Key Stakeholders |

### DEFINITION

Pocket guides are concise and simple information about critical steps or key decision points for hard-to-remember details in EBP recommendation.

### BENEFITS

- Useful and conveniently packaged information that is accessible at the point of care.
- Guides decisions/actions.
- Inexpensive and replaceable.

### PROCEDURE

- Review clinical practice guidelines and body of evidence.
- Collect information to include in the guide for local expert review.
- Identify critical steps and key decision points.
- Simplify information into quick-to-read phrases.
- Include visual cues (e.g., check box for action steps or infographics).
- Group information into logical sections and sequential steps.
- Print in pocket-size, foldable paper.
- Trial and seek user feedback for adapting content before larger rollout.
- Use as part of a bundle of implementation strategies.
- Update as needed.
- Clearly date revisions.
- Print on unique-color paper for easy identification and retrieval.
- Distribute and replace as needed.

### EXAMPLES

- Snellen pocket eye chart.
- Twelve lead ECG placement and interpretation card.

### CITATIONS

Ambroggio et al., 2013; Deuster, Roten, & Muehlebach, 2010; Gnanasampanthan, Porten, & Bissett, 2014; Page, Hardy, Fairfield, Orr, & Nichani, 2011; Popovski et al., 2015; Zwarenstein et al., 2014.

**PHASE 2**

## Strategy 2-3  Link Practice Change & Power Holder/Stakeholder Priorities

| PHASE | 2: Build Knowledge & Commitment |
| --- | --- |
| FOCUS | Connecting With Clinicians, Organizational Leaders, and Key Stakeholders |

### DEFINITION

Linking the practice change to stakeholder priorities explicitly connects the EBP change with identified stakeholder, leaders', and organizational mission, vision, strategic plan, and other objectives to support commitment to the EBP.

### BENEFITS

- Creates a sense of importance and urgency in adopting and integrating the practice change because of the value of stakeholders in influencing processes and outcomes.
- Helps stakeholders see the change as a potential benefit for the future of the organization.
- Builds on stakeholders' ability to act in the role of advocate, sponsor, partner, and agent of change.
- Prevents potential obstacles later in the implementation process if main concerns of stakeholders are acknowledged and addressed early.

### PROCEDURE

- Review evidence for anticipated outcomes of the practice change.
- Identify stakeholders for the practice change:
  - Evaluate the practice change and identify who may be affected by the change.
  - Stakeholders may be administrators or colleagues invested in a particular process.
- Determine the organization's priorities.
  - Review strategic plan, mission, vision, or recent senior leadership communications (e.g., newsletters, blogs, announcements).
  - Determine whether the practice change affects patients' experience, satisfaction, length of stay, readmission, or other key performance measures.
- Match anticipated outcomes from the EBP change to anticipated outcomes of stakeholder or organizational priorities.
- Determine relevance of process and outcome indicators based on stakeholder priorities.
- Develop an evaluation plan and tools for measuring these important process and outcome indicators.
  - Develop graphs and charts that concisely depict current performance (see Strategy 2-12).
- Demonstrate how the practice change may affect data.
- Consider cost or budget of the practice change.
  - Include resources needed from key stakeholders.
  - Recognize that cost may be a priority for many stakeholders.
- Demonstrate how the cost of the practice change creates a return on investment by meeting organizational goals.
- Structure practice change with a common goal that requires cooperation.

■ Present the evaluation results to stakeholders:

- Clearly articulate and repeat the common goal everyone is striving to achieve.
- Communicate important shared values and purpose.
- Organize reporting to be familiar with target audience (i.e., business plan, evidence synthesis report).
- Promote open communication.
- Allow time for stakeholders to ask questions and share concerns.
- Recognize that stakeholders who feel informed are more likely to advocate for the practice change.
- Acknowledge that this step may take several meetings and that additional information may be needed to target other stakeholders.
- Leave brief, written talking points and contact information with the stakeholder for later review.

■ Discuss stakeholder support with colleagues to begin building commitment for implementation.

■ Provide intermittent updates on practice change progress and results to stakeholders (see Strategy 2-23).

■ Facilitate stakeholder announcements (see Strategy 1-7) of support, rounding (see Strategy 3-19), and celebrations (see Strategy 4-1) for the EBP.

## EXAMPLE

Clearly articulate the EBP change and/or outcome along with the related strategic priority when discussing or reporting EBP work (see Tool 3.2). Once this link is clearly described, it will facilitate stakeholder announcements (see Strategy 1-7) of support, rounding (see Strategy 3-19), and celebrations (see Strategy 4-1) for the EBP. For example, hand hygiene is a priority for quality care. Consistent, frequent use of hand hygiene reduces hospital-acquired infections, length of stay, and cost. Use of hand hygiene matches value-based purchasing priorities and the organization's mission for providing quality care.

## CITATIONS

Bornbaum, Kornas, Peirson, & Rosella, 2015; *Harvard Business Review*, 2004; Ipsos MORI Social Research Institute, 2009; Kouzes & Posner, 2012; Langley & Denis, 2011.

**PHASE 2**

## Strategy 2-4   Change Agents: EBP Change Champion

| PHASE | 2: Build Knowledge & Commitment |
|---|---|
| FOCUS | Connecting With Clinicians, Organizational Leaders, and Key Stakeholders |

### DEFINITION

A change champion works in the clinical area where adoption of EBP is being promoted and is able to collaborate with the opinion leader, unit leaders, clinician, and colleagues to review evidence and plan implementation. This person commits to promoting a specific practice change, develops expertise on key aspects of the evidence, and guides the practice change based on his/her understanding of the evidence and the local context. The change champion uses social influence to work with a relatively small number of colleagues and may function within a core group to increase reach (Greenhalgh, Robert, Macfarlane, Bate, & Kyriakidou, 2004; Ploeg et al., 2010; Rogers, 2003; Titler, 2008).

### BENEFITS

- Uses informal influence within the existing social network for the clinical area.
- Assists the project leader as a local clinical expert committed to the practice change, who influences peers in a way that matches clinicians' preferred learning style.
- Uses strategies identified by knowing how the system works on his/her clinical area, whom to involve, and creatively crafts messages to support adoption of EBP.
- Span of influence is more local and is focused on the current EBP topic.

### PROCEDURE

Identify a change champion by looking for these characteristics:

- Connected with early adopters and has some degree of positive social influence through positive work relationships.
- Expert clinician who is consistently committed to high-quality care and passionate about the practice change; persuasive, credible, and influential clinical leader.
- Strong communication skills to share information and feedback.
- Identify one or more change champions committed to the EBP; determine the number needed based on needs (number of clinicians for sufficient local reach).

Define the roles of the champion:

- Include change champion in review of key evidence.
- Provide training and support to assist them throughout the EBP process.
- Outline change champions' role in training, troubleshooting, reinforcing the practice change, and recognizing colleagues adopting the practice change. Their role functions will require working beyond the usual shift work to function within the team and coordinate with the core group (see Strategy 2-5).
- Influence change at varying unit and organizational levels by attending key meetings and committees.

## PROCEDURE

- Assist with adapting practice recommendations and tailor the implementation plan and materials to fit the local setting.
- Share knowledge, rationale for the EBP, and resources with colleagues at the point of care.
- Train and demonstrate skills so that colleagues know how to adopt the EBP.
- Use and role-model the practice change (see Strategy 3-9).
- Provide just-in-time encouragement and troubleshooting (see Strategy 2-19 and 3-10) at the point of care.
- Provide continuous reinforcement.
- Report to team leaders or connect with opinion leaders on issues with implementation to work through revisions (see Strategy 2-6).
- Promote midstream corrections to keep momentum for adoption.
- Stay involved with interprofessional team members and attend stakeholder meetings.
- Change policy and documentation to support the EBP being incorporated into the system.
- May function within a core group, especially when working with a large group of clinicians, and use additional implementation strategies within the core group such as a gap analysis (see Strategy 2-12), academic detailing/educational outreach (see Strategy 2-9), reminders (see Strategy 3-1), or audit and feedback (see Strategies 3-12 and 3-13).

## EXAMPLES

- Clinicians who are valued for their clinical expertise and clinical leadership can work as a liaison to the EBP project director. As a change champion, they take responsibility for promoting adoption of the EBP by extending the work of the project director to reach more clinicians. They provide clinical expertise and serve as a resource beyond when the project director is available. Clinicians leading EBP through an internship or fellowship program need others committed to their EBP to provide expertise at the point of care.
- Soo, S., Berta, W., & Baker, G. R. (2009). Role of champions in the implementation of patient safety practice change. *Healthcare Quarterly, 12*(special issue), 123–128. doi:10.12927/HCQ.2009.20979

## CITATIONS

Abdullah et al., 2014; Fleuren, van Dommelen, & Dunnink, 2015; Greenhalgh, Robert, Macfarlane, Bate, & Kyriakidou, 2004; Hauck, Winsett, & Kuric, 2013; Kaasalainen et al., 2015; Ploeg et al., 2010; Rogers, 2003; Soo, Berta, & Baker, 2009; Titler, 2008.

## Strategy 2-5　Change Agents: Core Group

| PHASE | 2: Build Knowledge & Commitment |
|---|---|
| FOCUS | Connecting With Clinicians, Organizational Leaders, and Key Stakeholders |

### DEFINITION

The core group is a small group of clinicians representing all shifts and work days who are responsible for training, troubleshooting, and reinforcing the practice change with colleagues by expanding the reach to a group of clinicians (Titler, 2008).

### BENEFITS

- Matches clinician preference for receiving information from peers whom they perceive as having shared experiences, norms, and values.
- Established social networks can exert a powerful influence on peer group behavior.
- Increases the likelihood of reaching a critical mass more quickly to speed the practice change and sustainability.

### PROCEDURE

- Identify clinicians who have a positive influence promoting patient quality and safety.
- Determine which work shifts can be covered to ensure that a core group member is available throughout the initial "go live" and for several days or weeks afterward.
- Prepare core group members for key aspects of the evidence guiding the practice change (see Strategy 2-10):
  - Share and discuss key articles used to design the practice change.
  - Share how they can anticipate providing feedback to the team leaders.
- Assign the core group members to a small number of colleagues with whom to work as a training tree.
- Collaborate with the opinion leader (see Strategy 2-6), change champion, and unit leaders, such that core group members have ready access to experts.
- Define the roles of core group members in training, troubleshooting (see Strategies 2-19 and 3-10), reinforcing the practice change, and recognizing colleagues (see Strategy 3-11) adopting the practice change.
  - Lead adoption of the practice change to assigned colleagues.
  - Share knowledge with colleagues at the point of care.
  - Train and demonstrate skills so that colleagues know how to adopt the EBP (see Strategy 3-2).
  - Use and role-model the practice change (see Strategy 3-9).
  - Function as a knowledgeable resource for colleagues at the point of care.
  - Provide just-in-time encouragement and troubleshooting at the point of care (see Strategies 2-19 and 3-10).
  - Report to team leaders on issues with implementation and work through revisions and midstream corrections to keep momentum for adoption.
  - Provide regular check-ins (i.e., rounding) with team members to maintain momentum (see Strategy 3-19).

EXAMPLE

## Core Group Members' Interaction with the EBP Team and Colleagues

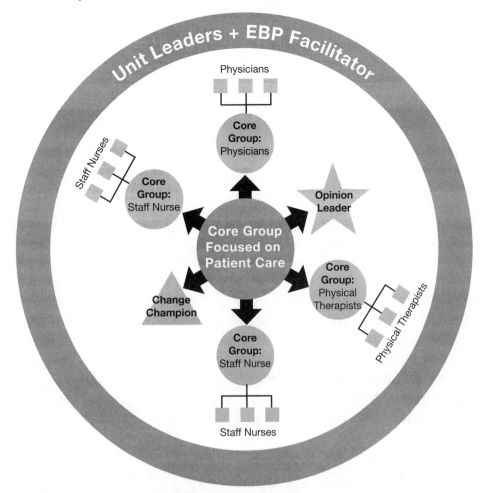

PHASE 2

CITATIONS

Adams & Barron, 2009; Dogherty, Harrison, Graham, Vandyk, & Keeping-Burke, 2013; Doyon et al., 2009; Estabrooks, Chong, Brigidear, & Profetto-McGrath, 2005; George & Tuite, 2008; Greenhalgh, Robert, Macfarlane, Bate, & Kyriakidou, 2004; Katz et al., 2016; Kortteisto, Kaila, Komulainen, Mäntyranta, & Rissanen, 2010; Marshall, West, & Aitken, 2013; Mold, Fox et al., 2014; O'Leary & Mhaolrúnaigh, 2012; Rogers, 2003; Thompson et al., 2001a; Thompson et al., 2001b; Titler, 2008.

## Strategy 2-6    Change Agents: Opinion Leader

| PHASE | 2: Build Knowledge & Commitment |
|---|---|
| FOCUS | Connecting With Clinicians, Organizational Leaders, and Key Stakeholders |

### DEFINITION

Opinion leaders are individuals whose ideas and behaviors serve as models to others. Opinion leaders screen evidence for fit in local setting, communicate messages to a group, influencing the attitudes and behaviors in the desired way. They are informal leaders promoting clinicians' use of evidence in clinical decision-making (Flodgren, Parmelli et al., 2011; 2011; Rogers, 2003).

### BENEFITS

- Influence others' opinions and behaviors because they are credible, likable, and trusted.
- Reduce uncertainty about a practice change.
- Set the standards for practice.

### PROCEDURE

- Different or multiple opinion leaders may need to be selected.
- Opinion leadership may be discipline-specific (i.e., for the interprofessional team) and may change over time.
- Combine opinion leadership with other effective strategies for greatest impact (e.g., academic detailing [see Strategy 2-9]).
- Select an opinion leader by one of the following methods:
  - Sociometric method: Self-report questionnaire identifying colleagues with influence and knowledge, and who are approachable.
  - Informant method: Ask individuals who is influential among the group of colleagues.
  - Self-designating method: Self-report of one's perceptions of their opinion leader activities.
  - Observation method: Someone independent of the team observes work activities and communication patterns among a group of colleagues.
- Define the role of the opinion leader:
  - Judge the fit and adapt evidence-based clinical recommendations based on local circumstances.
  - Endorse adoption of clinical practice recommendations.
  - Assist with determining a method for sharing information with peers (e.g., formal educational training [see Strategy 2-1], informal discussions, academic detailing or educational outreach [see Strategy 2-9], individualized feedback [see Strategies 3-22 and 4-2]).
  - Dispel misconceptions, provide actionable strategies and skills, and target actions that interfere with desired behavior or practice recommendations. Prepare by understanding the role and develop resources to influence colleagues (e.g., evidence summary [see Strategy 1-5], resource manual [see Strategy 2-16], presentation, logos or conversation starters).
  - Provide peer education with a personal touch, reassurance, and advice blending personal experience and evidence.
  - Discuss the role in implementation and provide ongoing training as needed.

**Opinion Leader Span of Influence**

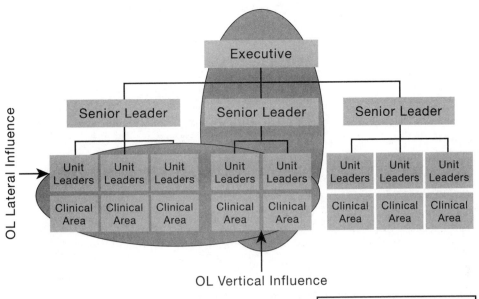

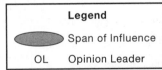

CITATIONS

Anderson & Titler, 2014; Breimaier et al., 2013; Carpenter & Sherbino, 2010; Farley, Hanbury, & Thompson, 2014; Flodgren et al., 2011; Lugtenberg, Burgers, Han, & Westert, 2014; Miech, 2016; Rogers, 2003; Rosen, Goodson, Thompson, & Wilson, 2015.

PHASE 2

## Strategy 2-7   Change Agents: Thought Leader

| PHASE | 2: Build Knowledge & Commitment |
|---|---|
| FOCUS | Connecting With Clinicians, Organizational Leaders, and Key Stakeholders |

### DEFINITION

A thought leader is "recognized as one of the foremost authorities in selected areas of specialization, resulting in its being the go-to individual or organization for said expertise" (Prince & Rogers, 2012).

### BENEFITS

- Increase in demand for the recommended practice.
- Attracts others to promote adoption of EBP.
- No research is yet available in healthcare to evaluate effectiveness of a thought leader.

### PROCEDURE

- Select a thought leader by looking for these characteristics:
  - Attractive to others (intelligent, charming, capable, connected, self-confident).
  - Drives high-volume use of the EBP.
  - Recognized by one's peers for his/her expertise and innovation in meeting needs of patients.
  - Sparks innovative ideas and a perspective for emerging trends and markets.
  - Mentions or relays information to help others.
- Define the thought leader role:
  - Demonstrate expertise.
  - Summarize the evidence or use evidence summaries (see Strategy 1-5) (e.g., given standard set of slides/materials to modify [see Strategy 2-16]).
  - Present to colleagues in a setting that will capture their attention (e.g., continuing education presentation over dinner [see Strategy 2-1]).
  - Listen to the needs of clinician users.
  - Identify and answer questions from clinician users.
  - Share insights as actionable and based on evidence.
  - Consistently provide value, benefit for others.
  - Keep things interesting.
  - Invite participation, inclusion.

### EXAMPLE

Bauer, E. (2003, November). Be a thought leader! [web log post] Retrieved from http://www.elise.com/blog/be_a_thought_leader

### CITATIONS

Agre, 2005; Bailyn, 2015; Brenner, 2014; Northcutt, n.d.; Prince & Rogers, 2012.

## Strategy 2-8    Change Agents: EBP Facilitator or Mentor

| PHASE | 2: Build Knowledge & Commitment |
|---|---|
| FOCUS | Connecting With Clinicians, Organizational Leaders, and Key Stakeholders |

### DEFINITION

The EBP facilitator or mentor is a leader with advanced EBP knowledge and skills who guides others through the EBP process. Their focus is on the mentee rather than on the project needs. The person may be internal or external to the organization (Abdullah et al., 2014; Lessard et al., 2016).

### BENEFITS

- Improves clinician knowledge, attitudes, skills, and confidence in adoption of EBP changes.
- Creates improvement in patient and organization outcomes.

### PROCEDURE

- Select an EBP facilitator or mentor by looking for these characteristics:
  - Provides a big-picture view of anticipated process and organizational and national agenda.
  - Demonstrates expertise with advanced EBP concepts and skills as well as mentoring behaviors.
  - Uses effective communication and interpersonal skills, and is politically savvy.
  - Demonstrates project management.
  - Uses technology for evidence, data management, and reporting.
  - Demonstrates persistence.
- Define the EBP facilitator or mentor role:
  - Seeks new evidence.
  - Identifies priority topics amenable to being addressed through the EBP process.
  - Promotes collaboration across disciplines and organizations to create an open, supportive, and trusting environment.
  - Provides or guides others in project management.
  - Provides constructive feedback and reassurance to guide others through the process.
  - Develops and provides educational sessions to build skills for adoption of the EBP and for the EBP process.
  - Creates a group identity.
  - Develops consensus, shares control, deals with conflict.
  - Identifies and develops skill sets of team members for coordination and division of project work.
  - Partners by providing consultation and leadership support for EBP project team.
  - Provides consultation for and serves as a liaison working within the organization.
  - Proactively addresses barriers to implementation of EBP.

*continues*

PHASE 2

## Strategy 2-8    Change Agents: EBP Facilitator or Mentor (Continued)

### PROCEDURE (Continued)

- Advocates and budgets for access to and use of resources for EBP.
- Develops and/or advises on development of an implementation plan and resources for implementation.
- Coordinates internal organizational dissemination (see Strategies 2-23, 3-8, and 3-20) to promote implementation, evaluation, and reporting.
- Develops and/or advises on steps in EBP process.
- Provides guidance for following organizational policies (e.g., approval and protecting patient confidentiality/data security) throughout evaluation and dissemination.
- Provides oversight and evaluation of the organization's EBP program to build EBP capacity; reports program metrics to senior leadership (see Strategy 2-23).
- Supports development of and leadership for an EBP program within the organization.
- Partners with unit managers and interprofessional team.
- Reports to senior leaders regarding EBP projects and program (see Strategy 2-23).
- Disseminates EBP within and outside the organization (see Chapter 12).
- Identifies opportunities for and supports novice presenters to disseminate externally to the organization.
- Creates a vision and leads strategic planning (see Strategy 4-9) efforts to expand delivery of evidence-based healthcare within the unit/clinic or organizational system.

■ Celebrates success of team (see Strategy 4-1).

**EXAMPLE**

**Job Title:** Evidence-Based Practice (EBP) Facilitator – Supervisory

**Basic Function and Responsibility**
To function as an EBP facilitator and change agent incorporating the primary role of implementation specialist and the supporting roles of consultant, clinician, educator, and administrator to support quality care and positive patient outcomes.

**Characteristic Responsibilities**

### Evidence-Based Practice
Assist clinicians to interpret research findings and provide leadership to incorporate research findings into practice.

Integrate research with quality improvement and safety activities to identify patient care problems, develop evidence-based standards and protocols, and evaluate changes in practice.

Collaborate with clinicians and other departments in planning and conducting evidence-based improvement activities.

Identify research needs and collaborate with research team to investigate clinical issues.

Assist others in the development of EBP grant proposals.

Assist others to communicate the results of EBP work through presentations and publications.

Promote and facilitate EBP activities that support departmental, divisional, and unit objectives.

Transform data into information for clinical and operational decision-making.

### Consultation
Provide consultation to facilitate use of clinical research and clinical practice recommendations for improving quality of care.

Serve as needed in a consultative and resource capacity to other divisions, the department, and the community.

**Qualifications**
A current license to practice nursing in this state.

A master's degree in nursing or a related field. A clinical doctorate (e.g., DNP) in nursing is preferred. If a master's degree is in a related field, a baccalaureate degree in nursing is required.

Demonstrated experience in EBP, education, and an area of clinical practice.

Written:     7/09
Revised:     12/13
Reviewed:    11/11

PHASE 2

*continues*

## Strategy 2-8    Change Agents: EBP Facilitator or Mentor (Continued)

### CITATIONS

Abdullah et al., 2014; Baskerville, Liddy, & Hogg, 2012; Berta et al., 2015; Cullen, Titler, & Rempel, 2011; Dogherty, Harrison, Graham, & Keeping-Burke, 2014; Dogherty, Harrison, Graham, Vandyk, & Keeping-Burke, 2013; Everett & Sitterding, 2011; Harvey & Kitson, 2016; Hauck, Winsett, & Kuric, 2013; Kitson & Harvey, 2016; Lessard et al., 2016; Magers, 2014; Morgan, 2012; Muller, McCauley, Harrington, Jablonski, & Strauss, 2011.

## Strategy 2-9   Educational Outreach/Academic Detailing

| PHASE | 2: Build Knowledge & Commitment |
|---|---|
| FOCUS | Connecting With Clinicians, Organizational Leaders, and Key Stakeholders |

### DEFINITION

Academic detailing (or educational outreach) refers to structured presentations designed to influence clinician adoption of a recommended practice (Soumerai & Avorn, 1990). Academic detailing is a communication method, based on pharmaceutical companies' specific approach for one-on-one individual discussion and presentation of evidence at the convenience of the clinician, which has been used to influence prescribing (Yeh, Van Hoof, & Fischer, 2016).

### BENEFITS

- Acceptable to clinicians and improves clinicians' knowledge, processes of care, and patient outcomes when combined with other strategies.
- Provides intended audience with evidence and how to apply it in practice.
- Convenient for clinicians, gives them positive reinforcement, and helps them to troubleshoot problems.
- Clinicians report academic detailing to be effective and feasible.

### PROCEDURE

- Identify who will be the messenger, to provide detailing visits (to individual or team); influence from a peer or someone with a similar background may be most effective.
- Select method of communication and duration of visit (10–60 minutes); in-person visits may be most effective, but other options include conference calls (over phone or computer webinar app), mail, or email.
- Provide the messenger with training on how to use academic detailing visits and how to tailor to specific clinician (e.g., convenient location for recipient, individual data, extent of evidence detailed, action steps to take as follow-up).
- Clearly articulate the goal.
- Reaffirm the individual's or team's support for reaching that goal (e.g., recognition for previous support and commitment).
- Identify one key indicator (e.g., swallow screening) from the practice recommendations to address in achieving the goal.
- Report the performance gap data (see Strategy 2-12) demonstrating an opportunity for improvement (e.g., percent of swallow screens completed within 24 hours of admission); may use clinician-specific data (see Strategy 4-2).
- Outline the evidence for the issue, including the extent of existing research supporting the practice recommendation and gaps in current knowledge (e.g., risk of aspiration pneumonia, need to do swallow screening, and challenges due to limited evidence about elevating the head of bed for bedside swallow screening in selected stroke patients).
- Identify current strategies in place to meet the indicator goal (e.g., standing orders [see Strategy 3-16] on admission, nursing assessment within 24 hours of admission, and referral as indicated).

*continues*

**PHASE 2**

**PHASE 2**

## Strategy 2-9    Educational Outreach/Academic Detailing (Continued)

### PROCEDURE (Continued)

- Provide challenging case examples.
- Admit to the challenges in meeting the goal (e.g., busy workloads and timely differential diagnosis for type of stroke) and troubleshoot solutions.
- Outline the unattractive alternatives to meeting the goal (e.g., uncomfortable nasogastric tube placement for oral intake and delayed administration of oral medications).
- State the desire to make the change systematic and with minimal impact on workload (e.g., template for orders to make the process easy for the clinicians).
- Provide clinical decision support (see Strategies 3-1 and 3-2) and/or patient educational materials (see Strategy 3-18) as needed.
- Brainstorm to identify innovative approaches to achieve the goal (e.g., preprinted orders).
- Develop an action plan (see Strategy 2-22) with next steps tailored to the clinicians' role, division of responsibility, and timeline.
- Again recognize efforts toward the goal (e.g., stroke certification) and reiterate group decisions; incentives (see Strategy 3-5) are optional.
- Plan for follow-up visits as a mechanism for reinfusion.

### EXAMPLE

Discussion related to stroke certification and swallow screening:

*Thank you for taking the time to meet face-to-face.*

*Our goal is to maintain stroke certification to improve patient care and patient outcomes.*

*You have previously provided important support and commitment to improving care for stroke patients.*

*An important indicator to improve care process for stroke patients is a focus on swallow screening.*

*Our current rate for swallow screening within 24 hours of admission is 64%, and our target is 90% documentation of completion.*

*Summarize evidence for risk of aspiration pneumonia, need to do swallow screening, and challenges due to limited evidence about elevating the head of bed for bedside swallow screening in selected stroke patients.*

*Current strategies are physician orders on admission, nursing assessment within 24 hours of admission, and referral as indicated.*

*A recent case example showed a delay in patients receiving medications when swallow screening was not done in a timely way.*

*You have a heavy workload and are busy with timely differential diagnosis for type of stroke.*

*The unattractive alternative is to insert a nasogastric tube for oral intake and delayed administration of oral medications, as in the case example.*

*Make the change systematic and with minimal impact on workload by having a template for orders to make the process easy for the clinicians.*

*Clinical decision support is built into the electronic record with standing orders for swallow screening and with easy-to-print patient educational materials.*

| EXAMPLE |
| --- |

*How can we make this easier to accomplish? What will help in your usual workflow (e.g., location of pre-printed orders within the documentation system)?*

*Let's develop an action plan with a few next steps tailored to your role, divide the responsibilities, and add a timeline.*

*I would like to recognize your leadership and ongoing support.*

*I will plan for a follow-up visit in a month to see how I can be helpful.*

| CITATIONS |
| --- |

Dyrkorn, Gjelstad, Espnes, & Lindbæk, 2016; Fischer, 2016; Morrow, Tattelman, Purcell, King, & Fordis, 2016; Moss et al., 2016; O'Brien et al., 2007; Soumerai & Avorn, 1990; Van Hoof, Harrison, Miller, Pappas, & Fischer, 2015; Yeh, Van Hoof, & Fischer, 2016.

## Strategy 2-10 Disseminate Credible Evidence With Clear Implications for Practice

| PHASE | 2: Build Knowledge & Commitment |
|---|---|
| FOCUS | Connecting With Clinicians, Organizational Leaders, and Key Stakeholders |

### DEFINITION

To disseminate credible evidence with clear implications for practice involves efforts to persuade the intended audience to adapt a practice using clearly written evidence that supports clinical decision-making.

### BENEFITS

- Gives power to evoke change when believing in the credibility of evidence.
- Influences attitudes when combined with other strategies (including short meetings, reminders, and audit and feedback).
- Offers a low-cost and feasible approach compared to other implementation strategies.

### PROCEDURE

- Examine clinicians' perceptions of evidence-based interventions as an initial step toward promoting adoption of a practice change. Perceptions can help to guide dissemination strategies aimed at clarifying effectiveness and risks.
- Focus on key steps that are critical to the practice change.
- Establish credibility by using guidelines from reputable and authoritative sources, such as guideline development groups (e.g., World Health Organization) and organizations that clinicians recognize as authoritative (e.g., American Academy of Pediatrics) rather than industry or consultants.
- Build credibility with clinicians by linking practices to patient outcomes, adapting recommendations to the setting, and considering other criteria (such as the balance of benefit and cost) in addition to the evidence.
- Involve clinicians in developing modes in which the evidence is presented.
- Make evidence accessible to clinicians in relevant and practical modes such as fact sheets, research or executive summaries (see Example 6.4), guidelines, and decision-making tools (see Strategy 3-2).
- Send a clear message about the proposed change.
  - Strong, simple recommendations are more likely to be adopted.
  - Use conditional statements.
  - Use concrete, actionable statements.
  - Justify any deliberate vagueness.
  - Use short sentences and proper punctuation.
  - Keep related information together.
  - Frame recommendations in terms of gains.
  - Focus on the risks of not doing the right thing, rather than on doing the wrong thing.
- Consider patient and clinician needs and perspectives, with attention to costs and benefits.
- Tailor strategies to demographic, structural, and cultural characteristics of subgroups.
- Use messages with appropriate style, imagery, and metaphors.
- Identify and use appropriate communication channels.
- Incorporate rigorous evaluation and monitoring of defined objectives and goals.
- Add reminders (see Strategy 3-1) and distribute written materials (see Strategy 2-16) at short meetings.

- Format the evidence to optimize attention of busy clinicians.
  - Use multiple formats.
  - Tailor to end users.
  - Highlight key features having the most impact for patient care.
  - Link key recommendations to more extensive resources.
  - Use graphics that best convey the information.
  - Use images for spatial structures, location, and detail.
  - Use simple words for procedural information and abstract concepts.

## EXAMPLE

Prescriptive practice changes disseminated through a sacred cow initiative to promote evidence-based care.

# MOOving Away From the Trough

Michele Wagner, MSN, RN, CNRN; Grace Matthews, MSN, RN-BC

A **sacred cow** that can be difficult to change is the traditional bedbath. Some falsely believe that quality care includes bathing patients with lots of soap using a basin and then toweling them dry. This practice may actually be harmful for patients (click here to see the evidence). **MOOve away from the trough and Go Basinless!**

- Basinless (bag) baths are in your store's catalog, # 923543. Warmers are free.
- Basinless baths use a pH balanced soap to protect the skin mantle.
- Basinless baths help to maintain skin moisture.
- Basinless baths are clean! No more reusing basins stored in drawers (or worse). Click here for examples of scripting this change for patients.

**Sacred cows** are old practices that are particularly resistant to change. UIHC Nursing is moving from tradition to evidence-based practices (EBP) and putting sacred cows to pasture.

Johnson, D., Lineweaver, L., & Maze, L. M. (200_). Patients' bath basins as potential source of infection: A multicenter sampling study. *American Journal of Critical Care, 18*(1), 31–40. doi:10.4037/ajcc2009968

Larson, E. L., Ciliberti, T., Chantler, C., Abraham, J., Lazaro, E. M., Venturanza, M., & Pancholi, P. (2004). Comparison of traditional and disposable bed baths in critically ill patients. *American Journal of Critical Care, 13*(3), 235–241.

Perry, G. J., & Kronenfeld, M. R. (2005). Evidence-based practice: A new paradigm brings new opportunities for health sciences librarians. *Medical Reference Services Quarterly, 24*(4), 1–16. doi:10.1300/J115v24n04_01

Rauen, C. A., Chulay, M., Bridges, E., Vollman, K., & Arbour, R. (2008). Seven evidence-based practice habits: Putting some scared cows to pasture. *Critical Care Nurse, 28*(2), 98–124.

*continues*

**Strategy 2-10    Disseminate Credible Evidence With Clear Implications for Practice (Continued)**

CITATIONS

Alanen, Välimäki, Kaila, & ECCE Study Group 2009; Cullen, L. & Adams, 2012; Greenhalgh, Robert, Macfarlane, Bate, & Kyriakidou, 2004; Grimshaw et al., 2004; Hanrahan et al., 2015; Haxton, Doering, Gingras, & Kelly, 2012; Jeffs et al., 2013; Kastner et al., 2015; Leslie, Erickson-Owens, & Cseh, 2015; Rashidian, Eccles, & Russell, 2008; Sidani et al., 2016.

## Strategy 2-11   Make Impact Observable

| PHASE | **2: Build Knowledge & Commitment** |
|---|---|
| FOCUS | **Connecting With Clinicians, Organizational Leaders, and Key Stakeholders** |

### DEFINITION

Observable impact is a visible or tangible effect that is clinically meaningful as a result of an EBP intervention (e.g., glow gel hand hygiene solution or photo of healing pressure ulcer) (Davies, Tremblay, & Edwards, 2010; Fishbein, Tellez, Lin, Sullivan, & Groll, 2011). Observability is "the degree to which the results of an innovation are visible to others" (Rogers, 2003, p. 258).

### BENEFITS

- Aids in creating links between clinical use and improved outcome.
- Highlights specific areas of improvement in practice so that clinicians understand its applicability to their practice and/or patients.
- Profoundly influences patients, clinicians, and the healthcare system, and has the potential to drive active implementation of change in practice.
- Makes use of the EBP more relevant, feasible, and, ultimately, beneficial for the patient.

### PROCEDURE

- Determine research findings or clinical practice recommendations to be implemented and their desired outcomes.
- Determine visual methods to demonstrate expected outcomes of proposed practice change (e.g., graphical display of patient data, trends, images, or photos).
- Prepare image or graph to highlight comparison and demonstrate a need for action. (If a visual image is not available, use a graphical display to demonstrate the need to act.)
- Gather positive data and develop them into a chart that is eye-pleasing and easy to read.
- Share visual outcomes that fit participants' roles and areas of interest.
- Display data where stakeholders can see them.
- Post or share the image or graph with educational resources (see Strategy 2-16).
- Reference data in staff meetings, pre-shift briefings or reports, and any department or facility publications.
- Review and reinforce the impact from practice change, matching evidence and visual outcome.
- Incorporate into ongoing evaluation to enhance sustainability of the practice change (see Chapter 11).
- Disseminate the findings to stakeholders (e.g., patients and clinicians) (see Chapter 12).

*continues*

**PHASE 2**

### Strategy 2-11    Make Impact Observable (Continued)

#### EXAMPLE

Some projects have an observable impact, or else data can be used to create an observable impact. One creative example was developed to promote pet visiting. To build buy-in, the nurse manager took photos during pet visits and created a small collection. The benefit was clearly visible, as expressed on participants' happy faces. Displaying a small collection of similar photos was strategic in demonstrating an impact to facilitate adoption.

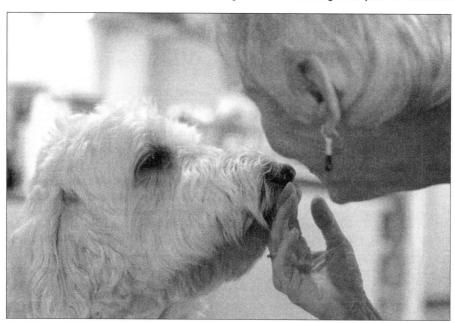

Acknowledgment: Sherry Lang, MA, RN, CPNP, NE-BC

(Cullen, Titler, & Drahozal, 1999; Cullen, Titler, & Drahozal, 2003; Titler & Drahozal, 1997)

#### CITATIONS

Bosch et al., 2016; Cullen, Titler, & Drahozal, 1999; Cullen, Titler, & Drahozal, 2003; Davies, Tremblay, & Edwards, 2010; Deochand & Deochand, 2016; Fishbein, Tellez, Lin, Sullivan, & Groll, 2011; Fleiszer, Semenic, Ritchie, Richer, & Denis, 2016a; Fleuren, van Dommelen, & Dunnink, 2015; Gerrish et al., 2011; Innis & Berta, 2016; Lee & Lee, 2014; Lehotsky et al., 2015; Overdyk et al., 2016; Putzer & Park, 2012; Rogers, 2003; Sehr et al., 2013; Snipelisky et al., 2016; Titler & Drahozal, 1997.

## Strategy 2-12    Gap Assessment/Gap Analysis

| PHASE | 2: Build Knowledge & Commitment |
|---|---|
| FOCUS | Connecting With Clinicians, Organizational Leaders, and Key Stakeholders |

### DEFINITION

Gap assessment/analysis demonstrates the difference between current practice or outcomes and the desired practice or outcome based on the best evidence.

### BENEFITS

- Clearly articulates the patient care improvement needed by comparing current practice to desired practice.
- Makes the need for change observable (see Strategy 2-11).
- Captures the attention of busy clinicians or executives in a short amount of time.
- Establishes a need that creates motivation for change.

### PROCEDURE

- Define the clinical issue and relevant practice recommendations.
- Capture insights about the practice and opportunities for improvement from stakeholders, including patients (e.g., SWOT/Strengths, Weaknesses, Opportunities, Threats analysis).
- Identify key process and outcome indicators (see Chapter 9).
- Select the two to three indicators with the strongest link to the goal.
- Collect data using a systematic process to ensure that they reflect current practice patterns and outcomes.
- Create a graphical display that highlights the percent or rate at which current practice matches or differs from the recommended practice.
- Report the graphical result (when possible) of performance gap to clinical or organizational leaders and key stakeholders.
- Qualitative data reporting is an alternative if graphical display is not appropriate (e.g., stories or case studies; see Strategy 2-17).
- If displaying multiple indicators, establish priorities among performance gaps based on:
  - The extent of relevance in a local setting
  - The magnitude of the problem
  - Patient priorities (see Strategy 3-21)
  - Amenability to change
- Propose next steps for performance improvement (e.g., members to join the task force, charge to the group).

*continues*

**Strategy 2-12    Gap Assessment/Gap Analysis (Continued)**

### EXAMPLE

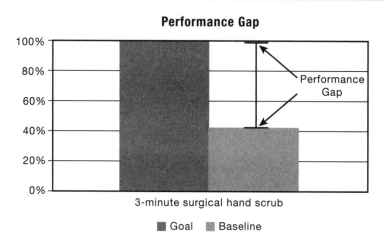

**Performance Gap**

3-minute surgical hand scrub

■ Goal    ■ Baseline

(Laurikainen, Rintala, Kaarto, & Routamaa, 2016)

### CITATIONS

Bosch et al., 2016; Bruno et al, 2014; Cahill, Murch, Cook, Heyland, & Canadian Critical Care Trials Group, 2014; Davis-Ajami, Costa, & Kulik, 2014; Laurikainen, Rintala, Kaarto, & Routamaa, 2016; McGregor et al., 2017; Mwaniki, Ayieko, Todd, & English, 2014; Ploeg et al., 2010; Rankin et al., 2016; Xu, Ren, Shi, & Jiang, 2013; Yam, Fales, Jemison, Gillum, & Bernstein, 2012.

## Strategy 2-13   Clinician Input

| PHASE | 2: Build Knowledge & Commitment |
|---|---|
| FOCUS | Connecting With Clinicians, Organizational Leaders, and Key Stakeholders |

### DEFINITION

Clinician input is the process of obtaining suggestions through shared decision-making from nurses and other professionals in the practice setting in order to improve the design of the practice change, implementation plan, or integration into clinical workflow.

### BENEFITS

- Identifies the need for an improvement in practice.
- Creates greater agreement with guideline recommendations and improves knowledge and adherence to guidelines.
- Helps identify potential barriers to the implementation of EBP to guide adaptations that increase the likelihood of successful adoption.
- Clinicians who are actively involved have a greater sense of empowerment, increased job satisfaction and performance, and they are more committed to adoption of the EBP.
- Intensifies feelings of ownership, shared mission, and goals.

### PROCEDURE

- Identify clinician end users who are credible and influential among their peers and who have varying clinical perspectives.
- Identify priority topics and needs from clinicians.
- Ask clinicians to review the EBP changes prior to implementation.
- Provide an opportunity for clinicians to ask questions regarding the practice change implementation process and possibilities for modification of the intervention to better meet their needs and the needs of the patient population they serve (see Strategy 2-15).
- Ask the clinicians for feedback regarding workflow, perceived barriers to implementation, perceived feasibility of the practice change, and perceived needs of and relevance to their patient population.
- Always brainstorm for solutions when identifying barriers.
- Incorporate feedback from all clinicians into the modification of both the design of the EBPs and implementation plan.
- Share with clinicians how their feedback was used to make changes.
- Create implementation tools or resources based on clinicians' suggestions.
- Involve clinicians in peer training as core group members (see Strategy 2-5).
- Ask clinicians to improve the effectiveness of the implemented interventions through continuous feedback with team and organizational leaders.

*continues*

PHASE 2

## Strategy 2-13    Clinician Input (Continued)

### EXAMPLE

Prior to implementation, a pilot phase was used to "test" use of the guideline recommendations in daily practice. Clinicians' input was sought by asking them to keep a patient log and record the time it took to use the guideline, resources needed, and obstacles with use of the guideline. Then clinicians and managers were interviewed to generate a list of barriers and facilitators. The practice recommendations were adapted for application in practice. Adaptation was made to 1) the guideline while retaining key elements essential to achieve improvements, and 2) the implementation plan to facilitate adoption of the EBP (Fleuren, Paulussen, van Dommelen, & Van Buuren, 2014; Fleuren, van Dommelen, & Dunnink, 2015).

### CITATIONS

Bahtsevani, Willman, Stoltz, & Östman, 2010; Bethel, Seitz, Landreth, Gibson, & Whitcomb, 2012; Brody, Barnes, Ruble, & Sakowski, 2012; Chou, Vaughn, McCoy, & Doebbeling, 2011; Davidson & Brown, 2014; Devalia, 2010; Fleuren, Paulussen, van Dommelen, & Van Buuren, 2014; Fleuren, van Dommelen, & Dunnink, 2015; Ireland, Kirkpatrick, Boblin, & Robertson, 2013; Johnson & May, 2015; Kastner et al., 2015; Kristensen & Hounsgaard, 2014; Taxman & Belenko, 2011; Thompson, McCaughan, Cullum, Sheldon, Mulhall, & Thompson, 2001a.

## Strategy 2-14   Local Adaptation & Simplify

| PHASE | 2: Build Knowledge & Commitment |
|---|---|
| FOCUS | Connecting With Clinicians, Organizational Leaders, and Key Stakeholders |

### DEFINITION

Local adaptation and simplify is making the practice change fit the setting and the workflow easy. Reinvention involves extensive adaption to suit the needs of the setting or to improve the fit to local conditions (Rabin, Brownson, Haire-Joshu, Kreuter, & Weaver, 2008).

### BENEFITS

- Matches the purpose of the EBP change with patient needs and resources; culturally appropriate care; organizational resources, equipment, and systems; and existing evidence-based protocols or policies.
- Makes innovations or EBP easier to adopt because they are understood and better match existing skills or workflow.
- Provides an opportunity to seek patient and family input.

### PROCEDURE

- Identify stakeholders and plan for communication with them to promote buy-in.
- Seek review or assistance from experts as needed throughout the process using a perspective of identifying solutions to match the local setting.
- Review research findings and clinical practice guidelines (CPGs) as needed to guide decisions in how to adapt and simplify CPG recommendations.
- Assess the fit of the CPG recommendations for the target patient population and cultural considerations.
- Assess the fit of the CPG for matches with local expertise and the organization's resources.
- Identify recommendations contradicting current organizational policies or contracts.
- Identify critical components that are essential for inclusion in the practice to achieve the desired outcome.
- Simplify recommendations to the fewest key steps that will improve outcomes (see Chapter 7).
- Assess tools for feasibility in practice and simplify as needed.
- Integrate with existing and related evidence-based protocols or policies.
- Revise the patient health record to match adapted and simplified local EBP protocol.
- Plan for trying/piloting the practice change to guide additional adaptations before integration or rollout (see Chapter 7).
- Develop messages and tools that are actionable and describe adaptations that are created.
- Identify key process and outcome indicators and tools for pilot evaluation to guide subsequent adaptation (see Chapter 9).
- Revise implementation and data collection tools to match key steps and expected outcomes from the localized practice protocol.

*continues*

**PHASE 2**

## Strategy 2-14   Local Adaptation & Simplify (Continued)
### EXAMPLE

#### Clinical Practice Recommendation
#### Standard 45. FLUSHING AND LOCKING
**Practice Criteria:** "Patency of arterial catheters used for hemodynamic monitoring is greater when heparin solution is infused, although existing studies are inconclusive due to variations in the catheter's location (peripheral versus pulmonary), duration of catheter use, and differences in patency measurement. The decision to use preservative-free 0.9% sodium chloride (USP) instead of heparin infusion should be based on the clinical risk of catheter occlusion, the anticipated length of time the arterial catheter will be required, and patient factors such as heparin sensitivities" (Infusion Nurses Society, 2011, p. S61).

#### Adapted Procedure for Practice: Organizational Procedure Manual Content
1. Explain the procedure to the patient.
2. Perform hand hygiene and wear gloves and face shield or goggles and face mask.
3. Assemble arterial line transducer:
   A. Obtain flush solution of heparinized saline or another solution per physician order. [5, 6]
      i. Heparinized normal saline is the standard-setup flush solution.
      ii. Normal saline is the flush solution of choice for patients determined to be at risk for heparin induced thrombocytopenia (HIT) or if the expected duration of the arterial line is less than or equal to 48 hours. [1, 2, 3, 4]
      iii. Consider other flush solutions for patients at risk for HIT and expected to require the peripheral arterial line for an extended duration. [4]
   B. Flush and calibrate transducer prior to insertion of the arterial line.
   C. Inflate pressure-monitoring bag to 300mm Hg.
   D. Level the transducer at the patient's mid-auxiliary line.

#### References
1. Assmann, A., Boeken, U., Feindt, P., Schurr, P., Akhyari, P., & Lichtenberg, A. (2010). Heparin-induced thrombocytopenia Type II after cardiac surgery: Predictors and outcome. *Thoracic and Cardiovascular Surgeon, 58*(8), 463–467. doi:10.1055/s-0030-1250184
2. Bloemen, A., Testroote, M. J., Janssen-Heijnen, M. L., & Janzing, H. M. (2012). Incidence and diagnosis of heparin-induced thrombocytopenia (HIT) in patients with traumatic injuries treated with unfractionated or low-molecular-weight heparin. A literature review. *Injury, 43*(5), 548–552. doi:10.1016/j.injury.2011.05.007
3. Caixeta, A., Dangas, G. D., Mehran, R., Feit, F., Nikolsky, E., Lansky, A. J.,…Stone, G. W. (2011). Incidence and clinical consequences of acquired thrombocytopenia after antithrombotic therapies in patients with acute coronary syndromes: Results from the Acute Catheterization and Urgent Intervention Triage Strategy (ACUITY) trial. *American Heart Journal, 161*(2), 298–306. doi:10.1016/j.ahj.2010.10.035
4. Cuker, A. (2011). Heparin-induced thrombocytopenia: Present and future. *Journal of Thrombosis and Thrombolysis, 31*(3), 353–66. doi:10.1007/s11239-011-0569-6
5. Halm, M. A. (2008). Flushing hemodynamic catheters: What does the science tell us? *American Journal of Critical Care, 17*(1), 73–76.
6. Infusion Nursing Society. (2011). Infusion Nursing standards of practice. *Journal of Infusion Nursing, 34*(Suppl 1), S61.

## CITATIONS

Alanen, Välimäki, Kaila, & ECCE Study Group, 2009; Baskerville, Liddy, & Hogg, 2012; Cullen, Smelser, Wagner, & Adams, 2012; Graan, Botti, Wood, & Redley, 2016; Harrison et al., 2013; Infusion Nurses Society, 2011; Kastner et al., 2015; Kis et al., 2010; Poulsen et al., 2010; Rabin, Brownson, Haire-Joshu, Krueter, & Weaver, 2008; Rogers, 2003; Veniegas, Kao, Rosales, & Arellanes, 2009; Weisner & Cameron Hay, 2015.

PHASE 2

## Strategy 2-15    Focus Groups for Planning Change

| PHASE | 2: Build Knowledge & Commitment |
|---|---|
| FOCUS | Connecting With Clinicians, Organizational Leaders, and Key Stakeholders |

### DEFINITION

Focus groups are small-group interviews used to identify how adoption of EBP has happened previously and to inform selection of implementation strategies. The combination of group interaction and facilitated discussion can guide revision and planning for acceptable and effective implementation strategies.

### BENEFITS

- A focus group is a cost-effective way to gain feedback on the usability of EBP and to provide a mechanism for clarification about how to guide selection of implementation strategies.

### PROCEDURE

- Define a clear purpose for the focus group (e.g., describe strategies that have been helpful in promoting adoption of EBP and to guide implementation planning).
- Develop several broad and open-ended questions to stimulate discussion and recall.
- Consider how data will be collected, participant identities protected, data reported, etc.
- Identify an objective facilitator who can probe for information and encourage participation by all group members and who is not a direct supervisor of group members.
- How to select participants:
  - Select participants to represent and share an understanding of the organizational context.
  - Identify a group (five to seven participants is optimal) who are representative of different shifts and will offer diverse perspectives.
- Arrange a focus group meeting.
- Conduct the focus group:
  - Communicate anonymity and/or confidentiality in reporting findings.
  - Provide introductions.
  - Ask and reframe questions to stimulate discussion and promote depth of understanding.
  - Seek clarification from participants, if needed.
  - Avoid leading questions and biases.
- Transcribe notes or recordings.
- Have two reviewers identify themes.
- Compare findings to seek agreement between reviewers.
- Develop a report of findings, maintaining confidentiality.

**PHASE 2**

| EXAMPLE |
|---|

**Introductory comments**
- Welcome participants.
- Complete introductions by stating the reason for participating and whom they represent.
- Define the purpose (e.g., to obtain feedback from clinicians regarding supportive systems and other changes that can help them implement central line infection prevention bundle).

**Describe procedure and guidelines to participants**
- Record the discussion for transcription and analysis.
- Request feedback from the group for validation of responses.
- Maintain confidentiality of responses, and do not list names in transcripts.
- Remind participants to keep conversations confidential (i.e., all comments "stay in the room").
- State that all feedback is welcome, specifically feedback that can lead to improvements in implementation planning. Request that participants take advantage of this opportunity to identify what is helpful for implementing improvements and strategies for moving forward. State that this session is not just for complaining. Identifying barriers is welcome when followed by brainstorming to identify helpful solutions.
- Encourage everyone to participate.

**Process**
- Start with a round robin approach and move to informal discussion.
- Several questions can help focus the discussion.
- After the focus group, transcribe the recordings.
- Plan to review the content with a team member to improve reliability of the interpretation.
- Ask participants to review transcripts for clarification or validation.
- Based on the ideas generated from the group, develop an implementation plan, and then summarize the focus group results and report them to the team and/or administration.

**Sample questions**
- Please identify examples of practice changes that were successfully implemented in your clinical area.
- What was helpful in getting these changes into practice?
- What implementation strategies were used?
- How were clinicians involved in planning?
- How were issues addressed proactively during the pilot?
- Which of these approaches would be helpful with this project?
- Do you have any other suggestions?

**Closing remarks**
- Again, recordings will be transcribed. Participants may be asked for their review of the content for clarification. An implementation plan will be developed. Results will be reported to the team and/or administration.
- Thank you for participating.

*continues*

## Strategy 2-15   Focus Groups for Planning Change (Continued)

### CITATIONS

Ashida, Heaney, Kmet, & Wilkins III., 2011; Dobbins et al., 2009; Fleuren, van Dommelen, & Dunnink, 2015; Fourney & Williams, 2003; Johnson & May, 2015; Kaasalainen et al., 2010; Kimber & Grimmer-Somers, 2011; Kristensen & Hounsgaard, 2013; Krueger & Casey, 2000; Lawton et al., 2016; Mader et al., 2016; Morrison & Peoples, 1999; Teela et al., 2015; Wingfield et al., 2015.

## Strategy 2-16    Resource Manual or Materials

| PHASE | 2: Build Knowledge & Commitment |
|---|---|
| FOCUS | Connecting With Clinicians, Organizational Leaders, and Key Stakeholders |

### DEFINITION

Use of resource manual or materials makes printed educational materials available that disseminate information and instructions on EBP. The purpose of these materials is to improve healthcare professionals' awareness, knowledge, attitudes, and skills regarding practice changes (Giguère et al., 2012). The success of printed materials in influencing the uptake of new practices is influenced by readability, content, organization, tone and language, illustrations, appearance and typography, and appeal (Williams, Caceda-Castro, Dusablon, & Stipa, 2016).

### BENEFITS

- Provides easy accessibility for clinicians.
- Lists concise instructions on the "how, when, where, and why" of a new practice.
- Assembles all relevant information into one source.
- Generally insufficient to change behavior but supplements other activities to influence uptake.

### PROCEDURE

- Plan the exact messages to include.
- Include only information that the reader needs to know. Consider national goal procedure for assessment and intervention, integration with other protocols, and considerations for special populations.
- Exclude information that the reader already knows.
- Begin with the most important information.
- Provide a list of resources (e.g., local experts).
- Limit the number of messages.
- Identify action steps.
- Limit paragraphs to 40–50 characters for ease of reading.
- Break up text with bullets.
- Pay attention to text appearance.
- Use visual elements to help explain the message.
- When showing graphics, number the images in logical order.
- Tell stories to place people in scenarios.
- Use common language and exclude jargon.
- Break manual into smaller parts or sections that can be absorbed quickly.
- Test for reading level and complexity before releasing to the audience.

*continues*

## Strategy 2-16    Resource Manual or Materials (Continued)

### EXAMPLE

**HYALURONIDASE FOR IV EXTRAVASATIONS IN PEDIATRIC PATIENTS**
**QUICK REFERENCE**

#### PATHOPHYSIOLOGY

Five mechanisms may activate tissue necrosis when an extravasation occurs: 1) direct cellular toxicity, 2) osmotic disturbances across the cell membrane leading to cell death, 3) ischemic necrosis, 4) mechanical compression, and 5) bacterial colonization. Consequences range from a short term inflammatory response to severe necrosis requiring surgical intervention and may cause long term disabilities. The extent of damage caused by

#### INDICATIONS FOR TREATMENT

• Stage 2 or greater extravasation
• Any amount of vesicant drug
• Some irritants, depending on concentration
• Any amount of blood products
• Agent specific recommendations- see Table 1.

ADMINISTRATION

**HYALURONIDASE FOR IV EXTRAVASATIONS IN PEDIATRIC PATIENTS**
**QUICK REFERENCE**

**AGENT SPECIFIC RECOMMENDATIONS FOR TREATMENT WITH HYALURONIDASE:**

| Treat<br>Use of hyaluronidase for this agent is supported by efficacy in two or more sources. | Consider Treatment<br>Efficacy of hyaluronidase for this agent is supported but evidence is limited, consider treatment.* | Explore other treatments<br>Use of hyaluronidase is contraindicated for these agents and/or other effective antidotes are available for treatment.** |
|---|---|---|
| Calcium solutions<br>Contrast media<br>Dextrose solutions (≥ 10%)<br>Docetaxel<br>Etoposide<br>Etoposide phosphate<br>Nafcillin<br>Paclitaxel (Taxol®)<br>Total Parenteral Nutrition<br>Vinblastine<br>Vincristine<br>Vinorelbine | Aminophylline<br>Carmustine<br>Chloramphenicol<br>Erythromycin<br>Hypertonic saline ≥ 3%<br>Mannitol (≥ 15% concentration)<br>Oxacillin<br>Penicillin<br>Phenytoin<br>Potassium solutions<br>Sodium tetradecyl sulfate<br>Teniposide<br>Theophylline<br>Tromethamine<br>Vancomycin | Carboplatin<br>Cisplatin<br>Cyclophosphamide<br>Dacarbazine<br>Dactinomycin<br>Daunorubicin<br>Dobutamine<br>Dopamine<br>Doxorubicin (Adriamycin®)<br>Epinephrine<br>Epirubicin<br>Fluorouracil<br>Idarubicin<br>Ifosfamide<br>Mechlorethamine<br>Mitomycin<br>Mitoxantrone<br>Norepinephrine<br>Oxaliplatin<br>Vasopressin |

\* Consider hyaluronidase for treatment of any large volume extravasation (EXCEPT when other treatments available, clear evidence of inefficacy, or contraindicated**).

**ADJUVANT THERAPIES:** Other therapies that may enhance the effectiveness of hyaluronidase.
**Positioning-** Elevate of the affected site for 24 to 72 hours to decrease edema and aid in normal absorption of extravasated fluids.

**Thermal modalities-** With the exception of vinca alkaloids, there is no clear evidence regarding the benefit of thermal modalities with hyaluronidase.

**Saline flushout-** Saline flushout is a technique that physically removes any extravasated material from the tissue. It may be indicated when there are multiple agents extravasated or for extravasations of large volumes or vesicant agents. Techniques for saline flushout vary from multiple incisions or stab wounds, with or without irrigation and manual expression, to subcutaneous

(Hanrahan, 2012)

### CITATIONS

CDC, 2010; Dalto, 2013; Federal Plain Language Guidelines, 2011; Giguère et al., 2012; Hanrahan, 2012; Williams, Caceda-Castro, Dusablon, & Stipa, 2016; Zwarenstein et al., 2014.

## Strategy 2-17    Case Studies

| PHASE | 2: Build Knowledge & Commitment |
|---|---|
| FOCUS | Connecting With Clinicians, Organizational Leaders, and Key Stakeholders |

### DEFINITION

A case study is the collection and presentation of detailed information about a particular participant or small group, including accounts for how EBP was helpful or would have been helpful for patient care. It has meaning only for that participant and only in that specific context. Case studies can consist of text, images, or a combination. These types of findings fit well in practice because clinical situations are embedded in context and characterize the complexity of real-world practice. As an implementation strategy, clinicians may be expected to respond to the case scenario with clinical decisions as a method to stimulate discussion or reflection for learning. Clinicians often use forms of analytical generalization that supports application of knowledge of past cases in new situations, with a goal to assess how this knowledge fits. Discussion or reflection is done in a way as to not impose prior knowledge onto the new case.

### BENEFITS

- Engage learners in reflection and brainstorming, identifies priorities and barriers to practice change, and determines the timing of implementation.
- Helps learners gain insight into real-life application.
- Increases confidence for application.

### PROCEDURE

- Identify a specific practice pattern or behavior impacting a clinical condition relevant to the EBP.
- Determine the correct audience and venue for reporting the case study or use of case-based training (e.g., informal inservice, committee meeting).
- Develop brief handout or audiovisual aid if appropriate.
- Schedule training session.
- Complete introductions, if appropriate.
- Establish ground rules about providing and receiving constructive feedback.
- Provide context for the case study, including sufficient information about patient, setting, and data collection to allow clinicians to understand the situation:
  - Background
  - Characteristics of the case scenario requiring attention
  - Unit or clinic where case occurred
  - Relevance of case to the EBP
- Provide patient description:
  - Patient demographics
  - Primary diagnosis and related conditions
  - Course of treatment
  - Relevant background information

*continues*

## Strategy 2-17   Case Studies (Continued)

### PROCEDURE (Continued)

- Review evidence guiding practice and recommended practices.
- Provide structured questions or prompts for discussion.
- Lead discussion about where practices did/did not match those recommended by EBP.
- Review critical steps in the practice procedure that are essential to achieve the desired outcome.
- Describe the result for the patient, including:
  - Any adverse event (actual or averted)
  - Opportunity costs to the patient (e.g., pain, longer length of stay, discharge to a location other than home)
  - Opportunity costs to the family (e.g, missed work days to care for patient, need for care assistance)
  - Opportunity costs to the organization (e.g., patient satisfaction, reportable measure, increased/decreased cost)
  - Opportunity costs to society (e.g., years of life gained)
- Review critical steps as actionable follow-up needed for practice improvement.
- Discuss results for their fit with previous knowledge, including direct experience with similar cases and previous research, guidelines, and theory.
- Determine whether change occurred and whether the change can be attributed to the intervention or whether it impacted the outcome.
- Plan for integration of the EBP (see Chapter 11).
- Provide a supportive learning environment and encourage participation in discussion.

### EXAMPLE

An EBP project related to nasogastric or feeding tube placement in critically ill patients could use the following case example of associated risks for this common procedure. This information could be used in an educational program and/or to gain commitment to increase use of a clinical procedure. Case studies from the unit or organization can be particularly meaningful in demonstrating an opportunity for improvement.

**Case of Misplaced Nasogastric Tube**

**Background**

Placement of nasogastric tubes is common in critically ill patients. Evidence-based protocols for placement verification are available. Multiple reports demonstrate that use of auscultation is not effective. Preventable mistakes still occur. Literature and case studies provide information regarding clinical sequelae. These case reports describe the pulmonary complications likely caused by misplacement of the nasogastric tube.

## EXAMPLE

### Case

A 60-year-old critically ill man was admitted to the critical care unit with respiratory distress and sepsis. He was intubated and needed enteral nutrition. NG placement failed on two attempts. A stiffened NG with stylet was inserted and 300 cc of clear yellow fluid aspirated. Auscultation after air insufflation was attempted but was ambiguous. An X-ray identified tube misplacement down the right bronchus and development of a new tension pneumothorax on the right side. After treatment, patient's condition improved, and the patient was then weaned from the mechanical ventilator.

### Discussion

- Current state of science/evidence for NG placement verification and risk of misplacement
- Relevance of this case to patient population
- Correct or alternative action available
- Related local policies (N-06.10, N-06.011)
- Updates to policy or practices needed?
- Follow-up planned

### Conclusion

NG placement is a common procedure for critically ill and hospitalized patients. The ability to aspirate fluid created a false positive. An abundance of literature describes practice recommendations and complications associated with use of nasogastric and feeding tubes. Use of these tubes continues, along with responsibility to improve common knowledge and ensure that practice guidelines and protocols are dependable and used consistently.

(Al Saif, Hammodi, Al-Azem, & Al-Hubail, 2015; Shah, Narayanaswamy, & Khobragade, 2016)

## CITATIONS

Al Saif, Hammodi, Al-Azem, & Al-Hubail, 2015; Becker et al., 1994-2012; Bhogal, Murray et al., 2011; Bruno et al., 2014; Drexel et al., 2011; Gnanasampanthan, Porten, & Bissett, 2014; Groot-Jensen, Kiessling, Zethraeus, Bjornstedt-Bennermo, & Henriksson, 2016; Maas et al., 2015; Salbach, Veinot, Jaglal, Bayley, & Rolfe, 2011; Shah, Narayanaswamy, & Khobragade, 2016; Tomatis et al., 2011

## Strategy 2-18    Teamwork

| STRATEGY | 2: Build Knowledge & Commitment |
| --- | --- |
| FOCUS | Building Organizational System Support |

### DEFINITION

Teamwork involves a group of people working collaboratively toward a common goal.

### BENEFITS

- Improves communication.
- Improves patient satisfaction and outcomes.
- Decreases costs.
- Improves clinician retention.
- Enhances workflow.

### PROCEDURE

- Define the scope of work for the team, with clear boundaries around charge to the group.
- Invite all stakeholders to participate in the team (see Strategies 2-3 and 2-13).
- Ensure that the goals of the team are shared by all members.
- Develop mutual trust among team members.
- Assign clear roles to each team member.
- Create communication mechanisms that can be conveniently accessed by all team members.
- Formulate measurable processes and action plan (see Strategy 2-22).
- Schedule meetings when team members can be present or join electronically/virtually.
- Secure sufficient resources to allow optimal team performance.
- Monitor the work of the team.
- Provide feedback toward achieving goals.

### EXAMPLES

- Agency for Healthcare Research and Quality (AHRQ). (2016b). TeamSTEPPS. Team strategies and tools to enhance performance and patient safety. Retrieved from http://www.ahrq.gov/teamstepps/index.html
- Brader, C., & Jaeger, M. (2014). *What makes an interdisciplinary team work? A collection of informed ideas, discussion prompts, and other materials to promote an atmosphere of collaboration, trust, and respect.* IPP/42. Retrieved from http://commons.pacificu.edu
- Royal College of Nursing. (2007). Developing and sustaining effective teams. Retrieved from https://www2.rcn.org.uk/__data/assets/pdf_file/0003/78735/003115.pdf

### CITATIONS

AHRQ, 2016b; Brader & Jaeger, 2014; Dow, DiazGranados, Mazmanian, & Retchin, 2013; Ezziane, Maruthappu, Gawn, Thompson, Athanasiou, & Warren, 2012; Murphy, 2015; Nancarrow et al., 2013; Royal College of Nursing, 2007; Taylor, Clay-Williams, Hogden, Braithwaite, & Groene, 2015.

## Strategy 2-19    Troubleshoot Use/Application

| PHASE | 2: Build Knowledge & Commitment |
|-------|----------------------------------|
| FOCUS | Building Organizational System Support |

### DEFINITION

Troubleshooting use and application is a problem-solving approach to identify challenges and solutions to implementing EBP changes in order to ensure compatibility with the local unit context and workflow.

### BENEFITS

- Engages point-of-care clinicians in identifying challenges and solutions.
- Tailors practice change to the context and needs of local settings.
- Creates a sense of local ownership among clinicians and improves application to patients.
- Provides ongoing support and constructive feedback.

### PROCEDURE

- Identify complex patients/scenarios that do not fit newly established workflow for use of practice recommendations.
- Determine factors that contribute to the complexity and complicate use of the recommendations.
- Review recommendations to verify that a true problem exists rather than simply resistance to change.
- Identify key components/principles from the practice recommendations.
- Review and reinforce clinician decision-making/thinking to target a solution.
- Use creative thinking strategies to identify possible solutions.
- Ask for clinician input (see Strategy 2-13).
- Reaffirm goal—application of recommendations to achieve outcomes.
- Revise workflow (e.g., policy) (see Strategy 3-2).
- Pilot/trial new approach (see Strategy 3-6).
- Determine effectiveness after pilot (see Chapter 9).
- Report results related to revised approach or workflow for use with other patients and team learning.

### EXAMPLE

Jankowski, I. M., & Nadzam, D. M. (2011). Identifying gaps, barriers, and solutions in implementing pressure ulcer prevention programs. *Joint Commission Journal on Quality & Patient Safety, 37*(6), 253–264. doi: 10.1016/S1553-7250(11)37033-X

### CITATIONS

Anas & Brunet, 2009; Baskerville, Liddy, & Hogg, 2012; Dogherty, Harrison, & Graham, 2010; Dogherty, Harrison, Graham, Vandyk, & Keeping-Burke, 2013; Fleuren, van Dommelen, & Dunnink, 2015; Hauck, Winsett, & Kuric, 2013; Jankowski & Nadzam, 2011; Liddy et al., 2015.

PHASE 2

## Strategy 2-20    Benchmark Data

| PHASE | 2: Build Knowledge & Commitment |
|---|---|
| FOCUS | Building Organizational System Support |

### DEFINITION

"Benchmarking in health care is defined as the continual and collaborative discipline of measuring and comparing the results of key work processes with those of the best performers in evaluating organizational performance. There are two types of benchmarking that can be used to evaluate patient safety and quality performance. Internal benchmarking is used to identify best practices within an organization, to compare best practices within the organization, and to compare current practice over time. The information and data can be plotted on a control chart with statistically derived upper and lower control limits. However, using only internal benchmarking does not necessarily represent the best practices elsewhere. Competitive or external benchmarking involves using comparative data between organizations to judge performance and identify improvements that have proven to be successful in other organizations" (Hughes, 2008b, Chapter 44, p. 2).

### BENEFITS

- Demonstrates priorities from performance comparison and standardized data using credible national or proprietary companies.
- Identifies quality indicators to use for benchmark comparison and improving care.
- Displays a clear comparison or gap in performance or successful outcome that provides direction for corrective action.
- Increases compliance with clinical practice recommendations when using strategies for competitions and data feedback (see Strategy 3-13).
- Gives immediate feedback on performance.
- Easy to implement and provides built-in evaluation.

### PROCEDURE

- Identify key process or outcome indicators that meet a local need (see Chapter 9).
- Review the organizational data for accuracy.
- Identify a comparison group (e.g., Press Ganey/set of local units) or organization.
- Determine comparability of local data to benchmark (e.g., case-mix).
- Graph the organizational data/comparison data on the same graph or type of graph.
- Determine whether organizational data exceed, meet, or are below comparison.
- Report results to clinical teams and include key processes or process indicators.
- Report results within QI (quality improvement) infrastructure.
- Use data for revision of EBP protocol, implementation, or reinfusion as indicated.

## EXAMPLE

Sample graph of quarterly data for one key indicator (bars) related to benchmark (line).

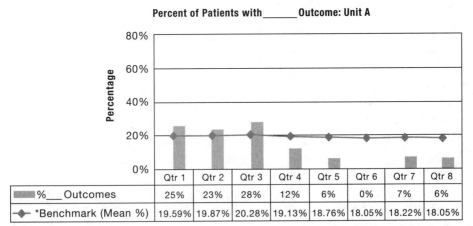

**Percent of Patients with _____ Outcome: Unit A**

| | Qtr 1 | Qtr 2 | Qtr 3 | Qtr 4 | Qtr 5 | Qtr 6 | Qtr 7 | Qtr 8 |
|---|---|---|---|---|---|---|---|---|
| %___ Outcomes | 25% | 23% | 28% | 12% | 6% | 0% | 7% | 6% |
| *Benchmark (Mean %) | 19.59% | 19.87% | 20.28% | 19.13% | 18.76% | 18.05% | 18.22% | 18.05% |

fictitious data

## CITATIONS

AHRQ, n.d.-a; Allegranzi, Conway, Larson, & Pittet, 2014; Ellis, 2006; Ettorchi-Tardy, Levif, & Michel, 2012; Gift & Mosel, 1994; Hughes, 2008b; Lovaglio, 2012; Medicare, n.d.-a; Medicare, n.d.-c; Michetti et al., 2012; Richardson & Tjoelker, 2012; Song et al., 2012; Vollman, 2013; Zachariah et al., 2014.

## Strategy 2-21    Inform Organizational Leaders

| PHASE | 2: Build Knowledge & Commitment |
|---|---|
| FOCUS | Building Organizational System Support |

### DEFINITION

Informing organizational leaders is a method of sharing EBP project accomplishments that are aligned with organizational priorities and outlining resources, if applicable, needed to accomplish next steps.

### BENEFITS

- Effective communication method.
- Increases project visibility with formal and informal leaders at all levels within the institution.
- Opportunity to clearly articulate resources (e.g., equipment, supplies, time) needed for implementation and integration of the practice change.

### PROCEDURE

- Decide which organizational leaders to target.
- Determine reporting frequency (e.g., quarterly, every 6 months).
- Choose the delivery method:
  - Email
  - Face-to-face
- Choose the reporting format:
  - Elevator speech (see Strategy 3-7)
  - Executive summary (see Example 6.4)
  - Reporting in the quality improvement (QI) system (see Strategy 3-20)
- Select content considering components from the EBP process:
  - Project title
  - Interprofessional team member names and credentials
  - Purpose statement
  - Rationale or background (see Strategy 2-14)
  - Synthesis of evidence
  - Practice change
  - Implementation strategies
  - Evaluation
  - Next steps
  - Conclusions and implications for practice
- Draft brief report with only essential information.
- Send or present EBP project information to targeted organizational leaders.

---

### EXAMPLE

**Progress Report:** Evidence-Based Nutritional Screening for Adult Oncology Patients in an Ambulatory Setting

**Project Director:** Amanda Poock, BSN, RN

**Team:** Geralyn Quinn, MSN, RN, OCN; Linda Abbott, DNP, RN, CWON, AOCN; Michele Farrington, BSN, RN, CPHON; Doug Robertson, RDN, LD; Bridget Drapeaux, MA, RDN, LD; Amy Lukas, RD, LD; Gloria Dorr, MA, RN-BC; Brack Bingham; Keith Burrell; and Kenneth Nepple, MD

The purpose of my EBP project is to revise, implement, and evaluate a nutritional screening tool for adult oncology patients in the Holden Comprehensive Cancer Center Clinic. The nutritional screening tool will be piloted with gastrointestinal cancer and breast cancer patients. I have already formed an interprofessional team composed of nurses, LIPs, and dietary services (names noted above).

This topic interests me as a staff nurse in the Cancer Center Clinic because we have many patients with nutritional needs, and it is important to both the patient and the healthcare team caring for them. The current nutritional screening tool does not enable the healthcare team to appropriately triage the nutritional needs of our patients. My hope is that the implementation of this new evidence-based screening tool will help both our patients and our healthcare team to feel confident that this important area of the patient's health and treatment plan is being addressed appropriately and promptly.

The team is now determining the scoring and algorithm that will coincide with the new screening tool. Two screening tools—the malnutrition universal screening tool (MUST) and the malnutrition screening tool (MST), which are supported for use in oncology patients—have been modified along with use of clinical expertise to develop an appropriate tool to better screen ambulatory adult oncology patients for nutritional needs.

Based on the score that the new tool generates for patients, an algorithm will be developed to indicate the next step that should be taken by the nursing staff (RNs or MAs). The algorithm will help nursing staff identify whether later re-evaluation is indicated, nutritional handouts and further patient education are appropriate, or if consultation with a dietician is the most appropriate action.

A project-specific staff questionnaire that addresses knowledge, perceptions, and behaviors was created and is being completed by RNs and MAs in the HCCC Clinic. Baseline nutritional patient data have been obtained from the patient health record and are being analyzed.

Poock, A. (2016, October). *Evidence-based nutrition screening for adult oncology patients in an ambulatory setting.* Presented at the Advanced Practice Institute: Promotion Adoption of Evidence-Based Practice, University of Iowa Hospitals and Clinics, Department of Nursing Services and Patient Care, Iowa City, IA.

### CITATIONS

Hauck, Winsett, & Kuric, 2013; Pryse, 2012; Pryse, McDaniel, & Schafer, 2014; Stetler, Ritchie, Rycroft-Malone, & Charns, 2014; Wang, Kao, & Lin, 2015.

## Strategy 2-22    Action Plan

| PHASE | 2: Build Knowledge & Commitment |
|---|---|
| FOCUS | Building Organizational System Support |

### DEFINITION

An action plan is a concise document outlining steps in the process with objectives, specific activities to accomplish the objectives, an estimated timeline, responsibility, and a method for tracking completed work. It is an outline of the project plan, breaking down tasks and responsibility into a smaller and actionable format (*Harvard Business Review*, 2004).

### BENEFITS

- Provides an easy method for planning for progress and tracking progress.
- Improves team and organizational focus on key activities.
- Increases involvement of clinicians and leaders, which ultimately contributes to better planning, follow-through, and patient outcome.
- Facilitates budget planning and acquiring resources early in planning.

### PROCEDURE

- Choose a planning tool (see Tool 4.2).
- Write the purpose or charge to the team.
- Write down the chair and team member names; involve key players.
- Bring team together for discussion, planning, and consensus building.
- Link to strategic priorities (e.g., mission, vision, values, and/or strategic plan).
- Identify key indicators of EBP project success or drivers (structures or processes) that need to be changed (see Chapter 9).
- Review performance data to identify key areas with opportunity for improvement.
- Identify key objectives to meet the goal/purpose (e.g., break down steps in the EBP process and project management milestones using an EBP process model as a guide). Keep list as short as possible to increase likelihood of completion (see Chapter 9).
- Identify activities or action steps to meet each objective. Have a clear idea of what each step looks like when completed.
- Determine resources needed (if any) for each action step.
- Determine who is responsible and write names on the action plan. Avoid listing a group to provide clear delineation of responsibility and division of work needed.
- Create an estimated timeline. The timeline may be modified later as work progresses.
- Set aside work sessions to have protected time to accomplish project management activities.
- Use the action plan as a team tool for agenda and minutes for team meetings.
- Review regularly and follow up or revise as conditions change.

**EXAMPLE**

Purpose: To outline specific components of a plan to promote pain assessment.

Team chair/co-chair:

Unit(s):

| Objective | Activities to Meet Objective | Materials or Resources Needed | Accountable Person | Projected Completion Date | Done |
|---|---|---|---|---|---|
| Identify new pain assessment tools | 1. Contact librarian<br>2. Conduct research<br>3. Retrieve articles | Librarian<br>60 minute meeting<br>Computer access | R. Smith/Pain committee<br>R. Smith/Librarian<br>AS Student | 7/1<br>7/6<br>7/7–7/10 | ☒<br>☒<br>☒ |
| Audit pain assessments | 25 audits | Audit tool | Pain champions<br>5 each X 5 | 8/1 | ☒ |

Action Plan Definitions

| | |
|---|---|
| Objective: | The goal or step in the EBP process to be addressed |
| Activities: | Actionable steps to be taken to achieve the objective |
| Materials or resources needed: | May include equipment, expertise, or personnel |
| Accountable person: | Name of one of or more specific people responsible for completing activities |
| Done: | Check box for indicating the step has been completed |

**CITATIONS**

AHRQ, 2015e; Bennett & Provost, 2015; Bruno et al., 2014; Cahill, Murch, Cook, & Heyland, 2014; Erasmus et al., 2010; Gifford, Davies, Tourangeau, & Lefebre, 2011; Haley et al., 2012; *Harvard Business Review*, 2004; Lowson et al., 2015; Mind Tools, 2016; Robinson et al., 2010; Schmidt, 2009; Shimizu & Shimanouchi, 2006; Vigorito, McNicoll, Adams, & Sexton, 2011.

## Strategy 2-23   Report to Senior Leaders

| PHASE | 2: Build Knowledge & Commitment |
|---|---|
| FOCUS | Building Organizational System Support |

### DEFINITION

Report to senior executives involves creating a brief summary of EBP work accomplished and includes a clear link to organizational priorities, national initiatives, and/or regulatory standards in order to guide decision-makers and resource allocation within the organization.

### BENEFITS

- Builds on senior executives' ability to influence change and their receptivity to local EBP.
- Maintains connection and commitment for the EBP by demonstrating value-add.
- May support structure or processes for EBP or lead to allocation of resources that benefit patient or organizational outcome.
- Provides an opportunity for executives to recognize the team and reinforce the value of EBP.

### PROCEDURE

- Determine the format for the report (e.g., memo, QI report, email).
- Keep document brief to promote readability.
- Include EBP purpose and background upfront to orient senior executive to the purpose of the document.
- Link to organizational priorities and recognize leadership support.
- Include accountable team members and a brief summary of activities.
- Describe the committee infrastructure used to support the EBP.
- Highlight evaluation results that are valued as organizational priorities (e.g., hospital-acquired conditions).
- Include actions taken, next steps, and dissemination plans with responsibility and timeline as appropriate.
- Attach additional information (e.g., graphs) if it provides brief supplemental information vital to improving interpretation.
- Develop an easy mechanism for executives to provide recognition as follow-up (e.g., schedule an event to celebrate success or send with email addresses).

**EXAMPLE**

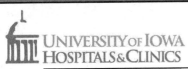

University of Iowa Health Care

*Department of Nursing Services and Patient Care*

*Nursing Research, Evidence-Based Practice and Quality*
*200 Hawkins Drive, T100 GH*
*Iowa City, IA 52242*
*319-384-9098*
*uihcnursingresearchandebp@uiowa.edu*
*www.uihealthcare.com*

**TO**: Chief Executive Officer
**FROM**: Laura Cullen, DNP, RN, FAAN
**DATE**: September 2016
**SUBJECT**: Impact of Nursing EBP at UIHC

Evidence-based practice (EBP) is making an impact at UI Hospitals and Clinics and beyond. *The Iowa Model Revised: Evidence-Based Practice to Promote Excellence in Health Care* outlines the systematic, interprofessional process. The Iowa Model has been requested more than 5,000 times and is widely recognized for its application in practice settings. A companion model (Cullen & Adams, 2012) is used to guide implementation of EBP changes to improve quality and safety and has been requested for use more than 2,250 times. The Nursing Research and EBP Committee and the Nursing Research, EBP, & Quality Office provide leadership for EBP within the department. A variety of programs promote adoption of interprofessional EBP.

EBP improves patient quality and safety, improves nurse satisfaction, reduces costs, and promotes innovative care. Examples of EBP initiatives, led UIHC staff nurse supporting UIHC strategic priorities are:

> Improved patient safety:
>> – Reduced ventilator-associated pneumonia (VAP) for adult and pediatric ICU patients.
>> – Thermoregulation in high-risk neonates and adult trauma patients.
>> – Bedside swallow screening for ischemic and hemorrhagic stroke patients supporting Joint Commission stroke certification.
> Improved patient satisfaction:
>> – Pet visiting.
>> – Planning for psychiatric crisis/exacerbation.
>> – Ketamine for opioid-tolerant orthopedic surgery patients.
> Reduced length of stay and costs:
>> – The MICU sedation management project resulted in an estimated cost avoidance of $1.9 million for the first 26 months following implementation.
>> – The incontinence-associated dermatitis team was able to reduce UIHC costs of more than $12,000/year by making product changes that reduce the use of multiple cleansers and lotions.
> Improved clinician satisfaction and safety:
>> – Reducing sharp injuries with double-gloving for operative procedures.
> Innovations in nursing practice:
>> – Eliminating auscultating bowel sounds for adults after abdominal surgery.
>> – NG placement verification in children and neonates.
>> – Eliminating "no fresh fruits and vegetables" restrictions for adult oncology patients.

A database of EBP projects captures nurse-led EBP projects and is updated annually. Results from the database are reported to the quality committee. The nursing department now has more than 40 active projects and many completed projects. A number of nursing EBP projects are published (attachment).

*continues*

PHASE 2

### Strategy 2-23    Report to Senior Leaders (Continued)

**CITATIONS**

Duffy, Culp, Sand-Jecklin, Stroupe, & Lucke-Wold, 2016; Estabrooks et al., 2015; Everett & Sitterding, 2011; Fleiszer, Semenic, Ritchie, Richer, & Denis, 2016b; Johnson et al., 2015; Lau et al., 2016; Lavoie-Tremblay et al., 2015; Lockett et al., 2014; Melnyk, 2016; Registered Nurses' Association of Ontario, 2013; Reich et al., 2015; Stetler, Ritchie, Rycroft-Malone, & Charns, 2014; Taylor, Clay-Williams, Hogden, Braithwaite, & Groene, 2015; ten Ham, Minnie, & van der Walt, 2016.

# Implementation Strategies for Evidence-Based Practice
## PHASE 3: PROMOTE ACTION & ADOPTION

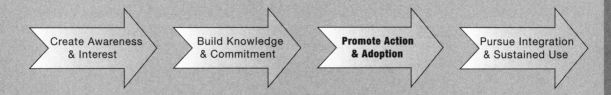

Create Awareness & Interest  →  Build Knowledge & Commitment  →  **Promote Action & Adoption**  →  Pursue Integration & Sustained Use

The most complex implementation strategies to perform are described. The evidence on how to use the procedures is provided to improve their effectiveness. Use in combination for a comprehensive implementation plan.

## Strategy 3-1   Reminders or Practice Prompts

| PHASE | 3: Promote Action & Adoption |
|---|---|
| FOCUS | Connecting With Clinicians, Organizational Leaders, and Key Stakeholders |

### DEFINITION

A reminder or practice prompt is a just-in-time cue to clinicians, provided at the point of care, to encourage use of EBP recommendations and to perform or avoid specific action. The notification can be in the form of paper or an electronic clinical-decision support and may include pocket cards, paper notes, decision algorithms, or practice alerts.

An electronic practice alert is a clinical decision support, provided to clinicians at the point of care, using an alert from the electronic documentation system or another electronic tool (e.g., hand-held device). The alert provides direction for actions by the clinician or patient. It may be an electronic "pop-up" signal or an audible alarm indicating a need for action, or an action to avoid, that involves a new or different practice.

### BENEFITS

- Provides clinicians with clinical decision support guiding the use of the practice recommendation before the practice has been integrated into their normal workflow.
- Offers timely cues to busy clinicians.
- Improves clinician performance and use of practice recommendations, reduces errors, and/or improves organizational system outcomes (e.g., reduce cost or length of stay).
- Provides real-time direction to the clinician or patient to address the clinical issue with the intent of avoiding an error or omission or influencing a behavior (e.g., smoking).

### PROCEDURE: General Alerts

- Identify which practice recommendations contribute to patient risk, improve patient outcomes, are new, or are easily forgotten by clinicians.
- Decide whether paper or electronic is best and create reminders.
- Use credible information on the reminder and include an explanation of the action.
- Provide space or the prompt or a mechanism for a clinician response.
- Include key messages in an easy-to-read format; keep it simple.
- Provide sufficient guidance about specific actions to accomplish the desired behavior change.
- Design for rapid and accurate interpretation. Keep format similar for ease of reading and interpretation; use visual cues where possible.
- Pilot test to work through integration into workflow.
- Place reminders in locations near where the practice will be performed (e.g., near computers for documentation within the patient health record or on the equipment used to set up a procedure).
- Consider varying placement for paper reminders to keep the reminder from becoming invisible and losing attention.
- Provide education about location and use of the reminder (see Stragegy 2-1).
- Evaluate for unintended consequences (e.g., lack of integration with other practice procedures or consideration of other patient conditions) and plan adjustments.

**PROCEDURE: Electronic Alerts**

- Determine functional abilities of the electronic patient health record.
- Determine who will be notified through the alert.
- Determine the trigger for the reminder/prompt by identifying potential low-volume and high-risk events (e.g., allergic reaction).
- Decide whether the electronic or paper option is best.
- Create an operational definition of the event that will trigger the electronic alert.
- Create a small trial with messages sent to one or two people, to work through details, before a larger pilot with a clinical team or area.
- Electronic alerts must be used carefully to avoid diluting the impact due to the sheer volume that clinicians encounter.
- Carefully consider the need for a suggested action (i.e., soft stop) versus a required action (i.e., hard stop) as a response in an electronic alert.
- Keep the format similar for all electronic alerts for ease of reading and interpretation; use visual cues (e.g., meaningful icons) where possible.
- When using an electronic prompt, create another small trial with limited recipients (i.e., five) before a larger pilot to trial the electronic alert for correct functioning of the trigger (i.e., correctly identifying the event and functioning of the alert with timely notification to the correct clinicians).
- Create a pilot plan or include in a larger project pilot as one of several implementation strategies.
- Provide education to clinical teams regarding the prompt, where to find the alert, functionality (e.g., soft stop, recommended action, or hard stop, required action), and response options.
- Evaluate for unintended consequences (e.g., treatment delay) and workarounds, and plan adjustments.

**EXAMPLE**

Flu vaccine electronic alert.

○ **Seasonal Flu Vaccine Screening**

Would you like a flu vaccine if there are no contraindications?   | **Yes** | **No/offered/refused** | **Previous dose in registry** |

*continues*

**PHASE 3**

**Strategy 3-1    Reminders or Practice Prompts (Continued)**

## CITATIONS

Arditi, Rège-Walther, Wyatt, Durieux, & Burnand, 2012; Bright et al., 2012; Fakhry, Hanna, Anderson, Holmes, & Nathwani, 2012; Förberg et al., 2016; Genco et al., 2016; Giguère et al., Gillaizeau et al., 2013; Institute for Safe Medication Practices, 2013; Johnson & May, 2015; Kosse, Brands, Bauer, Hortobagyi, & Lamoth, 2013; Morgan et al., 2015; Piscotty, Kalisch, Gracey-Thomas, & Yarandi, 2015; Sebastián-Viana et al., 2016; Shojania et al., 2009; Shojania et al., 2010; Smith et al., 2011; Szilagyi et al., 2015.

## Strategy 3-2   Demonstrate Workflow or Decision Algorithm

| PHASE | 3: Promote Action & Adoption |
|---|---|
| FOCUS | Connecting With Clinicians, Organizational Leaders, and Key Stakeholders |

### DEFINITION

Workflow demonstration is a method of mapping the steps in a procedure to guide integration of EBP recommendations into work routines. Workflow integration and mapping can be used to show the relationship between clinical scenarios and appropriate actions.

A decision algorithm is a flowchart to guide actions using patient data or risk to determine a course of action or interventions based on specific patient circumstances related to a clinical topic (e.g., advanced cardiac life support).

### BENEFITS

- Addresses workload concerns proactively.
- Breaks down decisions in an organized and progressive way when the clinical situation is complex, infrequent, or high risk.
- Provides a learning tool to guide and standardize clinical practice, when alternative treatments are available; improves integration into work routines.
- Readily available at the point of care.
- Available in multiple formats (e.g., paper, electronic).

### PROCEDURE: Workflow

- Identify key processes contributing to desired outcome reported in the literature.
- Determine baseline with process data regarding current practices.
- Consider incorporating LEAN procedure or human factors expert on the team.
- Observe current practice patterns.
- Gain insight by asking clinicians doing the work:
  - What are the steps in the care process?
  - Where are the bottlenecks?
  - What are the key steps or decision points?
  - Where does the process break down?
- Consider a focus group to identify and troubleshoot work processes that impact incorporating a new procedure into work routines.
- Map out the supplies, tasks, steps in the process, personnel involved, decision points, and environmental considerations for the current process (e.g., swim lane diagram).
- Identify opportunities to streamline:
  - Eliminate unnecessary steps.
  - Rearrange to improve ease of use.
  - Ensure consistent use.

*continues*

PHASE 3

## Strategy 3-2    Demonstrate Workflow or Decision Algorithm (Continued)

### PROCEDURE: Workflow

- Review impact on subsequent downstream steps and decisions.
- Review and revise work routines and come to agreement as a team.
- Design a brief, application-oriented description for use as a learning tool and/or as a clinical decision aid (e.g., care pathway, protocol).
- Distribute or display for easy access.
- Build into work routine using a team approach as a commitment to collective action to improve application in care processes.
- Make explicit changes in documentation, care rounds, and other practice prompts (see Strategy 3-1).
- Trial and revise as needed.
- Use key actions to develop process indicators for evaluation.

### PROCEDURE: Decision Algorithm

- Identify top-level clinical condition to address.
- Review evidence as a team to identify necessary steps or actions.
- Identify key processes contributing to desired outcome reported in the literature.
- Determine clinical criteria to use as a decision point for each intervention.
- Map out first-level clinical criteria for decision point.
- Identify priority order of choices among alternative treatments (e.g., most frequent first).
- Repeat process while developing subsequent downstream decisions.
- Use basic flowchart symbols within the algorithm as a visual cue indicating different actions:
  - Begin and end with an oval or a rounded rectangle.
  - An arrow shows the progressive flow of decision or information.
  - Decision points are diamonds.
  - Steps or actions are rectangles.
  - Data storage or data transmission uses a rectangle with concave end.
  - Other actions use different shapes; to find the right ones, use a resource such as www.wikihow.com/create-a-flowchart.
- Review and revise flowchart for consensus by the team.
- Distribute or display for easy access.
- Use as a learning tool and/or as a clinical decision aid (see Strategy 3-18).
- Consider building documentation system triggers using key actions (e.g., order sets [see Strategy 3-16], documentation templates [see Strategy 3-15]).
- Use key actions to develop process indicators for evaluation.

### EXAMPLE: Workflow

Robinson, S. T., & Kirsch, J. R. (2015). Lean strategies in the operating room. *Anesthesia Clinics, 33*(4), 713–730. doi:10.1016/j.anclin.2015.07.010

**EXAMPLE:** Algorithm

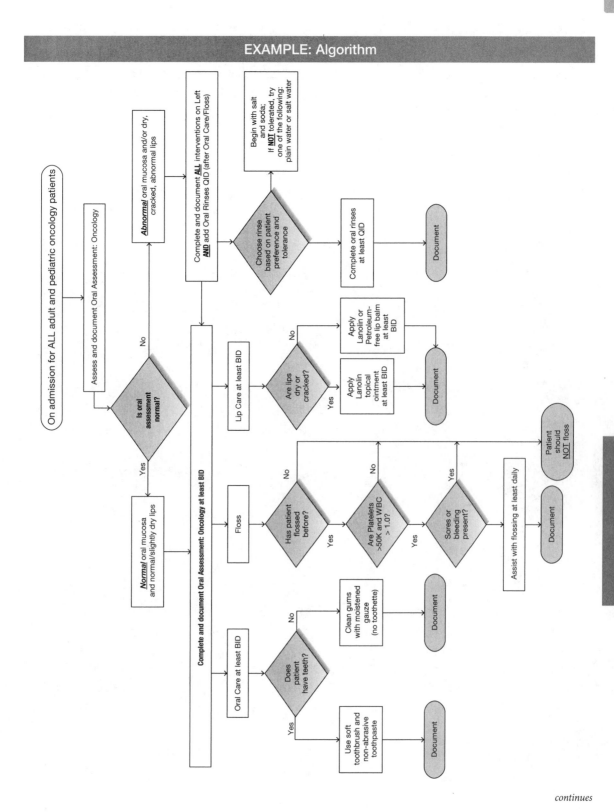

PHASE 3

*continues*

## Strategy 3-2  Demonstrate Workflow or Decision Algorithm (Continued)

### CITATIONS

Bosch et al., 2016; Brackett, Comer, & Whichello, 2013; Bright et al., 2012; Brummel et al., 2013; Carayon et al., 2014; Colón-Emeric et al., 2016; Deblois & Lepanto, 2016; Elsey et al., 2016; Fabry, 2015; Farrington, Cullen, & Dawson, 2013; Fleiszer, Semenic, Ritchie, Richer, & Denis, 2016a; Flowchart, n.d.; Gillespie & Marshall, 2015; Hefner et al., 2016; Johnson, Smith, & Mastro, 2012; Katz et al., 2016; Lang, 2012; Olsen et al., 2015; Portz & Johnston, 2014; Shalom, Shahar, Parmet, & Lunenfeld, 2015; Son et al., 2011; van Riet Paap et al., 2015; Wyatt et al., 2014; Yackel, McKennan, & Fox-Deise, 2010; Yanke et al., 2015.

## Strategy 3-3   Skill Competence

| PHASE | 3: Promote Action & Adoption |
|---|---|
| FOCUS | Connecting With Clinicians, Organizational Leaders, and Key Stakeholders |

### DEFINITION

Skill competence involves the psychomotor intellectual ability to carry out goal-directed actions with knowledge, attitudes, values, and abilities and with minimum expenditure of time and energy. Skill competence also includes judicious use of communication, professional judgment, clinical reasoning, and reflection. This competency is demonstrated for specific complex clinical situations found in daily practice for the benefit of the individual and the community being served (Bhatti & Ahmed, 2015; Fernandez et al., 2012; Panzarella, 2003; Schroeter, 2008; Windsor, Douglas, & Harvey, 2012).

### BENEFITS

- Enhances contribution by delivering professional services to meet explicit requirements under specific conditions that advance knowledge, increase adoption, ensure quality, reduce the likelihood of mistakes, and improve patient outcomes.
- Supports developmental progression that is facilitated through continuous, comprehensive formative assessment and feedback.
- Recognizes successes associated with the ability to deliver safe, quality healthcare services and allows for consistent, measurable expectations and abilities congruent with a particular setting.

### PROCEDURE

- Set learning goals by identifying knowledge/cognitive, attitudes/affective, skills/psychomotor, and other objectives (e.g., values, attributes) that are imperative to the EBP change and that reflect the "real world" of practice.
- Assess clinician knowledge and practices at baseline to determine needs.
- Optimize motivation and autonomy while expecting clinician to adapt practice, be flexible in learning, and be responsible for lifelong learning.
  - For motivated and interested learners, use:
    - ☐ Hands-on deliberate practice
  - For less interested learners, to generate motivation:
    - ☐ Identify early success through targeted practice.
    - ☐ Support learner in teaching individualized progress.
    - ☐ Observe rapid skill improvement.
    - ☐ Supervised practice with rapid feedback.

*continues*

**PHASE 3**

## Strategy 3-3    Skill Competence (Continued)

### PROCEDURE (Continued)

- Determine level of clinical reasoning required for identified objective (e.g., Bloom's taxonomy of cognitive domains and Miller's level of performance competence):
  - Remember/knows
  - Understand/knows how
  - Apply/shows how
  - Analysis
  - Evaluate/proficiently does
  - Create
- Deconstruct performance expectations into different functions or tasks of the procedure (e.g., outline elements into a procedure or checklist [see Strategy 3-14]).
- Incorporate contextual factors (e.g., local culture) relevant to clinical setting within performance procedures.
- Develop observable, formative, and summative assessment of competence with established reliability and validity.
- Determine evaluation criteria and number of repetitions required to reduce errors and "smooth" skill performance with economy of motion.
- Identify criteria for progressive milestones demonstrating accelerated expertise.
- Identify approaches that match different learning styles and performance goals:
  - Accommodating—concrete experience plus active experimentation
  - Diverging—concrete experience plus reflection
  - Converging—active experimentation plus abstract conceptualizing
  - Assimilating—abstract conceptualizing plus reflection
- Determine effective educational methods that match performance expectations:
  - Didactic
  - Vignettes or case studies (see Strategy 2-17) with think-aloud discussion for application
  - Observation or shadowing (e.g., clinical scenario, video)
  - Simulation (low- to high-fidelity)
  - Video snapshot or segment of practice
  - Standardized patient
  - Deliberate practice
  - Role model (see Strategy 3-9)
  - Online training
  - Interview or self report (least accurate)
- Identify training and development opportunities in the clinical setting to build expertise for new skills, alternative training opportunities, or needs.
- Provide faculty development to ensure reliable assessments.
- Establish inter-rater reliability for competency assessment to be completed by more than one data collector, if appropriate.

■ Provide standardized conditions for performance practice and assessment.

■ Promote self-directed practice through clinician's choice of schedule with access to training material.

■ Monitor performance on indicators at minimally acceptable level.

■ Provide robust feedback that:

  ● Occurs in real time

  ● Is constructive

  ● Provides positive reinforcement

  ● Guides performance during training to close performance gap

■ Establish ownership of mastery and responsibility for maintenance of practice.

■ Provide debriefing session with open-ended questions and discussion and objective evaluative data, if available; learners and teachers should provide insight and feedback.

■ Obtain clinician feedback and suggestions to improve training content and methods.

■ Reinforce and update skills or performance:

  ● Provide feedback for refinement and to confirm continued competence.

  ● Use educational outreach (see Strategy 2-9) for new practices and/or continuing education for updates on practices.

■ Assess ability to practice safely and effectively without the need for direct supervision.

■ Set clear expectations for employees, and reinforce behaviors that are consistent with the organization's mission.

■ Give incentives, awards, or recognition for maintaining essential performance (see Strategies 3-5 and 4-3).

■ Certify individuals with expertise in specialized areas.

| EXAMPLE | | | |
|---|---|---|---|
| **Components of Cultural Competency** | **Satisfactory** | **Unsatisfactory** | **Not Performed** |
| Conduct self-assessment of biases or stereotypes. | ☐ | ☐ | ☐ |
| Complete cultural health history—includes cultural beliefs and behaviors. | ☐ | ☐ | ☐ |
| Demonstrate use of translation resources. | ☐ | ☐ | ☐ |
| Facilitate cross-cultural collaboration in teamwork. | ☐ | ☐ | ☐ |

Employee: _____     Signature: _____
                (please print)

Evaluator: _____     Signature: _____
                (please print)

Date: _____     Date: _____

**PHASE 3**

*continues*

## Strategy 3-3    Skill Competence (Continued)

### CITATIONS

Aebersold, 2011; Arora et al., 2011; Bhatti & Ahmed, 2015; Caccia, Nakajima, & Kent, 2015; Fernandez et al., 2012; Forsberg, Ziegert, Hult, & Fors, 2014; Gattinger et al., 2015; Green & Aarons, 2011; Iowa State University, n.d.; Jansson et al., 2016; King et al., 2014; Kruglikova, Grantcharov, Drewes, & Funch-Jensen, 2010; Laibhen-Parkes, 2014; Lau et al., 2016; Lee, Huang, & Huang, 2016; Leicher & Mulder, 2016; Leung, Trevena, & Waters, 2014; Leung, Trevena, & Waters, 2016; Makic, Lovett, & Azam, 2012; Mann-Salinas et al., 2014; Marshall et al., 2011; Noordman, van der Weijden, & van Dulmen, 2014; Panzarella, 2003; Peltan, Shiga, Gordon, & Currier, 2015; Przybyl, Androwich, & Evans, 2015; QSEN Institute, 2012; Rassin, Kurzweil & Maoz, 2015; Reynolds, McLennon, Ebright, Murray, & Bakas, 2016; Reynolds, Murray, McLennon, & Bakas, 2016; Rosenzweig et al., 2012; Schroeter, 2008; Sheakley et al., 2016; Sprakes & Tyrer, 2010; Tolley, Marks-Maran, & Burke, 2010; Venkatasalu, Kelleher, & Shao, 2015; Wade & Webb, 2013; Watson, Stimpson, Topping, & Porock, 2002; Windsor, Douglas, & Harvey, 2012; Windt, 2016.

## Strategy 3-4    Give Evaluation Results to Colleagues

| PHASE | 3: Promote Action & Adoption |
|---|---|
| FOCUS | Connecting With Clinicians, Organizational Leaders, and Key Stakeholders |

### DEFINITION

Giving evaluation results to colleagues is the transmission of evaluative information by a team member that demonstrates use of desired practice or need for corrective action.

### BENEFITS

- Facilitates learning about EBP recommendations.
- Motivates clinicians through peer influence to embrace new EBP.
- Promotes innovative problem-solving.

### PROCEDURE

- Identify colleagues to whom results will be provided.
- Identify key indicators to report as feedback to clinicians regarding application of the EBP.
- Identify social networks (e.g., local chapter of a professional organization) for creative ideas that promote adoption of EBP to share.
- Provide performance monitoring (e.g., chart audit or see Strategy 3-12).
- Analyze practices or data.
- Determine how these results will be reported, in what setting, and using formal or informal approach (e.g., graphical display or verbal discussion).
- Report findings to colleagues.
- Discuss successes and opportunities for improvement.
- Discuss specific practice behaviors needed to achieve desired outcome (focus on few critical behaviors; see Strategy 3-13).
- Maintain respect and dignity for those who are being evaluated.
- Ensure closed-loop communication verifying receipt of the feedback (e.g., a simple nod or another nonverbal acceptance of feedback).
- Share approaches to adoption of the practice change found to be effective by other colleagues.
- Create mutually agreed-on action plan (see Strategy 2-22) for subsequent performance observation or data collection and anticipated follow-up with actionable feedback (see Strategy 3-13).
- Highlight the importance of goal-setting and regular evaluation of progress.
- Share learning from troubleshooting (see Strategy 2-19) with EBP team.

*continues*

## Strategy 3-4   Give Evaluation Results to Colleagues (Continued)

### EXAMPLE

Discussion with colleagues related to evaluation of pain practices.

*We are working to improve pain care for our post-operative patients. As part of the core group, let's review our practices.*

*We are working on several pain practices. Today, let's focus on using the patients' preferred pain-assessment scale. We regularly use the 0–10 numeric rating scale, and research shows that some patients prefer a different scale because it is easier for them to use. Older adults in particular may be better able to use the Iowa pain thermometer or verbal descriptor scale.*

*Our chart audit of the use of an EBP pain assessment for older post-operative adults using patients' preferred pain assessment scale shows:*

- *Seven of 10 patient charts audited identify the patient's identification of a preferred pain assessment scale.*

- *Six of 10 patient chart audits met the goal of consistently using the patients' preferred pain assessment scale.*

- *Assessment of a patient's pain consistently included self-reported acceptable pain intensity.*

*As follow-up, we have several items to share:*

- *These data demonstrate an improvement over last week.*

- *Each team member will complete additional data collection on each element of the pain assessment program.*

- *Use of patient-preferred pain assessment scale will be checked again next week.*

*Let's discuss how to assess a patient's preferences:*

- *When does it work best to determine the patient's preferred pain-assessment tool?*

- *Are there patient situations that make it difficult? How can we work through these situations?*

- *Can you suggest helpful resources or reminders so that we can consistently use the patient's preferred pain scale?*

- *What will help?*

*This EBP is showing progress.*

*I'd like to share your success with our colleagues. Keep up the good work.*

### CITATIONS

AHRQ, 2014; Anderson-Carpenter, Watson-Thompson, Jones, & Chaney, 2014; Fleiszer, Semenic, Ritchie, Richer, & Denis, 2016a; Forsner et al., 2010; Holleman, Poot, Mintjes-de Groot, & van Achterberg, 2009; Hysong, 2009; Hysong, Knox, & Haidet, 2014; Ivers et al., 2012; Ivers et al., 2014; Lee, Johnson, Newhouse, & Warren, 2013; Li-Ying, Paunova, & Egerod, 2016; Lowson et al., 2015; Maas et al., 2015; Payne & Hysong, 2016; Vachon et al., 2015; Ware et al., 2015.

## Strategy 3-5    Incentives

| PHASE | 3: Promote Action & Adoption |
|---|---|
| FOCUS | Connecting With Clinicians, Organizational Leaders, and Key Stakeholders |

### DEFINITION

Incentives are direct or indirect payments of money, commodities, or desired objects that are given to, or withheld from, an individual or a system in order to encourage behavioral change (Rogers, 2003).

An incentive is any factor (financial or nonfinancial) that provides motivation for a particular course of action or that counts as a reason for preferring one option compared to alternatives (Flodgren, Eccles, et al., 2011) and could be offered directly to individuals or groups of clinicians.

### BENEFITS

- Increases rate of adoption of an innovation and leads to adoption by individuals different from those who would otherwise adopt.
- Financial incentives are successful in mainstream industry for attainment of common goals and may increase EBP by clinicians.
- Nonfinancial incentives may include recognition or other rewards.
- Increases the degree of relative advantage of a new idea.
- Reduces barriers to change.
- Helps with persistence and mental effort.
- Significantly increases work performance if carefully implemented.
- Attracts, retains, motivates, satisfies, and improves performance.
- Encourages a learning environment by increasing information and reducing perceived differences between employees and executives:
  - Rewards employees for efforts in implementation of EBP.
  - Heightens commitment to organizational goals.
  - Increases acceptance of EBP.
- Incentives not only increase EBP implementation for individuals, but through professional organization recommendations, third-party payer requirements, and legislative mandates, entire organizations can be enticed into making implementation of EBP a priority.

### PROCEDURE

- Planning for incentives must occur early in the EBP implementation process in order to be effective and sustained.
  - Create pre-implementation communication plan about incentives.
  - Clinicians should have an opportunity to understand expectations prior to start of program.
- Determine the goal of adoption (e.g., trial of new idea, sustained adoption).
- Determine the desired adoptee (e.g., individual, organization).
- Establish reliability and validity of data used to set financial incentives.

*PHASE 3*

*continues*

## Strategy 3-5   Incentives (Continued)

### PROCEDURE (Continued)

- ▪ Determine magnitude of potential additional revenue or cost savings expected from providing EBP (e.g., increased number of patients, decreased unnecessary hospitalizations).
  - ● Consider publicly reportable metrics or transparency of data reporting for financial impact.
- ▪ Identify the budget for an incentive and validate its ability to both incentivize and meet budgetary cost effectiveness.
- ▪ Determine the method of incentive (e.g., positive, negative).
- ▪ Include clinicians in the determination of naturally occurring and nonfinancial incentives:
  - ● Autonomy (e.g., able to adjust work schedule or work assignment)
  - ● Self-efficacy or mastery of elevated skills (e.g., reflecting valued expertise)
  - ● Elevated sense of purpose to service that is larger than ourselves (e.g., increased number of partnership sites for practices, higher prestige, increased reputation for an institution, awards, and process performance feedback to clinicians)
- ▪ Consider characteristics of effective incentives:
  - ● Based on clear objectives linked to organizational priority
  - ● Realistic and deliverable
  - ● Reflective of clinicians' needs, values, preferences, motivators, perceived job satisfiers, or intent to stay in current job
  - ● Linked to process indicators within clinician's ability to influence
  - ● Well designed, strategic, and fits with the intended purpose
  - ● Contextually appropriate
  - ● Fair, equitable, and transparent
  - ● Timely
  - ● Measurable
  - ● Incorporates both financial and nonfinancial elements
- ▪ Determine how incentives will be granted (e.g., everyone who reaches the goal, person who reaches the goal first, individual or group challenge).
- ▪ Determine the time of payment or presentation (e.g., immediate, delayed).
- ▪ Monitor and communicate successes throughout project work.
- ▪ Include additional "smaller success" incentives.
- ▪ Broadcast reward or recognition in a way that stays visible and will continue to market the new practice or protocols that have been implemented.
- ▪ Evaluate the relationship of timely interventions to care processes and patient outcomes as well as sustained improvement over time.
  - ● Monitor for unintended consequences or altered resource allocation (e.g., reduced quality in processes that are not incentivized; diversion of time/appointments or attention to patients in incentivized care).

## EXAMPLES

A unit is seeking to improve identification and consistent use of the patients' preferred pain assessment scale, as an alternative to a 0–10 numeric pain-rating scale, for older adults when developing patient-centered pain plans and goals during the admission process. Possible incentives include:

**Award:** Everyone in the clinical area that meets or exceeds the desired criteria is entered into a drawing for an expenses-paid attendance at a professional development opportunity.

**Recognition:** Everyone in the clinical area who meets or exceeds the desired criteria receives a certificate of accomplishment and has their name displayed on a poster in the breakroom or is recognized in a ceremony by senior leaders.

**Financial reward:** Everyone in the clinical area who meets or exceeds the desired criteria receives a $50 bonus on their next paycheck.

**Other options:** Stickers, pins, small gift certificates, preferred work schedule, or designated parking near the hospital for a month.

## CITATIONS

Brocklehurst et al., 2013; Condly, Clark, & Stolovitch, 2003; Doebbeling & Flanagan, 2011; Edwards et al., 2007; Flodgren, Eccles et al., 2011; Frølich, 2012; Global Health Workforce Alliance, 2008; Grol & Wensing, 2004; Hsu, Chiang, Chang, Huang, & Chen, 2015; Hysong et al., 2012; Kane, Johnson, Town, & Butler, 2004; Kelly et al., 2011; Lau et al., 2016; Lugtenberg, Burgers, Han, & Westert, 2014; McGillis Hall, Lalonde, Dales, Peterson, & Cripps, 2011; Novak & McIntyre, 2010; Painter, 2013; Petersen et al., 2013; Rogers, 2003; Scott et al., 2011; Srigley et al., 2015; Stone et al., 2010; Walston & Chou, 2006; Wieck, Dols, & Northam, 2009; World Health Organization, 2000; Xian et al., 2010.

PHASE 3

## Strategy 3-6    Try the Practice Change

| PHASE | 3: Promote Action & Adoption |
|-------|------------------------------|
| FOCUS | Connecting With Clinicians, Organizational Leaders, and Key Stakeholders |

### DEFINITION

Trying the practice change is a small-scale and short-term trial of the EBP. It incorporates clinician and patient input into EBP adaptation, implementation strategies, or evaluation plan prior to a larger-scale use, integration, or rollout/scale-up. (Rogers, 2003; Walker, Mwaria, Coppola, & Chen, 2014).

### BENEFITS

- Facilitates identification of components of the EBP needing to be adapted, with suggestions for adaptation to improve feasibility.
- Provides opportunity to make the evidence-based intervention culturally appropriate.
- Provides information on feasibility of implementation tools/strategies and resource materials.
- Provides opportunity for feedback on evaluation or data collection tools.
- May provide early process and outcome data for establishing a gap analysis or trended evaluation.
- May improve fidelity of evidence-based intervention being implemented and thus improve outcomes.

### PROCEDURE

- Describe the purpose of the EBP change.
- Provide academic detailing/educational outreach (see Strategy 2-9) as an overview of the project.
- Encourage clinician and patient participation so that they can provide feedback from the pilot.
- Explain how the feedback will be collected and used for adaptation of the practice change to improve the fit in the workflow and local context; remind participants of their ability to influence practice changes impacting their work through early involvement.
- Develop an action plan (see Strategy 2-22) for piloting.
- Proceed with the pilot; it may be a small-scale, "table-top exercise" and/or a larger trial.
- Provide feedback from the pilot to the participating clinicians and patients about what was learned and how it will be used to adapt or roll out/scale up the EBP.
- Bring together experts from the clinical area and EBP experts for review of pilot data and decision-making about adaptation.
- Adapt the EBP, implementation strategies, resource materials, workflow and/or evaluation tools based on the pilot data to improve project integration and sustainability or to roll out to other areas.

## EXAMPLES

Hourly rounding can be difficult to implement with complex steps for an acute care setting, so trying the change may promote confidence with use.

▦ Research that examines issues with implementation of hourly rounding indicates that careful planning, communication, implementation, and evaluation are essential for effective adoption of the practice change.

▦ Assess adaption by and with clinician users, in particular early adopters who can be champions during implementation:

- Include unit-level clinicians and staff during all phases, including development and redesign.
- Consider workload and workflow in pilot planning.
- Identify meaningful outcomes as to why the implementation of the change is necessary.
- Create a larger, full pilot on the clinical area.
- Use project management and/or quality improvement process to support the re-evaluation of project.

## CITATIONS

Breslau, Weiss, Williams, Burness, & Kepka, 2015; Brosey & March, 2015; Cole, Esplin, & Baldwin, 2015; Dang et al., 2015; Deitrick, Baker, Paxton, Flores, & Swavely, 2012; Fabry, 2015; Farrington, Lang, Cullen, & Stewart, 2009; Innis & Berta, 2016; Knowlton et al., 2014; Liddy, Johnston, Nash, Irving, & Davidson, 2016; Mitchell, Lavenberg, Trotta, & Umscheid, 2014; Rogers, 2003; Rondinelli, Ecker, Crawford, Seelinger, & Omery, 2012; Toole, Meluskey, & Hall, 2016; Tucker, Bieber, Attlesey-Pries, Olson, & Dierkhising, 2012; Walker, Mwaria, Coppola, & Chen, 2014.

PHASE 3

## Strategy 3-7   Elevator Speech

| PHASE | 3: Promote Action & Adoption |
|-------|------------------------------|
| FOCUS | Connecting With Clinicians, Organizational Leaders, and Key Stakeholders |

### DEFINITION

An elevator speech refers to a persuasive "pitch," including a clear, brief description of the EBP, benefit to the organization, current progress, and potential impact shared with a leader that can be shared in 30–60 seconds (e.g., while riding the elevator) to secure funding or "sell" the idea that this work is special (Simpson, 2016).

### BENEFITS

- Captures the attention of a busy executive in a short amount of time.
- Summarizes the work, impact, and desired actions for follow-up.

### PROCEDURE

- Prepare ahead of time:
  - Define a clear purpose and goal (e.g., education, collaborate, sell an idea).
  - Define the audience and customer.
- Examine considerations for framing the content:
  - Be memorable, pique the interest of the audience, and reflect a burning issue.
  - Use a clear, concise, compelling "hook" that appeals to the listener's emotions.
- Identify yourself and establish credibility (share accomplishments that set you apart).
- Provide an introduction, and choose from options:
  - Ask a rhetorical question to synchronize beliefs.
  - Highlight a problem.
  - Use a four- to eight-word phrase that describes the value-add and challenge the audience to become involved.
- Content should:
  - Provide a brief summary of your work (don't overdo the details).
  - Focus on benefits, solutions, and results.
  - "Pitch" the EBP opportunity and answer "why" with proof, statistics, or supporting evidence (e.g., credentials, expertise, evidence).
  - Clearly identify decisions and who will make them.
  - Conclude and seek a commitment by adding an action request.
- Use voice, gestures, and demeanor to influence:
  - Be authentic.
  - Show your passion.
  - Provide a motivating or "bet the business on this" delivery method.

- Trial the pitch and practice on customers or colleagues.
- Adapt to reflect a spontaneous versus planned encounter and keep it conversational.
- Limit the pitch to 1 to 2 minutes maximum.
- Provide a business card, if appropriate.

## EXAMPLE

*Hello, I'm _____, a nurse in the cancer clinic and a member of the oral mucositis committee.*

*Oral mucositis hurts! It's like a canker sore, but worse! I see patients with this condition every day. In fact, cancer patients say that it's the most distressing side effect of cancer treatment. That's why this work is our top priority.*

*Consequences of oral mucositis can be severe, including serious infection and increased hospital costs.*

*Our committee's goal is to provide evidence-based care for cancer patients with difficult symptoms from their treatment.*

*So far, we've improved oral assessment and introduced cryotherapy. We're now focusing on oral care.*

*An interprofessional team made up of nurses, pharmacist, dentists, oncologists, speech pathologists, and dieticians are collaborating to develop interventions.*

*Our next strategy is to get our patients' oral care kits, and we are working with the College of Dentistry to access bulk supplies at a lower rate. We expect to have 65 oncology patients each month that could benefit. That means the cost of kits would be $10,000 annually. Can I count on you to help us achieve this?*

*Thank you for supporting our committee's efforts by providing time for our team to improve care.*

(Farrington, 2013).

## CITATIONS

Bycel, 2014; Denning & Dew, 2012; Fisher, 2014; Hughes, 2010; Kahle, 2016; Lawn, 2008; Peek, 2003; Simpson, 2016; Yaqub, 2014; Zorger, 2009.

PHASE 3

## Strategy 3-8    Report Progress & Updates

| PHASE | 3: Promote Action & Adoption |
|---|---|
| FOCUS | Connecting With Clinicians, Organizational Leaders, and Key Stakeholders |

### DEFINITION

Reporting progress and updates refers to sharing work accomplished and work to be completed with colleagues and interprofessional team members from a clinical area.

### BENEFITS

- Creates motivation for adoption and compliance with use.
- Provides an opportunity to troubleshoot how to address challenges.
- Fosters an opportunity to include consumer and clinician feedback in discussions and planning.

### PROCEDURE

- Decide what the audience wants to learn about and/or their information needs.
- Focus content on:
  - Applicability of the evidence and findings.
  - Engaging the specific audience.
  - Promoting collective action (selection and use of implementation strategies) to address feasibility.
  - Describing benefits and costs.
- Content should be brief and include only essential indicators (see Chapter 9).
- Grab clinicians' attention and create eye-catching information:
  - Make it fun.
  - Link information to purpose, advantage (see Strategy 1-1), and compatibility (see Strategy 1-2), and use a logo consistently across updates to help clinicians quickly connect with the specific initiative.
- Consider location and timing for discussion.
- Determine the type of discussion (e.g., face-to-face, asynchronous, oral, written).
- Ensure that information is easy to interpret (i.e., clinician can quickly skim to get key messages).
- Describe progress by linking to completed, current, and upcoming steps in the EBP process model.
- Make the progress observable, when possible (see Strategy 2-11).
- Determine frequency for discussions or information sharing.
- Adjust design of graphical display to spotlight or shift attention to details about the tasks to be completed to achieve desired improvement.
- Determine who will provide report (e.g., peer influence [see Strategy 4-5], team leader, change agent [see Table 8.1], organizational leader).
- During the discussion:
  - Describe how the audience will benefit from the information (i.e., "What's in it for me?").
  - Provide sufficient information to enhance credibility and reliability and gain trust from the audience.

## PROCEDURE (Continued)

- Trial the report and seek feedback for revisions.
- Recognize project team members.
  - Include a list of team member names, credentials, and contact information for key local experts.
  - Watch for additional opportunities to recognize the team and its work accomplished (see Strategies 3-11 and 4-3).
- Identify actions for progressive improvement (see Strategy 3-13), resources needed, and follow-up timeline.

## EXAMPLE

### The Stork Page
Feb 6 - Feb 12, 2016 - Issue 4

**Straight Talk-- EBP Catheter Project Update**
I just wanted to give everyone an update on my project and the catheter algorithm. First off, thanks for hanging with me during this long project; I couldn't do it without all your help! Second, you will start to see the new algorithms replacing the old ones in the catheter cabinets in the rooms. Thirdly, please fill out the post-survey if you haven't already or if you didn't at comps. (Yes this is the same survey as the first one!). Fourth, you will see a palpation row in the patient record to chart on in the next couple weeks, hopefully! Lastly, I wanted to show you how much of an effect you guys have had on our patients with this project! :)

-Abby Salton

L&D Catheter Queen

Average Foley dwell time: 376 minutes (pre) & 275 minutes (post)
10cm to birth interval with a foley: 89 minutes (pre) & 80 minutes (post)
Number of straight caths used: 5 (pre) & 25 (post)
10cm to birth interval with straight cath: 107 minutes (pre) & 84 minutes (post)

(Hiller, Farrington, Forman, McNulty, & Cullen, in press)

## CITATIONS

AHRQ, 2015a; AHRQ, 2015e; AHRQ, 2016a; Cullen, Greiner, Greiner, Bombei, & Comried, 2005; Cullen & Titler, 2004; Cullen, Wagner, Matthews, & Farrington, 2017; Gagliardi, Marshall, Huckson, James, & Moore, 2015; Gillespie & Marshall, 2015; Hiller, Farrington, Forman, & McNulty, in press; Kelly et al., 2011; Larson, Patel, Evans, & Saiman, 2013; Neufeld, Fernández, Christo, & Williams, 2013; Williams & Cullen, 2016.

## Strategy 3-9   Role Model

| PHASE | 3: Promote Action & Adoption |
|---|---|
| FOCUS | Connecting With Clinicians, Organizational Leaders, and Key Stakeholders |

### DEFINITION

A role model is an informal, unit-based member of the healthcare team who sets an example for colleagues by incorporating and demonstrating practice change recommendations in day-to-day care and as part of routine workflow.

### BENEFITS

- Can be used at all levels of the organization.
- Facilitates learning and informal discussion among colleagues about clinical decision-making.
- Sets expectation related to adopting practice change.
- Establishes a positive, familiar approach to providing support and assistance related to new recommendations and changes in work routines.

### PROCEDURE

- Select a role model; look for these characteristics:
  - Positive, respected clinician.
  - Committed and genuinely interested in topic and colleague success.
  - Openly shares information with colleagues.
  - Good listener.
  - Communicates effectively by speaking up and providing constructive feedback.
  - Humorous.
  - Patient.
  - Organized, flexible, and realistic.
  - Leads quietly from behind the scenes.
- Determine whether role models will participate as part of the core group (see Strategy 2-5) or serve as an extension of the core group:
  - If serving as an extension of the core group, identify a core group member who will be the link to the role models through regular communication.
- Develop resources for role models:
  - Educational materials.
  - Tools.
  - Description of role model expectations and activities to be completed.
- Arrange training sessions for role models by project leader.
- Outline the responsibilities of the role to provide consistency.
- What role models do, based on practice recommendations:
  - Share tools and resources consistently and with a clear description for use.
  - Demonstrate use of EBP recommendations in clinical practice, including:
    - ☐ Content—what practices to adopt and procedure for use.

## PROCEDURE

- ☐ Dose—when to provide the EBP recommendation (i.e., eligible patients, timing in care continuum, duration of intervention).
- ☐ Coverage—volume of population that fits target group of eligible patients.
- Discuss how to incorporate EBP recommendations into workflow.
- Demonstrate use of the practice change.
- Show and discuss how to engage patients, incorporate patient preferences, and incorporate family members/caregivers.
- Adapt to preferred learning style or information delivery method of mentee.
- Provide reminders to colleagues.
- Troubleshoot at point of care (see Strategy 2-19).
- Provide regular feedback that motivates progressive uptake of EBP recommendations.
- Describe adaptations that were effective for complex patient situations to colleagues.
- Coach colleagues through progressive adoption of EBP recommendations, creating a sense of team support.
- Foster skill development to promote independent practice related to integrating EBP recommendations.
- Provide just-in-time informal recognition at the point of care.
- Keep core group informed of activities, availability of needed supplies, progress, adaptation, and challenges.
- Assist core group to establish expectations for integration and consistent use of EBP recommendations.
- ▪ Report successes and adaptations used for group learning.
- ▪ Report results to project/unit leaders.
- ▪ Plan for withdrawal of role model support as progressive improvement is demonstrated through process evaluation.
- ▪ Provide role model recognition and appreciation.

## EXAMPLES

- ▪ Huis, A., Holleman, G., van Achterberg, T., Grol, R., Schoonhoven, L., & Hulscher, M. (2013). Explaining the effects of two different strategies for promoting hand hygiene in hospital nurses: A process evaluation alongside a cluster randomized controlled trial. *Implementation Science, 8*(41), 1–13. doi:10.1186/1748-5908-8-41
- ▪ Perry, S. B., Zeleznik, H., & Breisinger, T. (2014). Supporting clinical practice behavior change among neurologic physical therapists: A case study in knowledge translation. *Journal of Neurologic Physical Therapy, 38*(2), 134–143. doi:10.1097/NPT.0000000000000034

## CITATIONS

Badger & Cullen, 2015; Dogherty, Harrison, & Graham, 2010; Fleiszer, Semenic, Ritchie, Richer, & Denis, 2016a; Hauck, Winsett, & Kuric, 2013; Huddleston & Gray, 2016b; Huddleston, Mancini, & Gray, 2017; Huis, Holleman et al., 2013; Huis, Schoonhoven et al., 2013; Mahanes, Quatrara, & Shaw, 2013; Matthew-Maich, Ploeg, Dobbins, & Jack, 2013; McCormack et al., 2013; Perry, Zeleznik, & Breisinger, 2014; Stetler, Ritchie, Rycroft-Malone, & Charns, 2014; Taylor, Clay-Williams, Hogden, Braithwaite, & Groene, 2015; van der Zijpp et al., 2016; Warren, Montgomery, & Friedmann, 2016; Young, Rohwer, van Schalkwyk, Volmink, & Clarke, 2015.

PHASE 3

## Strategy 3-10   Troubleshooting at the Point of Care/Bedside

| PHASE | 3: Promote Action & Adoption |
|---|---|
| FOCUS | Connecting With Clinicians, Organizational Leaders, and Key Stakeholders |

### DEFINITION

Troubleshooting at the point of care is a problem-solving approach to identify barriers and solutions to implementing EBP changes in order to ensure applicability for complex patients.

### BENEFITS

- Engages point-of-care clinicians in identifying challenges and solutions.
- Tailors practice change to the context and needs of local settings.
- Creates a sense of local ownership among clinicians and improves application to patients.
- Provides ongoing support and constructive feedback.

### PROCEDURE

- Identify complex patient/scenario is not an exact fit for newly established work routines for use of practice recommendations.
- Determine factors that contribute to the complexity/complicating use of the recommendations.
- Review recommendations to verify that a true problem exists rather than simply resistance to change.
- Identify key components/principles from the practice recommendations.
- Review and reinforce clinician decision-making/thinking to target a solution.
- Use creative thinking strategies to identify possible solutions.
- Ask for clinician input (see Strategy 2-13).
- Reaffirm goal—application of recommendations to achieve outcomes.
- Revise workflow (e.g., policy) (see Strategy 3-2).
- Pilot/trial new approach or workflow (see Strategy 3-2).
- Determine effectiveness after pilot.
- Report results related to revised approach or workflow for use with other patients and team learning.

### EXAMPLE

Jankowski, I. M., & Nadzam, D. M. (2011). Identifying gaps, barriers, and solutions in implementing pressure ulcer prevention programs. *Joint Commission Journal on Quality & Patient Safety, 37*(6), 253–264. doi: 10.1016/S1553-7250(11)37033-X

### CITATIONS

Anas & Brunet, 2009; Baskerville, Liddy, & Hogg, 2012; Dogherty, Harrison, & Graham, 2010; Dogherty, Harrison, Graham, Vandyk, & Keeping-Burke, 2013; Fleuren, van Dommelen & Dunnink, 2015; Hauck, Winsett, & Kuric, 2013; Jankowski & Nadzam, 2011; Liddy et al., 2015.

## Strategy 3-11   Provide Recognition at the Point of Care

| PHASE | 3: Promote Action & Adoption |
|---|---|
| FOCUS | Connecting With Clinicians, Organizational Leaders, and Key Stakeholders |

### DEFINITION

Recognition at the point of care is providing just-in-time positive feedback or consequences to a person for a behavior or result (Larson, Patel, Evans, & Saiman, 2013; Nelson, 2016). Recognition identifies successful use of EBP during routine patient care through observation, informal audit, or report of practice patterns. Positive reinforcement is used as a behavior change strategy and may include praise or incentives. Based on the principle 'What is recognized or rewarded is repeated' (Nelson, 2016).

### BENEFITS

- Establishes EBP as the new standard for practice.
- Increases awareness of EBP benefits for healthcare professionals.

### PROCEDURE

- Identify critical practice behaviors from the evidence.
- Create a method for observing or collecting data on practice behaviors:
  - While rounding at the bedside
  - Observed behavior
  - Audit documentation of process indicators (see Strategy 3-12)
- Create a goal for identified behaviors.
- Identify when clinicians perform behaviors that surpass expectations.
- Provide just-in-time and informal positive reinforcement at the point of care or in work area soon after the observed behavior:
  - Identify the correct behavior.
  - Review how the behavior matches the evidence.
  - Describe how the practice closes the performance gap (see Strategy 2-12).
  - Learn how the clinicians are successfully incorporating the EBP.
- Consider alternatives to verbal/face-to-face when it is not feasible (e.g., electronic, by mail).
- Identify meaningful recognition that outweighs other disincentives that deter from adopting the EBP and reflect the natural focus on "what's in it for me."
- Plan ahead for recognition to be:
  - Closely tied to the specific, desired practice behavior
  - Timed as close to the action as possible
  - Frequently recognized until adoption becomes more routine
  - Informal to allow for spontaneous, "on the spot" recognition initially and can elevate to formal approaches
  - Private versus public, depending on preferences of the recipient
  - Personalized by the person providing recognition

**PHASE 3**

*continues*

## Strategy 3-11   Provide Recognition at the Point of Care (Continued)

### PROCEDURE (Continued)

- Given by a significant person in the organization or highly regarded peer
- Individualized to be valued by the recipient

■ Provide recognition or nonmonetary incentives first (employees want full appreciation, feeling "in" on discussion/decision, and interesting work), and then consider providing token rewards or incentive:
- Approval, appreciation
- Expressions of gratitude, thank you card, or certificate

■ Consider intangible or social recognition options:
- Acknowledgment
- Praise in public
- Involvement in decision-making
- Autonomy
- Perks in schedule, flexibility, or choice of work assignment
- First choice of lunch break for a week
- Opportunities to participate in interesting initiatives

■ Consider tangible recognition options:
- Certificate
- Trophy
- Paperweight or coffee mug

■ Consider rewards or monetary tokens in addition to recognition options:
- Treat for getting "caught" in the act of providing evidence-based care
- Perks for parking
- Small gift certificates
- Membership in a professional organization
- Attendance at a professional conference

■ Regularly provide recognition that is equivalent to the performance.

■ Be consistent with rewards.

■ Notify clinician's supervisor or enlist supervisor in recognition of positive performance.

■ Transition recognition from organizational leaders (if initiated at this level) to local unit leaders and then peers to develop ownership for the behavior.

■ Share positive behaviors among colleagues:
- Post or announce team members providing evidence-based care to provide social reinforcement.
- Nominate staff members for awards/drawings.
- Consider group celebrations as a mechanism for sustaining a practice change (see Strategy 4-1).

### EXAMPLE

Display an informational poster on the EBP that includes a photo of clinician "caught" using the EBP correctly in the past week and update regularly.

## CITATIONS

Al-Tawfiq, Abed, Al-Yami, & Birrer, 2013; Gillespie & Marshall, 2015; Kelly et al., 2011; Khan, Mehta, Gowda, Sacchi, & Vasavada, 2004; Larson et al., 2016; Larson, Patel, Evans, & Saiman, 2013; Mayer et al., 2011; Nelson, 2016; Neufeld, Fernández, Christo, & Williams, 2013; Srigley et al., 2015; Wigder, Cohan Ballis, Lazar, Urgo, & Dunn, 1999.

## Strategy 3-12    Audit Key Indicators

| PHASE | 3: Promote Action & Adoption |
|---|---|
| FOCUS | Building Organizational System Support |

### DEFINITION

An audit involves data collection of key indicators that will provide a summary of clinical performance collected over a specific time period, as a routine evaluation to improve performance or provision of evidence-based healthcare. Data may be collected at the clinician, team, or organizational level and are designed for local use, not necessarily generating generalizable data.

### BENEFITS

- Data collection can serve as a prompt and improve clinical processes and outcomes.

- Auditing improves clinical processes and outcomes.

### PROCEDURE

- Create evaluation plan delineating data elements, data location, formula (e.g., rate/1,000 patient days), reporting format (e.g., Pareto chart, run chart).
  - Identify key process indicators (see Chapter 9) (e.g., clinician knowledge, attitudes, and behaviors).
  - Identify key outcomes to impact (see Chapter 9) (e.g., reduced catheter-associated urinary tract infection).
  - Identify key structure indicators as appropriate (e.g., equipment or product availability, unit committee structure, level of staffing, or case mix).
  - Include indicators that may help explain or influence outcomes as balancing measures (e.g., length of stay may be influenced by level of physical activity during admission, duration of mechanical ventilation, or discharge destination).
  - Include indicators that represent potential barriers to adoption (e.g., access to equipment, ease of documentation), complexity that makes application difficult (e.g., interaction between multiple patient problems or competing practice recommendations), or workarounds from unforeseen pressure (e.g., high census leading to shortcuts in comprehensive assessment of critical comorbidities).
  - Identify indicators to include by visualizing how data will be used in feedback messages and recipient information needs.
  - Determine availability and access to electronic data (e.g., documentation from the electronic health record) or need for manual data collection.
  - Plan for protection of patient data (i.e., remove identifiers) and data security.
  - Plan for data management (i.e., data entry, cleanup, analysis, and report format).
- Submit request for data report or download, indicating that the work is EBP and linked to organizational priorities.
- Create forms for collecting needed data that are not available electronically (e.g., clinician knowledge assessment, observation, or chart audit form).
- Have clinical experts review forms and tools.
- Trial data-collection form for face validity and revise as needed.
- Train auditors for consistency in data collection.

- Collect data.
- Review and clean data as needed.
- Enter data for electronic management and analysis, if needed and/or available.
- Secure all data, especially data that could be relinked to re-identify individuals (e.g., patient record number).
- Create graphs for data reports that use consistent format for feedback so that sequential graphs are quickly interpretable.

## EXAMPLE

**Sample Inpatient Oral Assessment and Oral Care Chart Audit Form**

Patient record number: _____　　　　　　　　Area: _____

|  | Admission<br>Date:_____ | Day 1<br>Date:_____ | Day 4<br>Date:_____ |
|---|---|---|---|
| Oral assessment documented: at least once on the day of admission; at least two times on Day 1, if not discharged that day; and at least two times on Day 4, if still hospitalized. | ■ Yes<br>■ No | ■ Yes<br>■ No | ■ Yes<br>■ No |
| Oral assessment total score: | Score: _____ | Score 1: _____<br>Score 2: _____ | Score 1: _____<br>Score 2: _____ |
| Oral care documented: at least once on the day of admission; at least two times on Day 1, if not discharged that day; and at least two times on Day 4, if still hospitalized.<br><br>Mark interventions: | ■ Yes<br>■ No<br><br>■ Denture care<br>■ Floss<br>■ Gauze<br>■ Gel/Biotene | ■ Yes<br>■ No<br><br>■ Denture care<br>■ Floss<br>■ Gauze<br>■ Gel/Biotene | ■ Yes<br>■ No<br><br>■ Denture care<br>■ Floss<br>■ Gauze<br>■ Gel/Biotene |

## CITATIONS

Bowie, Bradley, & Rushmer, 2012; Cahill, Murch, Cook, Heyland, & Canadian Critical Care Trials Group, 2014; de Vos et al., 2013; Farrington, Cullen, & Dawson, 2013; Fleiszer, Semenic, Ritchie, Richer, & Denis, 2016a; Ivers et al., 2012; Ivers et al., 2014; Lahmann, Halfens, & Dassen, 2010; Landis-Lewis, Brehaut, Hochheiser, Douglas, & Jacobson, 2015; Lowson et al., 2015; Lugtenberg, Burgers, Han, & Westert, 2014; Mauger et al., 2014; Milat, Bauman, & Redman, 2015; Niederhauser et al., 2012; Payne & Hysong, 2016; Taylor, Clay-Williams, Hogden, Braithwaite, & Groene, 2015; van der Voort, van der Veer, & de Vos, 2012.

**PHASE 3**

## Strategy 3-13   Actionable and Timely Data Feedback

| PHASE | 3: Promote Action & Adoption |
|---|---|
| FOCUS | Building Organizational System Support |

### DEFINITION

Feedback is the reporting of organization, unit, or clinician-specific data back to clinicians or clinical teams. Data reported is a summary of clinical performance (e.g., based on charting audit/review, interview, questionnaire, or one-to-one observation of practice) to identify clinical behaviors needed to achieve the desired EBP improvement.

### BENEFITS

- Improves clinician involvement and goal-setting.
- Generates observability, with intensity and frequency of feedback impacting effectiveness.
- Feedback by a peer may promote increased engagement.
- Creates a positive culture for innovation and practice change, provides supportive messaging and rewards for a job well done, helps commit to the EBP, reduces cost, and helps with sustainment.
- Offers a reminder to perform the EBP, lets clinicians know whether their performance is adequate, increases ownership for using EBP, and provides evidence that actions are beneficial to patients.

### PROCEDURE

- Identify audience to receive feedback.
- Identify process and outcome indicators with opportunities for improvement or meeting/exceeding established goal or standards (see Chapter 9).
- Set target for process and outcome indicators.
- Audit performance by colleagues (when possible) (see Strategy 3-12).
- Tabulate audit results for display and easy interpretation to make the need for improvement observable (i.e., graphs) when offering feedback (see Strategy 2-11).
- Provide evidence supporting the desired performance on key indicators and impact of process indicators on patient, team, or organizational outcomes.
- Encourage and praise practices with high performance.
- Provide timely feedback.
- Provide specific/actionable suggestions about how to complete the task correctly.
- Adjust design of graphical display to spotlight or shift attention to details about the task to be completed to achieve desired improvement.
- Use consistent methods that are tailored to recipient.
- Use written form or post on clinical area.
- Ensure inclusion of all clinicians and other team members in team discussion of data feedback to facilitate team ownership and planning.
- Provide comparison from last measurement period (especially if trending data make recent changes less obvious) (see Strategy 4-10).
- Consider providing comparison data for individual performance to reference group (see Strategy 3-22).

## PROCEDURE

- Promote discussion of data and opportunities for improvement.
- Follow up discussion with written feedback.
- Create action plan based on reported findings (see Strategy 2-22).
- Provide feedback on regular or periodic basis to improve impact.
- Re-evaluate the goal for key indicators.

## EXAMPLE

- Nurse manager of unit implements EBP initiative to reduce patient falls by ensuring that all patients are mobile or ambulatory to the fullest extent.
- Process data tabulating unit use of ambulation are shared with discussion about how to promote use of safe-handling/ergonomics equipment, coordinate patient ambulation within the team, build ambulation into the patient care and unit workflow, obtain assistance from physical therapy, etc.
- Specific process data (e.g., risk assessments completed per policy; patient volume with mobility risk factor; volume of physical therapy referrals; frequency of clinician use of safe-handling/ergonomics equipment) are shared regularly with positive reinforcement and identified opportunities for continuous improvement in care processes.
- Review of data identifies clear actions clinicians can take to improve care processes (i.e., actionable feedback).

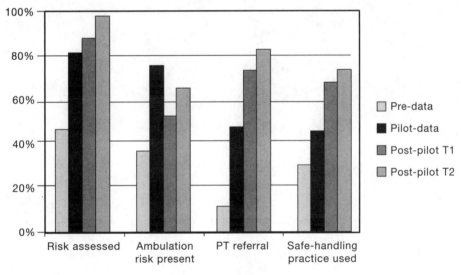

fictitious data

*continues*

PHASE 3

## Strategy 3-13    Actionable and Timely Data Feedback (Continued)

### CITATIONS

Armellion et al., 2013; Bruno et al., 2014; Fleiszer, Semenic, Ritchie, Richer, & Denis, 2016a; Fleuren, van Dommelen, & Dunnink, 2015; Hysong, Kell, Petersen, Campbell, & Trautner, 2016; Hysong, Knox, & Haidet, 2014; Hysong, Teal, Khan, & Haidet, 2012; Katz et al., 2014; Landis-Lewis, Brehaut, Hochheiser, Douglas, & Jacobson, 2015; Larson, Patel, Evans, & Saiman, 2013; Lugtenberg, Burgers, Han, & Westert, 2014; Mauger et al., 2014; Milat, Bauman, & Redman, 2015; Overdyk et al., 2016; Payne & Hysong, 2016.

## Strategy 3-14    Checklist

| PHASE | 3: Promote Action & Adoption |
|---|---|
| FOCUS | Building Organizational System Support |

### DEFINITION

A checklist is a simple cognitive tool designed to provide clinical decision support and promote task completion (Winters et al., 2009) that includes a list of items to be noted, checked, or remembered (AHRQ, 2013b) when performing a practice or procedure.

### BENEFITS

■ Provides a simple, reliable reminder for interprofessional communication.

■ Improves standardized use of key steps in a process.

■ Promotes team support for safe completion of care processes.

■ Provides a level playing field that empowers all team members to speak up.

### PROCEDURE

■ Identify a practice or procedure with practice variation that could impact outcomes:

- Consider practices or procedures where step-by-step procedure can be standardized without risking loss of key contextual information (e.g., variability in patient scenario or comorbidity) and where reliance on memory for the correct steps creates problems with practice variations that may negatively impact outcomes.

- Address simple or complicated procedures that can be broken down into manageable pieces that are repeatable for multiple patients or scenarios.

- If decision-making is required for complex problems when variable patient conditions exist that require different responses, consider other options (e.g., decision algorithm [see Strategy 3-2] or case studies [see Strategy 2-17] to describe their clinical course).

■ Obtain background information to use for content and design:

- Review the evidence for critical practice or procedure steps that are required to improve quality.

- Obtain any existing, relevant checklists already reported in the literature that can be adapted to match local needs and barriers while avoiding rework from duplicate development.

- Review local quality data and incident reports to identify potential issues to address within the checklist.

- Locate applicable content in existing, relevant organizational policies, procedures, or protocols.

■ Consider routine workflow during checklist development and implementation.

■ Obtain feedback from clinicians identifying challenges that contribute to variability in practice.

- Include interprofessional team members; recognize that provider leadership and participation may facilitate sustained use.

*continues*

**PHASE 3**

## Strategy 3-14    Checklist (Continued)

### PROCEDURE (Continued)

- Determine the type of checklist to develop.
  - Static parallel—list of read and do tasks completed by one person (e.g., emergency equipment checklist).
  - Static sequential with verification—list of tasks read by one person and completed by second person (e.g., central line insertion checklist).
  - Static sequential with verification and confirmation—list of tasks read by one person and completed by a variety of team members (e.g., operating room time-out).
  - Dynamic checklist with flowchart—includes multiple options for action that are decided on by team members (e.g., clinical decision algorithm [see Strategy 3-2]).
- Draft a list of critical steps or tasks.
  - Include only steps or tasks that need to be addressed and add value.
  - Address or consider phases of care separately (e.g., diagnosis, treatment, and monitoring; pre-, during, and post- intervention).
  - Divide checklists for multiple subprocedures or specific high-risk patient populations.
  - Steps or tasks should be simple, clear, concise, easy to comprehend, consistently interpreted, and actionable.
  - Simplify whenever possible.
  - Consider using a mnemonic (e.g., SBAR) to guide sequencing of steps and improve communication, if relevant.
- Indicate whether sequential task completion is essential for safety (e.g., patient identification before blood transfusion) and if any steps are optional.
- Clearly identify priority actions to be taken as follow-up steps (e.g., after completion of handoff checklist).
- Eliminate redundancy with existing documentation or data collection systems.
- Review checklist, by clinicians, for feasibility and clarity in order to facilitate use in practice.
  - Consider using a process (e.g., Delphi technique) to establish reliability and content validity (i.e., sufficiency, relevancy, and clarity of included items).
  - Establish a consensus threshold prior to seeking clinician input.
  - Continue development and revision until consensus is achieved.
- Ensure that correct equipment is readily available and conveniently accessible (e.g., procedure cart in a consistent location).
- Create a safety checklist briefing procedure to use consistently when completing the checklist.
  - Clearly identify role-specific actions associated with steps or tasks on the checklist.
  - Identify each team member's role at the beginning of the briefing in a way that is understood by everyone.
  - Establish clear consequences for not completing the checklist and briefing.

- Trial the checklist.
  - Consider a simulation-based trial prior to use in a clinical setting.
  - Encourage use of clinical judgment when patient-specific variation in practice is warranted.
  - Review when these scenarios should be incorporated in checklist revisions or when a decision algorithm would be useful (see Strategy 3-2).
  - Evaluate feasibility, usability, and unforeseen new risks created by use of the checklist.
- Revise the checklist as indicated based on evaluative data and clinician feedback.
- Monitor compliance with use of the checklist in daily practice.
- Evaluate comprehensiveness of item completion.
- Share case studies when use of the checklist prevented an error or adverse event.
- Provide real-time feedback to clinicians on checklist use.
- Evaluate checklist impact on care processes and outcomes; consider capturing avoided costs (e.g., reduced major complications).
- Develop a patient-friendly version to use as an educational resource to promote patient engagement.
- Regularly update checklist based on new evidence.

## EXAMPLE

World Health Organization. (2009). WHO surgical safety checklist. Retrieved from http://www.who.int/patientsafety/safesurgery/checklist/en

## CITATIONS

AHRQ, 2013b; Berenholtz et al., 2004; Bhogal, McGillivray et al., 2011; Borchard, Schwappach, Barbir, & Bezzola, 2012; Brunsveld-Reinders, Arbous, Kuiper, & de Jonge, 2015; Cavalcanti et al., 2016; Conroy, Elliott, & Burrell, 2013; Gagliardi, Marshall, Huckson, James, & Moore, 2015; Gawande, 2010; Gillespie & Marshall, 2015; Haynes et al., 2009; Henneman, Kleppel, & Hinchey, 2013; Hilligoss & Moffatt-Bruce, 2014; McDowell & McComb, 2014; McKee et al., 2008; National Public Radio Books, 2010; Pezzolesi et al., 2013; Treadwell, Lucas, & Tsou, 2014; Winters et al., 2009; WHO, n.d., 2008, 2009.

**PHASE 3**

## Strategy 3-15    Documentation

| PHASE | 3: Promote Action & Adoption |
| --- | --- |
| FOCUS | Building Organizational System Support |

### DEFINITION

Documentation uses an electronic or paper method to record care a patient receives from members of the interprofessional healthcare team.

### BENEFITS

- Improves interprofessional team awareness of practice changes.
- Improves compliance and sustainability of practice recommendations.
- Allows for efficient data recording and reporting.
- Facilitates team communication to enhance coordination and patient safety.

### PROCEDURE

- Review current documentation tools.
- Determine whether new documentation elements or revisions are needed to support practice recommendations:
  - Create user-friendly templates that are quick and easy to complete (e.g., check boxes, drop-down menus).
  - Ensure standardized location for documentation within the patient record.
  - Avoid the need for duplicate documentation.
  - Use smart phrases when possible
- Consider clinician for design.
- Garner stakeholder support or informatics governance support, if needed.
  - Seek user (e.g., frontline clinician) feedback on functionality, inclusiveness, and clarity of documentation elements.
- Consult institutional informatics team to request documentation changes.
- Consider placement of high priority and high frequency documentation near the top for easy access.
- Address or consider phases of care separately (e.g., assessment, treatment, and monitoring).
- Outline sequential documentation elements that are logical and enhance safety (e.g., patient identification before medication administration).
- Eliminate redundancy.
- Ensure easy access to equipment (e.g., computer for patient health record) and supplies (e.g., assessment tools).
- Allow time for clinician review.
- Trial the documentation.
- Prepare for undesirable consequences (e.g., check boxes lead to missed patient-specific details requiring a narrative note).
- Provide ongoing education about documentation processes/changes (e.g., orientation, inservices, annual competencies).
- Determine method and frequency to assess documentation compliance.
- Provide routine feedback to and from clinicians to improve documentation accuracy and completeness.

Oral Care Documentation for Oncology Patients

| | <Date> | | |
|---|---|---|---|
| | 0800 | 1200 | 2000 |
| Denture care | | | |
| Floss | X | | |
| Gauze | | | |
| Gel/Biotene® | | | |
| Gel/fluoride | | | |
| Lip care/lanolin | X | X | X |
| Rinse | X | X | X |
| Toothbrush/soft | X | | X |
| Toothpaste/Biotene | X | | X |
| Troxel syringe | | | |
| Washcloth | | | |
| Gum massage | | | |
| Independent | X | | X |
| Assistance of 1 | | | |
| Refused | | | |

**CITATIONS**

Byrnes et al., 2009; Eid & Bucknall, 2008; Fleiszer, Semenic, Ritchie, Richer, & Denis, 2016a; Ganz et al., 2013; Gunningberg, Fogelberg-Dahm, & Ehrenberg, 2009; Higuchi, Davies, Edwards, Ploeg, & Virani, 2011; Horn et al., 2010; Wuchner, 2014.

PHASE 3

## Strategy 3-16    Standing Orders

| PHASE | 3: Promote Action & Adoption |
|---|---|
| FOCUS | Building Organizational System Support |

### DEFINITION

A standing order is a prescribed set of actions to be taken based on policies, procedures, regulations, or other governing documents. Standing orders are usually generated by a clinical team using clinical practice guidelines and are built into the health record as an order set for decision support and may be in checklist format (McGreevey, 2013). They may include such prescriptive language as dose, route, schedule, or monitoring to be completed.

### BENEFITS

- Serves as decision support to increase standardization of treatments; reduces errors and treatment delays.
- Simplifies processes and improves efficiency and cost.
- Improves use of routine and preventive services (e.g., vaccinations).
- Patients report standing orders are acceptable.

### PROCEDURE

- Determine whether a standing order is the best approach for clinical decision support to address the practice issue by considering whether content is straightforward.
- Obtain leadership or informatics governance support to create specific standing orders.
- Involve clinical experts for evidence-based content and understanding of workflow.
- Identify pharmacologic, diagnostic, treatment, monitoring, or referral options supported by evidence.
  - Review evidence as a team to identify necessary actions or orders.
  - Decide criteria to be used for identification of eligible patients.
  - Review formulary, policies, or related documents for organizational restrictions or specific considerations.
  - Determine acceptable ranges for dose and frequency.
- Determine whether paper or an electronic system will be used and the method to trigger notification of initiation (e.g., health record triggers clinician notification as an alert [see Strategy 3-1], nurse-driven orders).
  - Allow time for programming or formatting.
- Draft a sample document demonstrating options and format of standing orders.
- Follow any organizational style guide to adhere to usability principles and to promote ease of interpretation across standing orders.
- Use design principles:
  - Arrange or group treatment options that are most important at the top
  - Place more commonly needed and desirable choices near the top or in a prominent manner
  - Group similar options or interventions needed at the same time (e.g., medication and lab draw for blood levels)
  - Arrange sequentially by time needed
  - Create or limit input required and harness existing data in health record (e.g., don't automate orders that would require a pregnancy test on male patients)

| PROCEDURE (Continued) |
| --- |

- • Consider default options carefully to avoid risk of error
- • Allow flexibility for individual patient needs
- ■ Create a standard associated with use of the standing orders.
- ■ Prepare for undesirable consequences (e.g., standing orders for hypoglycemia may lead to hyperglycemia).
- ■ Allow time for clinician review.
- ■ Use a logical naming convention for easy retrieval by busy clinicians.
- ■ Pilot/trial the standing orders.
- ■ Inform clinicians of the start date and the location of standing orders and how to use them.
- ■ Discuss rationale and inclusion/exclusion criteria for standing orders with clinicians.
- ■ Identify the role of each clinician in use of standing orders considering regulatory scope of practice standards.
- ■ Use clinician feedback and evaluative data to review and revise use of standing orders.
- ■ After piloting, obtain final approval/sign-off for standing orders.
- ■ Integrate standing orders into paper or electronic documentation system (e.g., computerized physician order entry, plan of care).
- ■ Establish efficient workflow for use of standing orders.
- ■ Engage patients and families/caregivers (e.g., publicize vaccines, decision aids [see Strategy 3-18]).
- ■ Monitor compliance with use of standing orders.
- ■ Establish a periodic review process for improvement and need for revision or reinfusion.

| EXAMPLES |
| --- |

**Example 1: Vaccinations**

Written orders stipulating that all persons meeting certain criteria (i.e., age or underlying medical condition) should be vaccinated, thus eliminating the need for individual physician's orders for each patient (CDC, 2015b).

**Example 2: Standing Orders for Ketamine Administration in Adults**

| ORDER SET |
| --- |

Ketamine for pain (adult) for use outside the OR, ASC, SICU

| MEDICATIONS |
| --- |

Ketamine/Lorazepam/Glycopyrrolate (Parenteral)

Ketamine/Lorazepam/Glycopyrrolate (Oral)

*continues*

PHASE 3

## Strategy 3-16 Standing Orders (Continued)

### EXAMPLES (Continued)

Precautions

- Assess blood pressure, heart rate, and respirations (rate, rhythm/pattern, effort, depth, presence of snoring, gurgling, etc); measure sedation via Riker/POSS.
- At baseline, every 15 minutes for 1 hour; then every 1 hour for 12 hours, then every 2 hours for 12 hours, then every 4 hours based on patient condition.

Oximetry, Continuous

- Continuous for first 24hrs, then prn Alarm High HR: 120
- Alarm Low HR: 50
- Alarm High SpO2: 100%
- Alarm Low SpO2: 90%
- Call H.O. if SpO2 less than or equal to: 90%

Oximetry, Spot Check

- PRN
- Tomorrow at __:__
- Call H.O. if SpO2 less than or equal to: 90%

Call Parameters

- Contact H.O./Primary Service if change in SBP greater than 20 mmHg or change in HR greater than or less than 20 beats per minute from baseline value, if respiratory rate is less than 12 breaths per minute, if Riker score is less than 3 or POSS score of 3 or 4 (exception: PACU refer to unit-based policy PS-PACU-06.003), if oxygen saturation at or below 90%, if increased secretions not responsive to glycopyrrolate.

(Farrington, Hanson et al., 2015)

### CITATIONS

Avery, O'Brien, Daddio Pierce, & Gazarian, 2015; Bedra, Hill Golder, Cha, Jeong, & Finkelstein, 2015; Bourdeaux, Davies, Thomas, Bewley, & Gould, 2014; Busby et al., 2011; CDC, 2015b; Chan et al., 2012; Dempsey et al., 2015; Farrington, Hanson et al., 2015; Hall, Montero, Cobian, & Regan, 2015; Immunization Action Coalition, 2015; Institute for Safe Medication Practices, 2010; Manley et al., 2014; May et al., 2014; McGreevey, 2013; Open Society Foundations, 2013; Pasero, Quinlan-Colwell, Rae, Broglio, & Drew, 2016; Sonstein, Clark, Seidensticker, Zeng, & Sharma, 2014; Tannenbaum et al., 2015; Weled et al., 2015; Zhang, Padman, & Levin, 2014.

## Strategy 3-17    Patient Reminders

| PHASE | 3: Promote Action & Adoption |
|---|---|
| FOCUS | Building Organizational System Support |

### DEFINITION

Patient reminders are a type of communication delivered to patients to prompt performance or avoidance of specific health behaviors from practice recommendations.

### BENEFITS

- Strengthens and reinforces communication between the patient and healthcare team.
- Fosters shared accountability and patient autonomy in managing their healthcare encounters.
- Encourages patients to incorporate evidence-based health behaviors into daily routines.
- Provides patients with timely, relevant, and personalized information.
- Offers a method to reach patients outside of regular clinical settings.

### PROCEDURE

- Determine when reminders would be beneficial.
- Determine type of reminders (e.g., health screenings, immunizations).
- Develop reminder content.
- Keep content easy to read.
- Consider information technology available to provide reminders that are acceptable and convenient for patients.
- Determine delivery method (e.g., electronic health record portal, text message, automated telephone call, paper mailing, brochure, email).
- Obtain patient feedback to evaluate acceptance and usefulness of reminders.
- Determine effectiveness of patient reminders on health outcomes.

*continues*

PHASE 3

## Strategy 3-17    Patient Reminders (Continued)

### EXAMPLE

Energy Through Motion©: An activity intervention for cancer-related fatigue in an ambulatory infusion center. Adult cancer patients undergoing chemotherapy participated in EBP to maintain or improve their cancer-related fatigue and quality of life:

- Participants were provided activity trackers, resistance bands, patient/family education (printed and video formats), secure text messages, and regular follow-up.

- Activity promotion was provided through patient reminders sent via secure text or email messages three times per week for 3 months.

- Encouraging messages and patient reminders from the program:

 **Message 1**

With moderate activity, you can still talk with those around you. Vigorous activity will make you take a breath after a few words. Hope you are enjoying the holiday weekend! Linda

 **Message 2**

Telling others about your commitment to take action can strengthen your willpower. Think about who you are going to tell. Linda

 **Message 3**

Think about how good you feel when you stay active regularly! Enjoy your weekend. Linda

(Abbott, 2016; Abbott & Hooke, in press)

### CITATIONS

Abbott, 2016; Abbott, & Hooke, in press; Frasure, 2014; Gerhardt, Schoettker, Donovan, Kotagal, & Muething, 2007; Maurer & Harris, 2014; Perri-Moore et al., 2016.

## Strategy 3-18    Patient Decision Aids

| PHASE | 3: Promote Action & Adoption |
|---|---|
| FOCUS | Building Organizational System Support |

### DEFINITION

Patient decision aids are tools to help patients participate in decisions that involve weighing the benefits and harms of treatment options (Stacey et al., 2014) and consider the best available evidence, taking into account patients' context, values, and preferences (Agoritsas et al., 2015).

### BENEFITS

- Increases knowledge and accurate understanding of risk perceptions.
- Assists selection of treatment option congruent with patient values.
- Lowers decisional conflict related to feeling uninformed and unclear about personal values; improves indecision about treatment options.
- Reduces selection of invasive procedures in favor of lower-risk options.

### PROCEDURE

- Form a group to select or develop a decision aid; include patient and/or family representative.
- Describe the health condition being targeted.
- Identify the needs and common questions of potential users.
- Identify the current standard evidence-based treatment options for the health condition.
- Examine the literature for existing decision aids:
  - Explore the fit for your organization, practice standards, patient population, and clinician preferences.
  - Determine key risks and benefits, along with reported occurrence.
- Use existing decision aid format to structure development of a new one, if needed.
- In new or existing aid, the following should be included:
  - List the positive features (benefits) and negative features (side effects, harms, disadvantages).
  - Display event rate probabilities and time period in plain language; consider primary language.
  - Include extent of key scientific uncertainties.
  - Consider use of graphics and pictures to convey message.
  - Outline patient values, preferences, resources, and options.
- Use the International Patient Decision Aid Standards (IPDAS) Collaboration checklist to ensure quality of the decision aid, available at http://ipdas.ohri.ca/IPDAS_checklist.pdf.

### EXAMPLES

- Agency for Healthcare Research and Quality (AHRQ). (n.d.-c). Effective health care program: Helping you make better treatment choices: Patient decision aids. Retrieved from https://www.effectivehealthcare.ahrq.gov/tools-and-resources/patient-decision-aids
- Centers for Disease Control and Prevention (CDC). (2016b). STEADI materials for your older adult patients. Retrieved from https://www.cdc.gov/steadi/patient.html

*continues*

**PHASE 3**

**Strategy 3-18    Patient Decision Aids (Continued)**

CITATIONS

AHRQ, n.d.-c; Agoritsas et al., 2015; Breslin, Mullan, & Montori, 2008; CDC, 2016b; Durand et al., 2015; Elwyn et al., n.d.; International Patient Decision Aid Standards (IPDAS) Collaboration, 2005; International Patient Decision Aid Standards Steering Committee, 2013; Stacey et al., 2014.

## Strategy 3-19 Rounding by Unit & Organizational Leadership

| PHASE | 3: Promote Action & Adoption |
|---|---|
| FOCUS | Building Organizational System Support |

### DEFINITION

Leadership rounds are routine, proactive visits to clinical areas to provide visible, continuous support for adopting and sustaining practice recommendations while recognizing individual and team activities to achieve the goal.

### BENEFITS

- Provides an opportunity to engage in face-to-face, interactive discussions with clinicians, patients, and families.
- Demonstrates attentiveness to daily unit or clinic function.
- Assists clinicians in integrating practice recommendations within complex care environments.
- Supports clinicians in connecting the practice change to patient outcomes.
- Promotes interactive learning.

### PROCEDURE

- Determine rounding intent; some examples include:
  - Improve the use of practice recommendations.
  - Provide a forum to maintain currency and competence.
  - Model expertise and leadership.
  - Recognize and acknowledge expertise.
  - Decrease clinician isolation.
  - Promote professional development.
  - Develop clinical decision-making, communication, and presentation skills.
- Choose the unit and/or organizational leaders who will participate.
- Determine the format (e.g., informal hallway conversations, breakroom discussions with food, formal presentations).
- Determine frequency (e.g., daily, weekly, monthly) when determining schedule.
  - Consider usual unit or clinic activity.
  - Ask about day and time preferences (consider altering days and times).
- Determine rounding length (e.g., 30 minutes, 1 hour).
- Schedule rounds and notify clinical areas.
- Provide positive feedback to clinicians during rounds.
- Obtain clinician feedback to adapt future rounds to meet the needs of individual units or clinics.

PHASE 3

*continues*

## Strategy 3-19   Rounding by Unit & Organizational Leadership (Continued)

### EXAMPLE

The following example is related to pain rounding by unit or organizational leadership.

### Introductory Comments

- Complete introductions with clinicians, patients, and/or families.
- Define the purpose (e.g., recognize individual and team activities and to achieve goals related to a new pain assessment scale).
- Ensure that participants know all feedback is welcome.

### Sample Questions—Clinician Audience

- How do you use whiteboards to communicate with patients and families about pain? Unit or organizational leaders could complete a visual compliance check regarding pain content on whiteboards.
- What do you use to complete a pain assessment?
- What patient and family education (e.g., verbal, written) is provided related to pain management?
- Is asking about pain a part of routine team rounding?
- Do you have any other comments or suggestions related to pain?

### Sample Questions—Patient/Family Audience

- What were your expectations about pain before you came to the hospital?
- What education (e.g., verbal, written) have you been given related to pain?
- Were you able to use the pain assessment scale you prefer?
- How are the whiteboards used to communicate with you about pain?
- Have you been able to get out of bed to the chair and go for walks with your pain sufficiently under control?
- Do you have any other comments or suggestions about pain?

### Closing Remarks

- Please feel free to contact me if you have additional feedback.
- Thank you for participating.

### CITATIONS

Aitken, Burmeister, Clayton, Dalais, & Gardner, 2011; Fleiszer, Semenic, Ritchie, Richer, & Denis, 2016a; Mahanes, Quatrara, & Shaw, 2013; Taylor, Clay-Williams, Hogden, Braithwaite, & Groene, 2015.

## Strategy 3-20 Report Into Quality Improvement Program

| PHASE | 3: Promote Action & Adoption |
|---|---|
| FOCUS | Building Organizational System Support |

### DEFINITION

Reporting into a quality improvement (QI) program is a statement of structures, processes, and outcomes related to an EBP improvement that is shared within the quality/performance improvement program and organizational infrastructure. Standardized content/forms or data elements addressing key steps using the organization's QI model are used.

### BENEFITS

- Strategically links EBP initiatives to QI program infrastructure and resources.
- Creates an efficient flow of information that notifies stakeholders and senior leaders of the impact.
- Facilitates clinician and stakeholder commitment to improving EBP.
- Avoids reporting duplication and confusion; supports sustainability because the existing infrastructure for QI is already resourced.
- Promotes senior leadership support for EBP adoption and sustainability.
- Establishes meaningfulness of clinicians' work.
- Relates EBP work to the mission and focus of institution's concurrent QI work, aligned with strategic department and institution goals.

### PROCEDURE

- Identify a clear purpose (see Chapter 2).
- Identify key process and outcome data to evaluate (see Chapter 9) and report (see Chapter 12).
- Report post-pilot data and plans for revision, integration, and/or rollout (see Chapter 11).
- Select paper, electronic, or both formats.
- Use the organization or department QI reporting template to share baseline data demonstrating an opportunity for improvement through EBP.
- Indicate that the project work is EBP.
- Be concise and organized when reporting process and outcomes.
- Link project work to organizational priorities.
- Make content readable, appropriate, and culturally sensitive.
- Submit the QI report to the department or organization's office for performance improvement.
- Determine key process and outcome indicators to track that support integration of the practice change (see Chapter 11) through continued QI monitoring.
- Report committee or infrastructure responsible for integration of the EBP into practice.
- Request feedback on report to ensure that content targets the appropriate audience.
- Update the QI report with activities implemented (e.g., quarterly) and trended data on a regular basis (e.g., every 6–12 months).

PHASE 3

*continues*

## Strategy 3-20   Report Into Quality Improvement Program (Continued)

### PROCEDURE (Continued)

- Submit updated QI reports as appropriate into QI program/system.
- Review reports of improvement for shared learning.
- Showcase improvements and provide senior leadership opportunities to recognize EBP teams (see Strategy 4-1).
- Set expectations for clinician ownership/accountability for improvement.
- Use findings to advocate for patients/clients and identify resource needs and report these to organizational leaders.
- Use findings to determine whether there is an opportunity to cycle to the top of the EBP process model for additional EBP interventions to expand on practice improvements.

### EXAMPLES

**Example 1: Reporting EBP Work Into QI**

Unit: CV step down
Division: ICU
Date: NA
Presenter: Laura Cullen, DNP, RN, FAAN

### Patient Preference for Pain Assessment Scale
### Nursing Quality Outcomes Report

Method:
❑ Quality Improvement
✓ Evidence-Based Practice
*(select one)*

**Define**: Use of NRS is hard-wired; patient preference for pain scale assessment can improve.

Goal: To provide evidence-based pain assessment matching patient preferences for older adults on a cardiac/cardiac surgery step-down unit. Used *The Iowa Model*.

**Measure:** Baseline data and data collected
- Patient report of use of their preferred pain scale; participation in pain management (pre = 53/98 or 54%; post = 45/100 or 45%)
- Trend patient satisfaction data
- Nurse feedback: pre = 31/59 or 53%; post = 22/53 or 42%

**Analyze:** Use of 0-10 NRS is hard-wired, yet research shows older adults often prefer a different scale. Even cognitively intact older adults are likely to prefer the VDS or Iowa Pain Thermometer. Nurses' pain assessments can improve with EBP.

**Improve:** Describe actions/solutions implemented (limit 4)
- Pocket cards with pain scale options in each room
- Core group journal club, reviewed actions of a change agent, planning implementation
- Rounding by NM and core group
- Weekly informal audit and actionable feedback

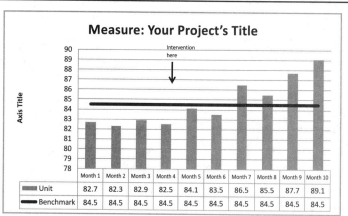

Shows steady improvement in patient satisfaction                 fictitious data

| | Month 1 | Month 2 | Month 3 | Month 4 | Month 5 | Month 6 | Month 7 | Month 8 | Month 9 | Month 10 |
|---|---|---|---|---|---|---|---|---|---|---|
| Unit | 82.7 | 82.3 | 82.9 | 82.5 | 84.1 | 83.5 | 86.5 | 85.5 | 87.7 | 89.1 |
| Benchmark | 84.5 | 84.5 | 84.5 | 84.5 | 84.5 | 84.5 | 84.5 | 84.5 | 84.5 | 84.5 |

**Control:** Follow-up
- Ongoing monitoring of patient satisfaction data
- Nurse residency reinfusion and education
- Replace pocket cards as needed
- Plan regular reinfusion by core group members
- Core group will report poster at national EBP conference

PHASE 3

**Example 2: Performance Improvement Quality Report**

**Date submitted:**                    **Submitted by:**

**Center/department/division/unit or clinic:**

**Project title:**

**Project team members:**

**Status:** ☐ **Complete** ☐ **In progress**

**Project source (check all that apply):**

☐ Core data, unit, chart audits, etc.        ☐ Patient satisfaction
☐ Benchmarking                              ☐ Sentinel/adverse event
☐ Other data source                         ☐ Interprofessional project
                                            ☐ Evidence-based practice

**Area of improvement (check all that apply):**

☐ Quality (clinical outcomes)        ☐ Cost         ☐ People (staffing/credentialing)
☐ Service (efficiency—internal process)   ☐ Growth (new or expanding service)

**Problem statement (in terms of primary metric):**



**Anticipated improvement (in terms of primary metric):**



**Intervention description and date implemented:**



**Realized improvement (with supporting data):**



**Follow-up plans—how long will the intervention be monitored:**

*continues*

**PHASE 3**

**Strategy 3-20　Report Into Quality Improvement Program (Continued)**

CITATIONS

AHRQ, 2015b, 2015c, 2015e, 2016a; Barnsteiner, Reeder, Palma, Preston, & Walton, 2010; Bosch et al., 2016; Cullen, Greiner, Greiner, Bombei, & Comried, 2005; Cullen, Hanrahan et al., in press; Cullen, Wagner, Matthews, & Farrington, 2017; Dückers, Wagner, Vos, & Groenewegen, 2011; Ford II, Krahn, Wise, & Oliver, 2011; Gruen et al., 2008; Hulscher, Schouten, Grol, & Buchan, 2013; Leone, Standoli, & Hirth, 2009; Lindamer et al., 2009; Nordqvist, Timpka, & Lindqvist, 2009; Registered Nurses' Association of Ontario, 2013; Stetler, Ritchie, Rycroft-Malone, & Charns, 2014; Titler, 2010; VanDeusen et al., 2010.

## Strategy 3-21   Link to Patient/Family Needs & Organizational Priorities

| PHASE | 3: Promote Action & Adoption |
|---|---|
| FOCUS | Building Organizational System Support |

### DEFINITION

Creating a link to patient/family needs and organizational priorities connects the EBP change to value outcomes.

### BENEFITS

- Improves awareness, knowledge, and attitudes regarding the importance (value) of the practice change for patients.
- Improves patient satisfaction with and engagement in their healthcare experience.
- Builds clinician confidence and competence in aligning with patient/family needs that also match organizational priorities.
- Enhances allocation of resources to successfully implement the practice change.
- Contributes to achievement of organizational goals including fiscal goals through reimbursement incentives.

### PROCEDURE

- Include frontline clinicians with appropriate interprofessional patient and/or family representation in practice change decision.
- Provide data about the practice, supporting evidence, value, and benefits for patients, their families, the organization, and clinicians.
- Ensure and demonstrate how the practice is aligned with patient/family needs and/or organizational priorities and supported by key senior leaders.
- Engage the team in discussion about organizational priorities, how they are linked to reimbursement incentives, and regulatory requirements.
- Engage key leaders in the practice change and obtain commitment to:
  - Articulate and model how the practice change is consistent with the vision for an EBP culture that emphasizes patient needs as a key priority.
  - Communicate to senior leaders and back to team members.
  - Ensure routine auditing and provision for ongoing feedback regarding effects on patient symptoms, satisfaction, and fiscal and clinical outcomes.
  - Engage clinicians in the practice change and coach them as needed.
  - Offer opportunities for professional development (e.g., education [see Strategy 2-1], journal clubs [see Strategy 1-4], conferences) to strengthen links to patient needs and organizational priorities.
- Ensure that information technology resources are available (including literature search databases) to retrieve key indicator data from health records and other databases (e.g., patient satisfaction or experience, financial disincentives and incentives, clinical outcomes).
- Discuss links to patient/family needs and organizational priorities when sharing key data with frontline clinicians.

*continues*

**PHASE 3**

## Strategy 3-21    Link to Patient/Family Needs & Organizational Priorities (Continued)

### EXAMPLES

Adequate patient pain management

■ Patient satisfaction ratings include how well their pain was managed while hospitalized.

■ Patient satisfaction is a measure of the patient experience that is also part of the healthcare reimbursement programs with fiscal implications for organizations who perform well or poorly.

Chlorhexidine gluconate (CHG) bathing to reduce/prevent hospital-acquired conditions (HAC)

■ Important patient need that requires a team approach and partnership with patients.

■ A key outcome for fiscal implications as healthcare reimbursement includes incentives and disincentives for HAC, including central-line-associated bloodstream infections.

### CITATIONS

CMS, 2017; Fleiszer, Semenic, Ritchie, Richer, & Denis, 2016a; Foy et al., 2002; Grol & Grimshaw, 2003; Innis & Berta, 2016; Katz et al., 2010)

## Strategy 3-22  Individual Performance Evaluation

| PHASE | 3: Promote Action & Adoption |
|---|---|
| FOCUS | Building Organizational System Support |

### DEFINITION

An individual performance evaluation uses a systematic, standardized process to compare work behavior to a preset standard and is completed at least annually by an employee's supervisor. The aim is to establish the employee's work contribution, quality of work compared to the standard, and potential for advancement (Nemeth, 2014, p. 399). It provides an opportunity to identify individual actions that accomplish EBP priorities for the clinical area.

### BENEFITS

- Provides an opportunity to develop and recognize expertise, desired attitudes, and behaviors.
- Improves performance, motivation, and communication about expectations framed as a learning opportunity.
- Reinforces positive behaviors or practices that are aligned with EBP priorities.
- Provides a systematic approach to incorporate individual clinician goals and coaching about clinical priorities.

### PROCEDURE

- Include EBP components within each job description (e.g., chief nurse executive, chief executive officer, clinician).
- Include EBP performance criteria for each role in performance tools and step in the clinical ladder or other professional development program.
- Review and revise performance criteria based on feedback from appropriate groups and representatives of that role to include appropriate EBP criteria.
- Identify organizational or unit needs related to EBP priorities (e.g., indicators used for Magnet recognition or Centers for Medicare & Medicaid Services hospital compare public reporting).
- Communicate to clinician at orientation about EBP priorities and practices as the routine approach.
- Provide notice of performance review to allow for collection of relevant information on use of EBP.
- Schedule a suitable time and location for discussion to reflect opportunities for routine provision of EBP (e.g. when caring for patient related to current EBP initiatives).
- Listen to and determine EBP goals.
- Discuss strengths related to job responsibilities where use of EBP is apparent.
- Determine level of participation in EBP or QI activities related to clinical practice priorities. Include sufficient detail outlining specific decisions and actions related to recommended practice to guide future action.

*continues*

PHASE 3

## Strategy 3-22    Individual Performance Evaluation (Continued)

### PROCEDURE (Continued)

- Keep feedback observable, actionable, timely, and specific to EBP priorities.
- Link decisions and actions to evidence supporting recommended practice.
- Ask questions to understand clinician perspective about providing evidence-based care to troubleshoot challenges and recognize provision of evidence-based care.
- Discuss link between benefits to clinician and patient from use of practice recommendation.
- Have clinician identify two actions to take to promote EBP addressing a relevant quality indicator.
- Use SMART (specific, measurable, actionable, realistic, time bound) format for writing EBP goals.
- Create agreement regarding expected EBP performance objectives and timely feedback.
- Review EBP performance regularly and provide just-in-time verbal and written feedback.
- Set incremental and progressively more advanced performance goals for EBP mastery.

### EXAMPLE

**EBP Performance Goals**

In the next 6 months, I will complete the following unit activities:

- Create a unit educational poster of pain-assessment methods for older adults with dementia.
- Complete a monthly chart audit of first 10 admissions with a diagnosis of dementia related to the following process indicators: frequency of pain assessment, self-report versus nonverbal assessment methods, pain scale used, patient report of acceptability of pain intensity, charting of pain quality and locations, interventions used when pain is rated "not acceptable," and monitoring for risk of sedation.

### CITATIONS

Fleiszer, Semenic, Ritchie, Richer, & Denis, 2016b; Fleuren, van Dommelen, & Dunnink, 2015; Hageman, Ring, Gregory, Rubash, & Harmon, 2015; Hysong, Kell, Petersen, Campbell, & Trautner, 2016; Hysong, Knox, & Haidet, 2014; Ivers et al., 2012; Ivers et al., 2014; Lehotsky et al., 2015; Maas et al., 2015; Medicare, n.d.-b; Nemeth, 2014; Raja et al., 2015; Stetler, Ritchie, Rycroft-Malone, & Charns, 2014.

# Implementation Strategies for Evidence-Based Practice
## PHASE 4: PURSUE INTEGRATION & SUSTAINED USE

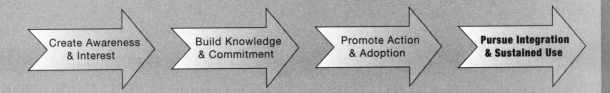

The most complex implementation strategies to perform are described. The evidence on how to use the procedures is provided to improve their effectiveness. Use in combination for a comprehensive implementation plan.

## Strategy 4-1    Celebrate Local Unit Progress

| PHASE | 4: Pursue Integration & Sustained Use |
|---|---|
| FOCUS | Connecting With Clinicians, Organizational Leaders, and Key Stakeholders |

### DEFINITION

Celebrations are events or presentations to share and acknowledge local unit progress regarding impact and sustainability of an EBP change.

### BENEFITS

- Demonstrates interest and value from unit and organizational leaders.
- Acknowledges success; recognizes and celebrates achievements.
- Encourages clinicians to maintain their momentum related to practice change recommendations.
- Focuses energy on achieving the goal of a sustained practice change.
- Produces positive influences on clinicians (e.g., job satisfaction, commitment to the organization).
- Bestows confidence and enthusiastic energy.

### PROCEDURE

- Determine purpose of celebration:
  - Single or multiple topics
  - Individual or team progress
- Decide on the type of setting for the celebration (e.g., grand rounds, social gathering).
- Decide whom to invite (be inclusive and strategic).
- Determine the moderator or speaker for the event (e.g., senior leader).
  - Provide the moderator/speaker with information in advance for preparation.
- Choose the date and time; consider repeating the event for night and weekend clinicians.
- Determine the best location (e.g., in or near work setting) and reserve space.
- Determine the space layout and specific setup; reserve equipment.
- Select a theme.
- Estimate the available budget for food, awards or prizes, and decorations.
- Advertise the event or presentation within the organization (e.g., email broadcast, flyer) and/or to external or community representatives.
- Create and order awards or prizes (e.g., plaque, certificate).
- Order food.
- Arrange or set up site to be used.
- Decorate and arrange displays (e.g., posters [see Strategy 1-6]).
- Take photos before, during, and after the celebration.
- Send thank you notes to those involved (e.g., moderator or speaker, presenters, individuals, teams).
- Write a brief report regarding the celebration to share internally and/or externally (e.g., news release, blog, digital displays in public areas).

EXAMPLE

# EBP Staff Nurse Internship Celebration

Nursing Research & EBP Committee and Office of Nursing Research, EBP & Quality
Department of Nursing Services and Patient Care

UNIVERSITY OF IOWA
HOSPITALS&CLINICS
University of Iowa Health Care
Department of Nursing Services
and Patient Care

University of Iowa
Stead Family
Children's Hospital
Changing Medicine. Changing Kids' Lives.®

## Purpose

- To celebrate the success of the most recent EBP Staff Nurse Interns and teams

## Frameworks

- The Iowa Model Revised: Evidence-Based Practice to Promote Excellence in Health Care (Iowa Model Collaborative, 2017)
- Implementation Strategies for EBP (Cullen & Adams, 2012)

## EBP Interns

- Kristina Ehret, MSN, RN, CCRN
- Robin Enfield, BSN, RN, CNRN
- Shannon Greene, BSN, RN
- Seth Jackson, BSN, RN
- Amy Lage, BSN, RN, C-NPT
- Lori Oberbroeckling, BSN, RN, CEN
- Amanda Poock, BSN, RN
- Abby Salton, BSN, RNC-OB

## Acknowledgements

- Partial funding from the Office of Nursing Research, EBP & Quality
- Nurses and teams who supported each project

Invitation

### Superman Initiative: Prone Therapy for Severe ARDS in MICU

Intern: Kristina Ehret, MSN, RN, CCRN
Staff Nurse Mentor: Amy Bowman, BSN, RN, CCRN
Team: Cheryl Bonder, MSN, RN, CCRN; Joe Greiner, BSN, RN, CPN2;
Lynn Comried, MA, RN, CCRN; Melissa Forsythe, RRT; Dana Foster,
ARNP; Rhonda Barr, DPT; Sue Little, RD; Gregory Schmidt, MD; Kevin
Doerschug, MD; Michele Farrington, BSN, RN, CPHON; Laura Cullen,
DNP, RN, FAAN

### Defining an Evidence-Based Practice for Seizure Recognition and Management

Intern: Robin Enfield, BSN, RN, CNRN
Staff Nurse Mentor: Colleen Finnegan, BSN, RN
Team: Dan Le, BSN, RN; Michele Wiegel, MSN, RN, CNRN; Kelly Petrulevich, BSN,
RN, OCN; Gloria Dorr, MA, RN-BC; Laura Cullen, DNP, RN, FAAN

### Lymphedema Patient Education

Intern: Shannon Greene, BSN, RN
Team: Carmen Kealoha, MA, RN; Linda Abbott, DNP, RN, CWON, AOCN;
Stephanie Cummings, BSN, RN; Wei Chen, MD, FACS; Angela Williams,
MA; Megan Zarifis, CMA; Karisa Schnieders, BSN, RN; CMSRN; Ericka
Larson, BSN, RN; Jean Arnett, MA, RN, CBCN, AOCN; Becca Miner, DNP
RN-BC, CNML; Jody Martin, OTR/L, CLT; Michele Farrington, BSN, RN,
CPHON

### Spore No More: C. Diff in MICU

Intern: Seth Jackson, BSN, RN
Staff Nurse Mentor: Amy Bowman, BSN, RN, CCRN
Team: Cheryl Bomber, MSN, RN, CCRN; Karen Stenger, MA, RN, CCRN;
Lynn Comried, MA, RN, CCRN; Laura Cullen, DNP, RN, FAAN

### Improving Critical Thinking Skills in Newer Nursing Staff with Preceptor Led Strategies

Intern: Amy Lage, BSN, RN, C-NPT
Team: Jeanna Hampton, RN, MBA, RNC-NIC; Stephanie Stewart, MSN,
RNC-NIC; Emily Spellman, MSN, RNC-NIC; Michele Farrington, BSN, RN, CPHON

### Multidisciplinary Approach to Reduce Return Visits to the ED

Intern: Lori Oberbroeckling, BSN, RN, CEN
Team: Laura Vahnke, MSN, RN, CNRN; Greg Bell, MD; Alycia Rarsjem, MSW; Katy
Demeulenaere, MSW; Melanie Berry, BA; Peggy O'Neill, BSN, RN, ACM; Sharon Tucker, PhD,
RN, PMHCNS-BC, FAAN; Anita Fagerlund, RN; Stacy Davis, BSN, RN, Joanne Grey, MSN, MA,
RN; Nancy Hall, BSN, RN; Vivian Oviluda, MBA, MSN, RN; Lauren Yapp, BSN, RN; Ryan
Faustino, ASN, RN, RNEMT-P, CCP, BA; Casaundra Ellis, BSN, RN, CEH; Amelia Godfrey-Love,
BSN, RN; Michele Farrington, BSN, RN, CPHON

### Nutritional Screening Tool for Outpatient Adult Oncology Patients

Intern: Amanda Poock, BSN, RN
Team: Geralyn Quinn, MSN, RN, OCN; Linda Abbott, DNP, RN, CWON, AOCN;
Doug Robertson, RDN, LD; Bridget Drapeaux, MA, RDN, LD; Amy Lukas, RD, LD;
Gloria Dorr, MA, RN-BC; Bracii Bingham; Kenth Burrell; Kenneth Nepple, MD;
Michele Farrington, BSN, RN, CPHON

### Intrapartum Bladder Care

Intern: Abby Salton, BSN, RNC-OB
Team: Amy Salton, BSN, RN, C-EFM; Jessie Forman, MSN, RN, RNC-OB;
Hilary Mann, MSN, RN, RNC-OB; Lynn Hinmeitoch, MPH, ARNP, CNM; Jenny
Driscoll, BSN, RN; Tracy Finke, NA; Kelly Ward, MD; Michele Farrington,
BSN, RN, CPHON

PHASE 4

*continues*

## Strategy 4-1    Celebrate Local Unit Progress (Continued)

### CITATIONS

Berenson & Rice, 2016; Dogherty, Harrison, & Graham, 2010; Dogherty, Harrison, Graham, Vandyk, & Keeping-Burke, 2013; Frasure, 2014; Kouzes & Posner, 2012; Odedra & Hitchcock, 2012; Sveinsdóttir, Ragnarsdóttir, & Blöndal, 2016; van der Zijpp et al., 2016.

## Strategy 4-2   Individualize Data Feedback

| PHASE | 4: Pursue Integration & Sustained Use |
|---|---|
| FOCUS | Connecting With Clinicians, Organizational Leaders, and Key Stakeholders |

### DEFINITION

Individualized data feedback is the communication of collected data related to an individual's performance, reported back to the individual and/or the team to demonstrate one's improvement or need for improvement over time, compare individual to group performance as a motivator, or show a direct impact on results.

### BENEFITS

- Motivates clinicians positively when a nonpunitive, learning approach is used.
- Offers individual access to EBP results as it directly relates to one's personal contribution and provides direction for how to improve one's own performance.
- Allows individuals to feel part of a team and encourages participation in other EBP improvements.
- Monitors practice in real time.
- Can be used with limited resources.
- Improves the learning environment for systematic change by providing data to show trends.

### PROCEDURE

- Use a systematic approach for both evaluation and feedback.
- Select only a few critical indicators for data collection and reporting that are perceived as credible by end users (see Chapter 9):
  - Consider reliability, validity, and representativeness of data.
  - Consider individual competence skill levels and behaviors (see Strategy 3-3).
  - Identify the comparison (e.g., individual to team, data reported in clinical practice guidelines or research reports, within group comparison).
- Determine benchmarks for comparison (see Strategy 2-20).
- Determine method of data collection (e.g., chart audit [see Strategy 3-12], video surveillance).
  - Determine where to locate the data for data retrieval (e.g., acceptable documentation).
  - Create a monitoring tool or data report of the few critical indicators with operational definitions for consistent data analysis.
- Determine the sample and time frame for data collection.
- Establish credibility with clinician recipients or have data feedback provided by a credible local leader/ champion (see Strategy 2-4).
- Make performance observable (see Strategy 2-11); display (e.g., graph) results to demonstrate unit average, acceptable benchmarks (see Strategy 2-20) or high performers compared to individual clinician.
- Identify clinicians consistently performing better than average and determine their workflow for shared learning.
- Provide each individual with a personalized document detailing the effect of his or her contribution to the results.

*continues*

## Strategy 4-2    Individualize Data Feedback (Continued)

### PROCEDURE (Continued)

- Provide timely, nonpunitive feedback based on data collected.
  - Begin by asking for insights:
    - ☐ How have you attempted to use the practice change?
    - ☐ Are you satisfied with your use of the practice change?
    - ☐ Can you point out important steps that were missed?
  - Respond.
  - Provide descriptive feedback about specific recommended tasks or procedures:
    - ☐ Describe what was done correctly.
    - ☐ Provide suggestions for how to make improvements.
    - ☐ Link to the practice recommendation.
    - ☐ Display the data.
    - ☐ Reinforce correct and incorrect practices.
    - ☐ Discuss the situations when appropriate practices were difficult to follow or did not occur.
    - ☐ Review documentation as a learning tool.
  - Ask for additional insights:
    - ☐ Do you feel a need to improve?
    - ☐ How do you prefer to receive information on your performance?
  - Respond.
  - Ask for suggestions:
    - ☐ Was this discussion helpful?
    - ☐ What will help you apply this knowledge in practice?
  - Respond with question-and-answer discussion, and develop an action plan (see Strategy 2-22).
- Allow for individual review, then anonymous review and discussion, prior to publicly reporting individual clinician data compared to better performers or the group mean.
- Discuss data using a learning-and-improvement approach that is professional, objective, fair, and nonpunitive:
  - Identify relevance to desired outcome.
  - Describe strategies to improve performance.
  - Plan for reporting data within quality improvement program.
  - Plan for additional rounds of data collection and reporting.
- Make subsequent decisions based on the data that focus on a few key behaviors.
- Offer appreciation for participating in the EBP change as a means of encouraging future involvement and interest in projects.
- Continue data feedback (see Strategy 3-13) to promote sustained change.

**EXAMPLE**

**EBP Compliance by Clinician**

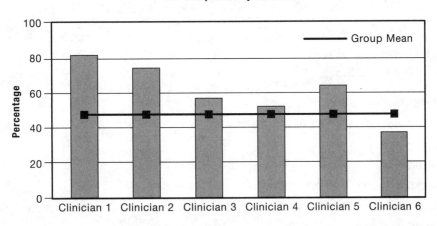

fictitious data

**CITATIONS**

Aggarwal, Singh, Sharma, Singh, & Bansal, 2016; Beaty et al., 2013; Bradley et al., 2004; Conway et al., 2014; Crowe et al., 2015; de Visser, 2015; Huis, Holleman et al., 2013; Larson et al., 2016; Larson, Patel, Evans, & Saiman, 2013; Levchenko, Boscart, & Fernie, 2014; Luke & Alavosius, 2011; Maas, van Dulmen et al., 2015; Ofek Shlomai, Rao, & Patole, 2015; Pusic et al., 2016; Raja et al., 2015; Spence, Derbyshire, Walsh, & Murray, 2016.

## Strategy 4-3    Public Recognition

| PHASE | 4: Pursue Integration & Sustained Use |
|---|---|
| FOCUS | Connecting With Clinicians, Organizational Leaders, and Key Stakeholders |

### DEFINITION

Public recognition acknowledges individual or interprofessional team success with EBP change.

### BENEFITS

- Engages interprofessional team.
- Increases feeling of value among the healthcare team.
- Improves team morale.
- Provides support.
- Promotes a positive, healthy work environment.
- Establishes expectations and norms for return on investment from support during work time or financial resources provided.

### PROCEDURE

- Determine frequency of recognition (e.g., weekly, monthly, quarterly) and ensure that it is provided in a timely manner.
- Determine whom to recognize (e.g., individual, interprofessional team) and how they can be identified or nominated.
- Determine recognition type and format (consider available technology):
  - Verbal (e.g., local press, the DAISY Award®, patient or family recognition opportunities, celebration event, "employee of the month")
  - Nonverbal (e.g., newspaper release, website announcement, social media, blog, digital displays in public areas, newsletter, kudos or thank-you board in clinical area public space)
  - Award or incentive (e.g., plaque, certificate) (see Strategy 3-5)
  - Nomination:
    - ☐ Local, state, or national professional organization
    - ☐ Local organization (e.g., Nurses' Week, Nursing Recognition Day)
  - Assist with abstract writing or development of an oral presentation, poster presentation, or publication.
- Decide who will provide the recognition (e.g., senior leader, nurse manager, physician, peer, administrator, retention and recognition committee).

## PROCEDURE

- Considerations for recognition event:
  - Determine whom to invite (be inclusive and strategic).
  - Decide who will provide the recognition (e.g., patient/family, peer, senior leader).
  - Choose date and time; consider repeating the event so that team members working nights and weekends can participate.
  - Determine best location and reserve space.
  - Determine whether food will be provided and place order.
  - Advertise event within organization (e.g., email broadcast, flyer) and/or to external or community representatives.

## EXAMPLE

The DAISY Foundation. (2017). What is the DAISY Award? Retrieved from https://www.daisyfoundation.org/daisy-award

## CITATIONS

Barnes, Barnes, & Sweeney, 2016a; Barnes, Barnes, & Sweeney, 2016b; Frasure, 2014; Ganz et al., 2013; Huddleston & Gray, 2016a; Huddleston & Gray, 2016b; Huddleston, Mancini, & Gray, 2017; Kouzes & Posner, 2012; Nayback-Beebe et al., 2013; Sung, Chang, & Abbey, 2008; Sveinsdóttir, Ragnarsdóttir, & Blöndal, 2016; Taylor, Clay-Williams, Hogden, Braithwaite, & Groene, 2015; Turck, Silva, Tremblay, & Sachse, 2014; van der Zijpp et al., 2016.

## Strategy 4-4  Personalize the Messages to Staff Based on Actual Improvement Data

| PHASE | 4: Pursue Integration & Sustained Use |
| --- | --- |
| FOCUS | Connecting With Clinicians, Organizational Leaders, and Key Stakeholders |

### DEFINITION

Personalized messages are tailored communication and discussion related to the benefits and improved outcomes associated with practice recommendations for individual clinicians or groups of clinicians.

### BENEFITS

- Emphasizes advantages from adhering to practice recommendations.
- Promotes collaboration.
- Emphasizes shared accountability.
- Enhances self-motivation.

### PROCEDURE

- Determine method to systematically monitor and report ongoing use of practice recommendations (see Strategy 3-8) and associated outcomes.
  - Ensure that local data are readily available and timely.
  - Consider the type of data display (e.g., improvement needs to be clear, visible to all clinicians).
- Determine frequency of dialogue with clinicians (e.g., monthly, quarterly).
- Determine timing of discussions (e.g., daily huddle, shift change):
  - Needs to be consistent, regular, and meaningful.
  - Include all shifts (e.g., days, evenings, nights, weekends).
- Decide on type of interaction to provide follow-up and timely feedback to the interprofessional team (e.g., nurses, rehabilitation therapy, pharmacy, providers):
  - Individual or small group.
  - Informal or formal.
  - Face-to-face or discussion-based versus email or passive.
- Outline components of the message to be shared (e.g., improved or maintained patient outcomes, benefits to patients, benefits to clinicians, relevance to clinicians):
  - Frame and tailor the message to the characteristics of an individual or select group (e.g., not one size fits all, congruent with motivation).
  - Describe the benefits (e.g., "what's in it for me").
  - Ensure message aligns with context of clinical area, patient population, and clinical realities.
  - Provide rationale.
  - Indicate actions that individuals or groups can take to create further improvements.
- Consider creating a friendly competition between clinical areas if they are addressing the same practice change (e.g., hand hygiene, surgical-site infections).
- Determine whether rewards (see Strategy 3-11) or incentives (see Strategy 3-5) are available for high-performing areas.

| EXAMPLE |
| --- |

Formatted as sound bites (see Strategy 1-3) related to an EBP project on double-gloving for surgical procedures (Stebral & Steelman, 2006):

- Implementation of double-gloving decreased sharps injuries by 23.5%.

- Double-gloving saved time by decreasing the amount of required paperwork and need for a work-up in the employee health clinic if a sharps injury occurred.

- Use of double-gloving decreased the viral load exposure if a sharps injury did occur.

| CITATIONS |
| --- |

Caminiti, Scoditti, Diodati, & Passalacqua, 2005; Fleiszer, Semenic, Ritchie, Richer, & Denis, 2016a; Fleuren, van Dommelen, & Dunnink, 2015; Ireland, Kirkpatrick, Boblin, & Robertson, 2013; Pelletier & Sharp, 2008; Stebral & Steelman, 2006.

## Strategy 4-5   Peer Influence

| PHASE | 4: Pursue Integration & Sustained Use |
|---|---|
| FOCUS | Connecting With Clinicians, Organizational Leaders, and Key Stakeholders |

### DEFINITION

Peer influence involves interpersonal interaction and communication used by trusted, respected, credible colleagues to motivate incorporating practice recommendations as the new "norm" or standard for care delivery.

### BENEFITS

- Peers are often readily available and easily accessible.
- Builds trust and confidence in decision-making.
- Enhances open and bidirectional communication.
- Promotes teamwork.
- Advice tailored to the EBP change and the local clinical area context that increases knowledge and understanding for application.

### PROCEDURE

- Develop strategies to provide influence within social networks versus across social networks using established clinical experts.
- Characteristics:
  - Determine the type of healthcare team members (e.g., nurse, physician, housekeeper, front desk staff) to provide peer influence based on the practice change.
  - Choose motivated, persuasive individuals.
  - Find individuals positive about the change, dedicated to the topic, and respected and trusted by colleagues.
- Outline the responsibilities of the role to provide consistency.
- Decide on the method for peer influence (e.g., demonstration, observational learning, direction and guidance, experiential knowledge, simple clinical tips).
  - Multiple, interactive approaches are more successful than single approaches for integrating and sustaining practice changes.
- Deliver message as a peer for "just-in-time" discussion.
  - Choose 1:1 or group session.
  - Focus on interactive and coaching approach to interpersonal communication.
  - Tailor feedback to individual clinician requesting assistance and support to incorporate EBP change into work routine and in complex patient situations (see Strategies 2-19 and 3-10).
  - Adapt message to counter individual, organizational, and environmental barriers to the practice recommendations.
- Some alternatives to face-to-face discussion for an asynchronous approach include email, national newsletter or magazine, state or local announcement (see Strategy 1-7), and LISTSERV.
- Calculate reach (will depend on the delivery method selected and span of influence).
- Consider the use of competition to enhance practice improvements among individual clinicians or between clinical areas.

| EXAMPLES |
| --- |

**Formal Peer Influence:**

Nurse A: *As you know, I represent the unit on the Nursing Pain Committee as part of shared governance. At the committee meeting today, we discussed updates regarding pain management with nasogastric (NG) tube insertion for pediatric patients.*

Nurse B: *Oh, what's new?*

Nurse A: *Let's look at the policy. Page 2 has suggested strategies to reduce pain and fear with NG tube insertion that will benefit our pediatric patients. Research evidence supports the use of distraction before procedures to help with both fear and pain. A childlife specialist will first talk with the patient and family to determine the best approach based on the patient's needs. Here is how you can contact them. Atomized lidocaine is located in the medication-dispensing cabinet, and the dosing table is on the supply cabinet door. Do you have any questions about this?*

Nurse B: *Not right now, but I may have questions when I place my next NG tube.*

Nurse A: *Please let me know when you next take care of a patient with an order for NG tube placement. I would be happy to go with you to help* [see Strategies 3-9 and 3-10].

**Informal Peer Influence:**

Nurse A: *Can you help me with something?*

Nurse B: *Sure. What do you need?*

Nurse A: *I need to insert a nasogastric (NG) tube on the 5-year old patient in Room 2, but I have not done it in a while.*

Nurse B: *Let's look at the policy first. It has good information.*

Nurse A: *Give me 5 minutes to read this, and then I will come find you.*

(5 minutes later)

Nurse B: *Let's quickly discuss pain and fear management before we see the patient.*

Nurse A: *I need to obtain atomized lidocaine from the medication-dispensing cabinet, and the dose will be _____ because my patient weighs _____.*

Nurse B: *What do you think could also be done to help manage the patient's fear?*

Nurse A: *I am thinking about use of distraction by a childlife specialist.*

Nurse B: *Research evidence supports the use of distraction before procedures to help with both fear and pain. A childlife specialist will first talk with the patient and family to determine the best approach based on the patient's needs. Here is how you can contact them: _____.*

Nurse A: *Great. This is really helpful. Do you have any other tips?*

Nurse B: *I would be happy to go with you to help* [see Strategies 3-9 and 3-10].

(Farrington, Bruene, & Wagner, 2015)

**PHASE 4**

*continues*

## Strategy 4-5    Peer Influence (Continued)

### CITATIONS

Alkhateeb & Doucette, 2009; Bosch et al., 2016; Farrington, Bruene, & Wagner, 2015; Gainforth et al., 2014; Hoke & Guarracino, 2016; Huis, Holleman et al., 2013; Johnson, Ford II, & McCluskey, 2012; Kaasalainen et al., 2015; Lau et al., 2016; Maas, van der Wees et al., 2015; Magers, 2014; Mold, Aspy et al., 2014; Ploeg et al., 2010; Pronovost et al., 2013; Rangachari et al., 2014; Taylor, Clay-Williams, Hogden, Braithwaite, & Groene, 2015; Thompson et al., 2001b.

## Strategy 4-6    Audit and Feedback

| PHASE | 4: Pursue Integration & Sustained Use |
|-------|---------------------------------------|
| FOCUS | Building Organizational System Support |

### DEFINITION

Audit and feedback refers to a collection and reporting of "any summary of clinical performance of health care over a specified period of time" that includes data or key indicators with actionable steps to take that will contribute to improvement (Ivers et al., 2012, p. 7).

### BENEFITS

- Clearly describes how to improve clinical outcomes for patients based on key structure, process, and outcome indicators.
- Improves clinician involvement through goal-setting.
- Most effective when large improvement is needed.
- Creates a learning culture.
- Reduces cost.
- Helps sustain a practice change.

### PROCEDURE

- Select indicators (see Strategy 3-12).
  - Use pilot data (see Chapter 9) to determine which key indicators to continue to evaluate for sustaining EBP.
  - Narrow to key structure, process, and outcome indicators (see Chapter 11).
  - Obtain input from clinical experts to select key indicators.
  - Continue to include balancing indicators that may help explain or influence outcomes (e.g., length of stay may be influenced by level of physical activity during admission, duration of mechanical ventilation, or discharge location).
- Plan data collection and management.
  - Determine availability and access to existing data (e.g., documentation in the health record) or need for manual data collection.
  - Plan for protection of patient identity (i.e., remove identifiers) and data security (e.g., data storage).
  - Plan for data management (i.e., data entry, cleanup, analysis, report format).
  - Submit request for data report or download, indicating that the work is EBP.
  - Collect and clean data.
  - Enter data for electronic analysis and establish reliability with minimum (e.g., 10%) recheck.
- Establish a goal or threshold for process and outcome indicators.
- Create graphs for data reports using a consistent format for display and easy interpretation (see Chapters 9 and 11) to make the need for improvement observable (see Strategy 2-11).
  - Adjust graphical display to spotlight or shift attention to details about the task to be completed that will help to achieve desired improvement.

**PHASE 4**

*continues*

## Strategy 4-6   Audit and Feedback (Continued)

### PROCEDURE (Continued)

- Provide timely, specific/actionable suggestions about how to improve. Link indicators to supporting evidence.
- Encourage and praise practices with high performance or demonstrated progress.
- Provide feedback in written form or post in clinical area.
- Ensure data are used in team discussions to facilitate ownership and action planning (see Strategy 2-22).
- Provide trend for comparison data from last measurement period (especially if trending data make recent changes less obvious) (see Tool 11.2).
- Determine frequency that provides regular, periodic actionable feedback (i.e., frequent, timely feedback improves impact) (see Strategy 3-13).
- Re-evaluate target for key indicators.

### EXAMPLES

Example 1: Fall Prevention Audit

| Record Number | Admit Date | Unit | Fall Risk Assessment Completed Daily | Physical Activity Impairment Present | PT/OT Referral | Safe-Handling Practices Used | Ambulation at Lease BID | Fall |
|---|---|---|---|---|---|---|---|---|
| | | | ☐ Yes<br>☐ No | ☐ Yes<br>☐ No | ☐ Yes<br>☐ No | ☐ Yes<br>☐ No | ☐ Yes<br>☐ No | ☐ Yes<br>☐ No |
| | | | ☐ Yes<br>☐ No | ☐ Yes<br>☐ No | ☐ Yes<br>☐ No | ☐ Yes<br>☐ No | ☐ Yes<br>☐ No | ☐ Yes<br>☐ No |
| | | | ☐ Yes<br>☐ No | ☐ Yes<br>☐ No | ☐ Yes<br>☐ No | ☐ Yes<br>☐ No | ☐ Yes<br>☐ No | ☐ Yes<br>☐ No |
| | | | ☐ Yes<br>☐ No | ☐ Yes<br>☐ No | ☐ Yes<br>☐ No | ☐ Yes<br>☐ No | ☐ Yes<br>☐ No | ☐ Yes<br>☐ No |
| | | | ☐ Yes<br>☐ No | ☐ Yes<br>☐ No | ☐ Yes<br>☐ No | ☐ Yes<br>☐ No | ☐ Yes<br>☐ No | ☐ Yes<br>☐ No |
| | | | ☐ Yes<br>☐ No | ☐ Yes<br>☐ No | ☐ Yes<br>☐ No | ☐ Yes<br>☐ No | ☐ Yes<br>☐ No | ☐ Yes<br>☐ No |
| | | | ☐ Yes<br>☐ No | ☐ Yes<br>☐ No | ☐ Yes<br>☐ No | ☐ Yes<br>☐ No | ☐ Yes<br>☐ No | ☐ Yes<br>☐ No |
| | | | ☐ Yes<br>☐ No | ☐ Yes<br>☐ No | ☐ Yes<br>☐ No | ☐ Yes<br>☐ No | ☐ Yes<br>☐ No | ☐ Yes<br>☐ No |

Example 2: Falls Data for Feedback

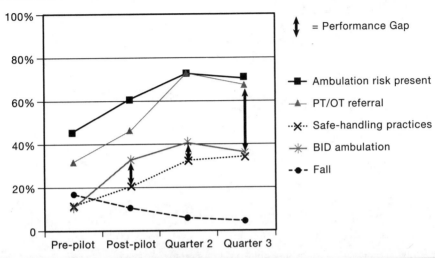

CITATIONS

Armellion et al., 2013; Cahill, Murch, Cook, & Heyland, 2014; de Vos et al., 2013; Fleiszer, Semenic, Ritchie, Richer, & Denis, 2016a; Hysong, Kell, Petersen, Campbell, & Trautner, 2016; Hysong, Knox, & Haidet, 2014; Hysong, Teal, Khan, & Haidet, 2012; Ivers et al., 2012; Ivers et al., 2014; Landis-Lewis, Brehaut, Hochheiser, Douglas, & Jacobson, 2015; Larson et al., 2016; Larson, Patel, Evans, & Saiman, 2013; Lowson et al., 2015; Lugtenberg et al., 2014; Milat, Bauman, & Redman, 2015; Overdyk et al., 2016; Payne & Hysong, 2016; Taylor, Clay-Williams, Hogden, Braithwaite, & Groene, 2015; van der Voort, van der Veer, & de Vos, 2012; WHO, 2010.

PHASE 4

## Strategy 4-7   Revise Policy, Procedure, or Protocol

| PHASE | 4: Pursue Integration & Sustained Use |
|---|---|
| FOCUS | Building Organizational System Support |

### DEFINITION

Revising a policy, procedure, or protocol is to update a written standard for practice that outlines steps to follow and is based on current evidence. Procedural elements may be edited based on lessons learned during the pilot.

### BENEFITS

- Improves standardization and provides direction for safe EBP.
- Improves processes and outcomes.
- Reduces litigation claims.
- Incorporates the practice change into the infrastructure to promote sustainable change.

### PROCEDURE

- Determine the need for a written protocol (see Tool 7.1).
  - Not every nursing practice can or should have a written protocol.
  - Identify whether a written protocol exists or a new one will need to be developed.
  - Consider the organizational context.
- Notify the committee responsible for protocol development and approval of your plans for revisions.
- Seek practice questions and feedback from key stakeholders; include patient preferences.
- Format protocol revisions according to organizational standards and submit for review and approval.
  - Outline key components of practice and cite associated evidence.
  - Outline the procedure steps required to perform the practice or consider partnering with a commercial vendor for an electronic evidence-based procedure manual.
  - Include explanatory information, if needed (e.g., key points from the evidence).
  - Specify applicable patient populations and frequency of assessments, interventions, or monitoring.
  - Consider including a description of how to document the practice (e.g., screen shots).
  - Add resource links, if available.
  - Add the development, review, and/or revision dates.

- Integrate practice change into the workflow (see Strategy 3-2).
  - Coordinate with informatics for order sets (see Strategy 3-16), documentation (see Strategy 3-15), or alerts (see Strategy 3-1) included in the protocol.
  - Create supplemental tools (e.g., checklist [see Strategy 3-14] and/or an algorithm [see Strategy 3-2]) that facilitate implementation of the practice change.
- Include the written protocol in education and competency testing.
- A simulation experience that uses the written protocol increases the likelihood that clinicians will use the EBP in providing care. Ensure that the necessary resources, equipment, and supplies are readily available.
- Disseminate the protocol to stakeholders:
  - Use the organizational committees and infrastructure.
  - Communicate the protocol to clinicians using additional strategies (e.g., academic detailing [see Strategy 2-9] and unit champions [see Strategy 2-4]).
- Identify other implementation strategies to combine with this one; revising the protocol alone does not ensure adherence.
- Monitor effectiveness of the protocol by collecting point prevalence data (e.g., audit [see Strategy 3-12] and provide actionable feedback to stakeholders [see Strategies 3-13 and 4-6]).

*continues*

**Strategy 4-7    Revise Policy, Procedure, or Protocol (Continued)**

EXAMPLE

AC-01.02.500

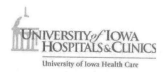

**Policy and Procedure Manual**

**Department of Nursing Services and Patient
Ambulatory Care Standards of Practice**                          AC- 01.02.500

---

**SUBJECT/TITLE:**    Pain Management in the Ambulatory Setting

**PURPOSE:**    To provide standardized pain management.
To describe assessment and documentation standards for patients in the
ambulatory setting.

**POLICY:**

1. Patients who routinely receive any component of a nursing screening/assessment (e.g., vital
   signs) will be screened for pain[R1, N1] which will be documented in the electronic health
   record.
   a. Positive screening results for pain will be communicated to the licensed independent
      practitioner (LIP) for follow-up.

2. If an intervention for pain is provided (including non-pharmacologic interventions), the
   patient and/or family will receive education regarding pain management[R2-R5, L1-L3] and an
   assessment of pain will be completed at baseline and peak effect of the intervention, if the
   patient remains in the clinic at the peak effect time of the intervention.
   a. If the patient is able to provide a self-report of pain, assessment may include pain
      intensity or a value from another self-report scale.
   b. If the patient is unable to provide a self-report of pain, pain assessment will include
      use of an appropriate pain scale based on the patient's age.

3. If an opioid medication is ordered by the LIP for pain or prior to a procedure that does not
   include procedural sedation:
   a. Complete and document the following with each dose administered:
      i.  Sedation assessment using the Modified Pasero Opioid-Induced Sedation
          Scale (POSS)[N2]
      ii. Respiratory assessment[N2]
          a) Rate
          b) Rhythm/Pattern

Pain Management in the Ambulatory Setting
Page 1 of 3

PHASE 4

| EXAMPLE |
|---|

AC-01.02.500

    c) Effort

    d) Depth

    e) Airway Characteristics

b. If the patient will be discharged prior to the initial reassessment (timing based on peak effect of opioid, patient activity, risk factors for sedation, and previous exposure to opioids) after opioid administration, the patient/family will be instructed on what to watch for and report to the LIP.

c. If the patient remains in the clinic at the time of the initial reassessment (timing based on peak effect of opioid, patient activity, risk factors for sedation, and previous exposure to opioids), the following are completed and documented:

    i. Sedation assessment using the Modified POSS[N2]

    ii. Respiratory assessment[N2]

        a) Rate

        b) Rhythm/Pattern

        c) Effort

        d) Depth

        e) Airway Characteristics

4. Follow policy SS-A-01.19 for opioid medications administered as part of procedural sedation.

## PRECAUTIONS, CONSIDERATIONS, AND OBSERVATIONS:

1. Administration of an opioid medication is communicated (e.g., ticket to ride, verbal report) when a patient is transferred to another clinic or inpatient unit.

2. Special consideration is given when certain medications (e.g., benzodiazepines, antiemetics, antiepileptics, antihistamines) are administered in addition to an opioid medication since these medications may potentiate sedation.

## RELATED DEPARTMENT OF NURSING STANDARDS:

AC-01-.01.060 Intake of Patients for Outpatient Visit
N-02.401 Pain Management for Adults: Inpatient
N-02.402 Monitoring for Unintended Sedation in Patients Receiving Opioids for Pain Management - Inpatient
N-CWS-PEDS-02.080 Pain Management for Infants and Children

## RELATED HOSPITAL WIDE POLICIES:

SS-A-01.19    Procedural Sedation and Analgesia Program

*continues*

PHASE 4

**Strategy 4-7   Revise Policy, Procedure, or Protocol (Continued)**

**EXAMPLE (Continued)**

AC-01.02.500

## REFERENCES:

R1   Rhodes, D.J., Koshy, R.C., Waterfield, W.C., Wu, A.W., & Grossman, S.A. (2001). Feasibility of quantitative pain assessment in outpatient oncology practice. *Journal of Clinical Oncology, 19*(2), 501-508.

R2   Dewar, A., Craig, K., Muir, J., & Cole, C. (2003). Testing the effectiveness of a nursing intervention in relieving pain following day surgery. *Ambulatory Surgery, 10*(2), 81-88.

R3   Good, M., Albert, J. M., Anderson, G. C., Wotman, S., Cong, X., Lane, D., & Ahn, S. (2010). Supplementing relaxation and music for pain after surgery. *Nursing Research, 59*(4), 259-269.

R4   Tracy, S., Dufault, M., Kogut, S., Martin, V., Rossi, S., & Willey-Temkin, C. (2007). Translating best practices in nondrug postoperative pain management. *Nursing Research, 55*(2 Suppl.), S57-S67.

R5   Wong, E. M., Chan, S. W., & Chair, S. Y. (2010). Effectiveness of an educational intervention on levels of pain, anxiety, and self-efficacy for patients with musculoskeletal trauma. *Journal of Advanced Nursing, 66*(5), 1120-1131.

N1   American Pain Society. (2008). *Principles of analgesic use in the treatment of acute pain* (6th ed.). Glenview, IL: American Pain Society.

N2   Jarzyna, D., Jungquist, C. R., Pasero, C., Willens, J. S., Nisbet, A., Oakes, L., . . . Polomano, R. C. (2011). American Society for Pain Management Nursing guidelines on monitoring for opioid-induced sedation and respiratory depression. *Pain Management Nursing, 12*(3), 118-145.

L1   Pasero, C., & McCaffery, M. (2011). *Pain assessment and pharmacologic management.* St. Louis, MO: Mosby, Inc.

L2   Wells, N., Pasero, C., & McCaffery, M. (2008). Improving the quality of care through pain assessment and management. In R.G. Hughes (Ed.), *Patient safety and quality: An evidence-based handbook for nurses* (pp. 1-29). Rockville, MD: Agency for Healthcare Research and Quality.

L3   Pasero, C. (2009). Assessment of sedation during opioid administration for pain management. *Journal of PeriAnesthesia Nursing, 24*(3), 186-190.

Date created:  2/01
Source:  PNP
Date approved:  2/01
Date effective:  2/01
Date Revised:  8/01, 7/04, 7/07, 10/10, 10/13, 03/14, 12/16
Date Reviewed:

PHASE 4

## CITATIONS

Aebersold, 2011; Aldeyab et al., 2011; Alexander & Allen, 2011; Bosch et al., 2016; Bray, Cummings, Wolf, Massing, & Reaves, 2009; Delmore, Lebovits, Baldock, Suggs, & Ayello, 2011; Devalia, 2010; Dixon & Keasling, 2014; Duff, Walker, & Omari, 2011; Farrington, Cullen, & Dawson, 2010; Krill, Staffileno, & Raven, 2012; Long, Burkett, & McGee, 2009; Melnyk, Fineout-Overholt, Gallagher-Ford, & Stillwell, 2011; Moore, 2014; Oman, Duran, & Fink, 2008; O'Rourke et al., 2011; Qaseem, Snow, Owens, Shekelle, & Clinical Guidelines Committee of the American College of Physicians, 2010; Rodriguez et al., 2014; Squires, Moralejo, & Lefort, 2007; Wagner, Matthews, & Cullen, 2013; Weddig, Baker, & Auld, G., 2011.

## Strategy 4-8    Competency Metric for Discontinuing Training

| PHASE | 4: Pursue Integration & Sustained Use |
|---|---|
| FOCUS | Building Organizational System Support |

### DEFINITION

A competency metric for discontinuing training refers to clinical performance at a preset goal indicating successful learning and performance of essential skills. This provides an opportunity to discontinue training, as the target for achievement indicates sufficient performance such that loss of sustainment is unlikely, and monitoring may be less frequent or done informally.

### BENEFITS

- Sets basic competency standard for provision of evidence-based care.
- Provides direction for development of educational or other implementation strategies to promote EBP without use of unnecessary resources.
- Allows for identification of expertise that translates to minimum expenditure of time and energy by clinicians.

### PROCEDURE

- Identify learning goals by reviewing knowledge/cognitive, attitudes/affective, skills/psychomotor, and other objectives (e.g., values, attributes) that are imperative to the EBP change and reflect the 'real world' of practice.
- Develop operational definitions for key indicators and relevant time frame for attainment and evaluation.
- Determine method of data collection:
  - Chart audit (see Strategy 3-12)
  - Observation
  - Video recording
  - Patient interview
  - Clinician interview or self report (least accurate)
  - Incident reports
- Identify or create assessment tools for key indicators that capture maximum information for performance but balance with feasibility.
- Validate measurement of behavior/practice performance measures.
- Set target for acceptable performance measures.
- Provide faculty development to ensure reliable assessments.
- Establish inter-rater reliability for competency assessment to be completed by more than one data collector, if appropriate.
- Provide standardized conditions for performance practice and assessment.
- Monitor performance (see Strategy 4-6) on indicators at a minimally acceptable level.

- Reassess performance to determine performance retention and provide feedback (see Strategy 3-13) on key indicators as needed to clinicians, trainees, or students.
- Discontinue competency assessment when target performance achieved.
- Stay attuned for identified need to reinforce or revise competency training and assessment.

## EXAMPLE

Knowledge and skill competency assessment is used to track individual or group competency to established goals. These assessments should be used to determine readiness to move away from continued training toward more advanced skill acquisition. In this example, monitoring patient response to pain medications includes monitoring for sedation and respiratory status (Chou et al., 2016; Fishman et al., 2013; Herr et al., 2015).

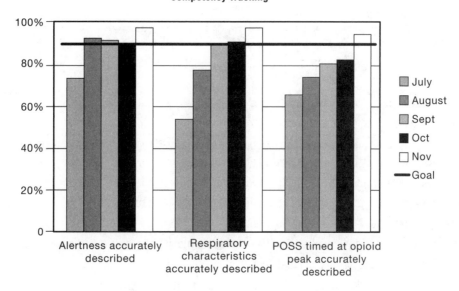

**Competency Tracking**

fictitious data

## CITATIONS

Bhatti & Ahmed, 2015; Chou et al., 2016; Clinkard et al., 2015; Fishman et al., 2013; Fleuren, van Dommelen, & Dunnink, 2015; Gattinger et al., 2015; Herr et al., 2015; Leung, Trevena, & Waters, 2014; Leung, Trevena, & Waters, 2016; Panzarella, 2003; Reynolds, McLennon, Ebright, Murray, & Bakas, 2016; Reynolds, Murray, McLennon, & Bakas, 2016; Salaripour & Perl, 2013; Sprakes & Tyrer, 2010; Wishart, Warwick, Pitsinis, Duffy, & Britton, 2010.

PHASE 4

## Strategy 4-9    Strategic Plan

| PHASE | 4: Pursue Integration & Sustained Use |
|-------|----------------------------------------|
| FOCUS | Building Organizational System Support |

### DEFINITION

The strategic plan is a document used to outline how to actualize the organization's mission. Strategic planning for EBP is done at the organizational, departmental, and clinical team level.

### BENEFITS

- Improves CEO commitment.
- Promotes development of organizational infrastructure.
- Improves outcomes and financial performance.

### PROCEDURE

- Arrange time to review internal needs and external pressures (e.g., national agenda).
- Involve clinicians.
- Identify key priorities (e.g., clinical outcomes, cost savings).
  - Consider strength of body of evidence for each priority.
- Identify existing strengths and opportunities that can leverage clinician skills and competitive advantage while also addressing performance gaps (see Strategy 2-12).
- Scan horizon for opportunities with the perspective of the ideal future or desire for change.
- Address organizational characteristics necessary to facilitate provision of EBP:
  - Provide protected time, free of clinical responsibility.
  - Regular discussion and implementation of EBP in order to motivate leaders and clinicians' contributions.
  - Provide easily accessible information and educational resources.
  - Create mechanisms for empowering and involving clinicians to enact change that will contribute to organizational goals and break down hierarchical structures.
  - Align professional goals with organizational goals (i.e., clinical outcomes versus fiscal constraints).
  - Build a sense of professional autonomy that allows flexibility to address the clinical need, within flexible protocols and without fear of "blame."
  - Include mechanisms that support recognition (see Strategy 4-3) and dissemination (see Chapter 12).
- Create stretch goals that capture where you want to be in 2–3 years and that align with a view toward future developments:
  - Stretch goals for focal areas (e.g., pain management) essential for achieving the organizational mission.
  - Stretch goals for clinicians' work beyond existing roles.

■ Link goals to existing or needed committees or infrastructure to promote persistent commitment.

■ Provide clear steps that make implementation actionable.

■ Include evaluative component for demonstrating that the goal was accomplished.

■ Create a business case that will "sell" an idea beyond describing it as a "patient need."

■ Communicate the strategic plan broadly.

■ Regularly review and discuss, with organizational leaders, including EBP initiatives, developments, progress, and outcomes.

■ Include reporting of EBP metrics (e.g., EBP initiatives, outcomes, and reach) to the CEO and governing board.

■ Regularly review, update, and renew commitment to the plan.

■ Seek CEO and leadership renewed commitment to the strategic plan.

## EXAMPLE

Elements of an organizational strategic plan for resources and EBP:

Invest in development of organizational experts:

■ Select an EBP process model for consistent use.

■ Provide grand rounds describing how to use the Iowa Model.

■ Lead discussions during performance-improvement committee meetings using two to three example EBP initiatives (e.g., pressure injury prevention) currently active, and match the steps used with the Iowa Model.

■ Recruit clinicians and leaders with EBP experience.

Provide internal and external programs:

■ Provide 4-hour continuing education program describing steps in the Iowa Model.

■ Create a mechanism for addressing clinician-identified issues.

■ Identify two annual national/international CE programs and budget for staff attendance; submit abstracts for paper or poster presentation.

Identify resources:

■ Add librarian as a member of the nursing practice committee.

■ Create and update an internal portal with links to resources.

■ Locate existing printed materials (see Strategy 2-16) (e.g., guidelines, toolkits) on topics now underway (e.g., pressure injury prevention).

■ Locate faculty from local school of nursing with interest in EBP to serve as mentor.

Celebrate success with high-profile recognition and rewards:

■ Provide EBP award ceremony during Nurses' Week.

■ Recognize teams achieving exceptional clinical outcomes during CEO announcements or award ceremony.

*continues*

## Strategy 4-9    Strategic Plan (Continued)

### CITATIONS

Aarons, Ehrhart, Farahnak, & Sklar, 2014; Alleyne & Jumaa, 2007; Bernstein et al., 2009; Boyal & Hewison, 2016; Brandt et al., 2009; Chang, 2014; Cullen, Greiner, Greiner, Bombei, & Comried, 2005; Drenkard, 2012; Flodgren, Rojas-Reyes, Cole, & Foxcroft, 2012; Hauck, Winsett, & Kuric, 2013; Ingersoll, Witzel, Berry, & Qualls, 2010; Jeffs, MacMillan, McKey, & Ferris, 2009; Kaissi & Begun, 2008; Puetz, 2014; Schifalacqua, Shepard, & Kelley, 2012; Shirey et al., 2011; Shoemaker & Fischer, 2011; Stetler, Ritchie, Rycroft-Malone, & Charns, 2014; Stichler, 2007; Ubbink, Guyatt, & Vermeulen, 2013; Upenieks, & Sitterding, 2008; Williams, Perillo, & Brown, 2015.

## Strategy 4-10    Trend Results

| PHASE | 4: Pursue Integration & Sustained Use |
| --- | --- |
| FOCUS | Building Organizational System Support |

### DEFINITION

Trended results are a method to routinely and consistently display evaluation results and outcomes from a practice change in order to target subsequent feedback, suggestions, and implementation strategies to meet established goals.

### BENEFITS

- Demonstrates sustained gains, incremental improvements, or need for reinfusion.
- Provides transparency and visibility of results.
- Allows interprofessional team to set future goals based on results.
- Encourages shared accountability (e.g., clearly identify and address poor performance, recognize and reward high performance).
- Provides long-term follow-up of both clinical indicators and contextual factors.

### PROCEDURE

- Determine method to obtain accurate and credible results for process and/or outcome indicators related to the practice change:
  - Choose a few key indicators (see Chapter 9).
  - Determine economical and professional resources needed.
  - Decide how data will be retrieved (e.g., automated report from patient health record, manual documentation chart audits).
  - Determine how results will be calculated.
  - Consider the type of data display (e.g., run chart, statistical process control chart, [see Tools 11.3 and 11.4]).
  - Ensure that results are clear and easy to interpret.
- Determine frequency of data collection (e.g., weekly, monthly).
- Decide total time frame for data collection (e.g., 1 year, 2 years, ongoing).
- Regularly share results with, and seek feedback from, the interprofessional team, key stakeholders, and senior leaders.
- Include actionable feedback (see Strategy 3-13).
- Report results within the institutional quality improvement program (e.g., quarterly, twice a year) (see Strategy 3-20).

*continues*

## Strategy 4-10    Trend Results (Continued)

### EXAMPLE

Trended Outcome Data

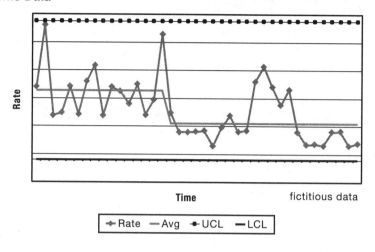

Time                                fictitious data

Rate — Avg — UCL — LCL

Avg = Average
UCL = Upper control limit
LCL = Lower control limit

### CITATIONS

Benneyan, 1998a; Benneyan, 1998b; Benneyan, Lloyd, & Plsek, 2003; Caminiti, Scoditti, Diodati, & Passalacqua, 2005; Carey & Lloyd, 2001; Fleuren, van Dommelen, & Dunnink, 2015; Higuchi, Davies, Edwards, Ploeg, & Virani, 2011; Mohammed, Worthington, & Woodall, 2008; Smith, 2014; Taylor, Clay-Williams, Hogden, Braithwaite, & Groene, 2015.

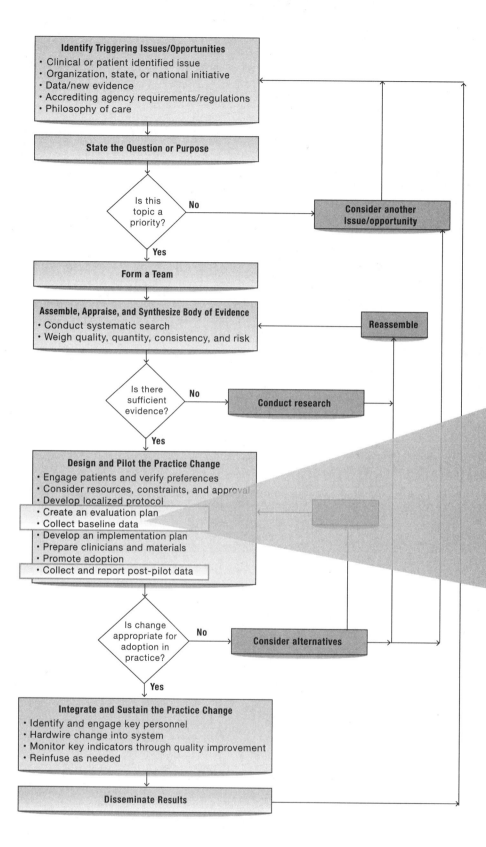

# EVALUATION

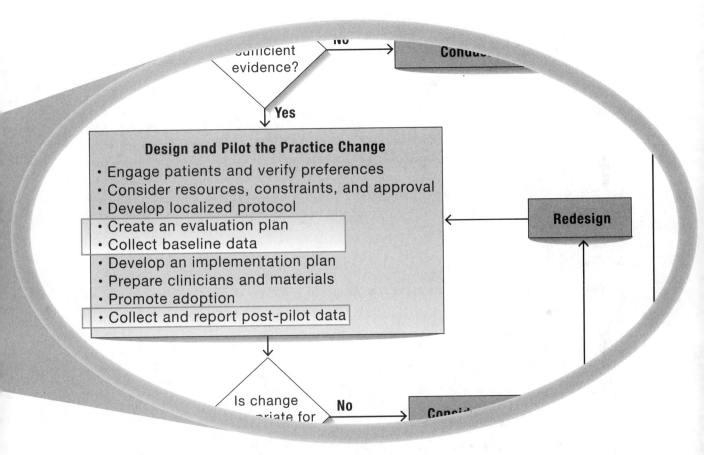

...ficient evidence?

No → Condu...

Yes

**Design and Pilot the Practice Change**
- Engage patients and verify preferences
- Consider resources, constraints, and approval
- Develop localized protocol
- Create an evaluation plan
- Collect baseline data
- Develop an implementation plan
- Prepare clinicians and materials
- Promote adoption
- Collect and report post-pilot data

Redesign ←

Is change ...riate for → No → Consi...

*"You may never know what results come of your action, but if you do nothing there will be no result."*

–Mahatma Gandhi

**N**urses are often eager to start implementing practice changes found through critique and synthesis of the evidence. Taking time to collect baseline data before implementation is critical in order to later identify whether the practice change worked as intended, to identify how well the implementation strategies worked, and to demonstrate an impact through improved outcomes.

# Baseline Data Collection

It is important to create a comprehensive evaluation plan for the pilot and to collect baseline data prior to implementing any practice change (Puterman et al., 2013; Russell, Wallace, & Ketley, 2011). Evaluation is meant to maximize the benefits of a change process and reduce unnecessary harm (American Evaluation Association, 2012). Evaluation of evidence-based practice (EBP) usually contrasts baseline with post-implementation data (i.e., pre-/post-comparison) from the pilot and also includes trended process and outcome measures for integration and sustainability.

# Sample Size

An important decision when planning for evaluation is to determine the sample size. Elements of the project purpose statement include the specific patient population and pilot unit, clinic, or setting. It is helpful to know approximately how many patients the pilot area typically treats with the clinical condition related to the topic. The pilot group may be a subset of those patients. Consider the patient volume typically seen in a reasonable amount of time (e.g., one month). The following questions should be considered when planning the pilot evaluation:

- Which patients from the unit, clinic, or setting should be included in the sample?
- What data or indicators are critical to collect?
- How will those indicators be operationalized (i.e., how are the indicator defined and measured)?
- Is the measure sensitive to the practice change?
- How will the data be collected (i.e., data source) so that the data are sensitive to the practice change?
- How long will the pilot last?
- How frequently will data be collected?
- How frequently will data be reported back to clinicians?
- What is the goal (i.e., what value indicates success)?

A sample of at least 25–50 patients is desirable for each pre- and post-implementation group. However, the sample size must be feasible (Puterman et al., 2013; Russell et al., 2011). Completing the pilot in a timely manner will help maintain the team's interest (Russell et al., 2011).

## Sample Plan

Using consecutive patients for the sample will help capture typical patients or a representative group from the unit or clinic and the usual variability of patients receiving care without oversampling unusual patients (Puterman et al., 2013). For example, collecting data every Wednesday on an inpatient unit may include the same patient for more than one data collection point. If the typical length of stay is relatively short (several days), the data may oversample patients with unusually long lengths of stay. The sample may not be representative and may impact interpretation of results.

The sample size may need to be adjusted based on patient volume during the pilot period. If the patient volume is small (e.g., highly specialized procedure), consider extending the data collection period and reducing the sample size (Cullen, Dawson, & Williams, 2010). If the volume is high (e.g., operating room), consider sampling with fewer patients at appropriate intervals (e.g., first 10 patients or alternate days) (Dolezal, Cullen, Harp, & Mueller, 2011) or random sampling (e.g., every fifth patient).

## Components to Evaluate

A comprehensive evaluation plan includes both process and outcome data. EBP evaluation should include the following components (Bick & Graham, 2010; Gardner, Gardner, & O'Connell, 2014; Parry et al., 2013):

- Knowledge
- Perceptions or attitudes
- Behaviors or practices
- Outcomes
- Balancing measures

Clinician knowledge, perceptions or attitudes, and practice behaviors are process measures that impact the desired outcomes (Fleuren, van Dommelen, & Dunnink, 2015; Gardner et al., 2014; Russell et al., 2011; Sleutel, Barbosa-Leiker, & Wilson, 2015; Smitz Naranjo & Viswanatha Kaimal, 2011). Likewise, patient and family knowledge, perceptions, and health behaviors will also impact outcomes. A sustained improvement in an outcome can be achieved only by changes in the process of care delivery. The process measures provide direction for implementation planning and reinfusion (see Tools 9.1 and 9.2).

**RESOURCE: Individual Evaluation Plan Outline**

This downloadable comprehensive planning tool was developed by the Centers for Disease Control and Prevention (CDC, 2016) as a template to facilitate planning of health programs. Tool content, available through http://www.cdc.gov/asthma/program_eval/guide.htm, includes:

- Introduction and stakeholder engagement
- Description of what you are evaluating
- Evaluation design
- Gather credible evidence
- Data analysis and interpretation
- Use and communication of evaluation findings
- Evaluation management

## Knowledge Assessment

Clinician knowledge should be assessed before and after the practice change is piloted (Siriwardena & Gillam, 2014). The knowledge assessment seeks to determine the education needs of clinicians and to guide informational sessions during implementation.

The knowledge assessment must be project-specific with regard to the topic and practice change. Keep the number of items on the questionnaire reasonable (e.g., 10–15) to facilitate completion and return (Kirchhoff, 2009; Sleutel et al., 2015; Spurlock & Wonder, 2015). Content for the knowledge assessment should include this information:

- Why the EBP change is important (e.g., incidence, severity of the condition)
- What clinicians need to know to be able to perform the EBP change
- What the expected impact will be

Analysis of results is easier if questions are multiple choice, true-false, or matching instead of open-ended (Korhonen et al., 2015; Spurlock & Wonder, 2015). However, one open-ended question may be included to capture elements not identified in the other knowledge items (Kwok, Callard, & McLaws, 2015). It is helpful to have a few clinicians review the knowledge assessment for clarity before distributing the questionnaire. Knowledge assessments for local use can also be developed building on continuing-education articles found in the literature (Cohen et al., 2016; Denenberg & Curtiss, 2016; Schweickert et al., 2016).

## Perception or Attitude Assessment

The same clinician questionnaire can include a separate section on perceptions or attitudes about the EBP change (see Examples 9.1 and 9.2). Clinician perceptions should be sought related to both the EBP change and implementation. Use a simple scale with response options such as 1 = Strongly Disagree to 4 = Strongly Agree (Likert, 1932). Avoid use of a midpoint response option to make interpretation of findings easier. Keep the questionnaire short to ensure easy administration and improve the response rate (Kirchhoff, 2009; Sleutel et al., 2015; Spurlock & Wonder, 2015).

## Behavior or Practice Assessment

Evaluation of behavior or practice performance is useful in determining whether the EBP protocol is being used as intended (Korhonen et al., 2015). Key behaviors for the intervention that impact the outcome are identified and evaluated (Korhonen et al., 2015).

Tools for monitoring key indicators can be developed for a variety of data collection methods:

- Manual review of documentation in the patient health record (see Example 9.3 and Tool 9.3). (Bowie, Bradley, & Rushmer, 2012; Gardner et al., 2014; Kenny, Baker, Lanzon, Stevens, & Yancy, 2008; Korhonen et al., 2015; Kwok et al., 2015; Puterman et al., 2013; Siriwardena & Gillam, 2014).

- Observation of current practices (Fleuren et al., 2015; Korhonen et al., 2015; Kwok et al., 2015; Russell et al., 2011; Siriwardena & Gillam, 2014).

- Clinician self-report using a questionnaire of current practices (Fleuren et al., 2015; Russell et al., 2011; Spurlock & Wonder, 2015 [see Examples 9.1 and 9.2 and Tool 9.4]).

- Interview of clinicians reporting most recent practices in an appropriate patient situation (Balla, Heneghan, Glasziou, Thompson, & Balla, 2009; Bowie et al., 2012; Fleuren et al., 2015; Russell et al., 2011; Puterman et al., 2013; Siriwardena & Gillam, 2014).

Time, resources, and data availability will help determine the data collection method. Baseline data collection should include key indicators based on the proposed practice change, resources and support for implementation, and data that will also be needed post-pilot (Kirchhoff, 2009; Korhonen et al., 2015; Russell et al., 2011). Develop the practice protocol and then identify key process indicators to include in the evaluation. Additional examples are available in the literature (Brown, Wickline, Ecoff, & Glaser, 2009; Burkitt et al., 2010; Chan, Ho, & Day, 2008).

## Outcomes

Outcomes are evaluated to demonstrate an impact. Outcomes may also indicate a need to revise the practice change or implementation plan and may be used to determine whether rollout of the practice change to other areas is appropriate. Outcomes may address patient, family, clinician, or organizational perspectives. Patient or family outcomes will be based on clinical data related to a patient event (e.g., nosocomial infection), whereas clinician outcomes include operational data (e.g., work-related injuries). Organizational outcomes may include length of stay or cost, structure or environmental indicators (e.g., airflow in the operating room or therapeutic milieu), or human resource and talent management (e.g., retention).

## Balancing Measures

Outcome measures should also include relevant balancing measures (Institute for Healthcare Improvement, 2017; Russell et al., 2011). Balancing measures are used to explain outcome variation (e.g., impact of varying census on reported outcomes), but more importantly to reflect avoidance of undesirable consequences from competing practice recommendations (e.g., determining how far to elevate the head of bed to reduce aspiration risk while avoiding increased risk of pressure injury).

# Patient and/or Family Feedback

Chapter 7 describes engaging patients in the pilot phase of the EBP process. Feedback from patients and/or families also remains essential to incorporate their experiences during evaluation. Knowledge is foundational to improving patient health behaviors (Jones & Coke, 2016; Menendez et al., 2017; Stacey et al., 2017). Patients' perceptions have been shown to impact health behaviors and patients' use of healthcare services (Holt et al., 2016). Thus, patient knowledge, attitudes, health behaviors, and health outcomes are important components of a comprehensive evaluation plan. As an example, patient feedback was collected about their knowledge, attitudes, and health behaviors related to oral care for oral mucositis (see Example 9.4). Feedback was sought using questionnaires adapted from several tools reported in the literature (Gussgard, Jokstad, Hope, Wood, & Tenenbaum, 2015; Kartin, Tasci, Soyeur, & Elmali, 2014; Kushner et al., 2008; Rosenthal et al., 2008). Patient feedback provided support for an evidence-based oral care intervention to reduce oral mucositis (Cullen, Baumler et al., in press).

# Data Analysis and Interpretation

Methods for data analysis in EBP should be simple and meaningful to clinicians. Descriptive statistics such as frequency, range, and mean are often used for data analysis to demonstrate clinically meaningful improvements (Fleuren et al., 2015). EBP reports using simple descriptive statistics show practice improvements (Cullen, Hanrahan et al., in press; Madsen et al., 2005; Neis, 2015; Sehr et al., 2013). Statistically significant changes are the goal of experimental research, not necessarily for EBP, though inferential statistics may be possible for EBP. Examples are cited to highlight differences in reporting research and EBP, and between EBP reports (Cheifetz et al., 2014; Huether, Abbott, Cullen, Cullen, & Gaarde, 2016; Schmitdiel et al., 2017). As an alternative, EBP addressing cancer-related fatigue used inferential statistics and shows a statistically significant improvement (Huether et al., 2016).

Evaluation results should be summarized for easy interpretation by clinicians (Russell et al., 2011; Smith, 2014).

**RESOURCES: How to Display Comparative Information People Can Understand and Use**

| Resource | Description | Source |
|---|---|---|
| Robert Wood Johnson Foundation | Comprehensive information for clinicians when determining how best to display information. Advantages and challenges are clearly explained, with guidance to increase clarity. | http://www.rwjf.org/content/dam/farm/reports/reports/2010/rwjf69342 |

# Results

Results should be reported in a way that will facilitate interpretation and actionable feedback trending (see Strategies 3-13 and 4-6) by clinicians (see Figure 9.1) (Abela, 2013; American Institutes for Research, 2017; Robert Wood Johnson Foundation, 2010). Report results that demonstrate both successes and opportunities for improvement (Russell et al., 2011). Include data reported in the literature and how pilot data compare, because they may be critical to achieve the desired outcome. Discuss the data so that feedback is actionable and clinicians will know what they must do to maintain or achieve the selected outcomes (Duff, Walker, & Omari, 2011; Hysong, 2009).

After the pilot is complete, the evaluative data are used to help determine next steps for the project. If the desired outcomes have been achieved, planning for integration in the pilot area and rollout of the practice change to other appropriate areas will follow. If the desired outcomes are not achieved, critical analysis of processes and implementation strategies is warranted.

Results should be reported within the institution's quality improvement (QI) infrastructure (see Example 9.4). Reporting in the QI program supports integration and notification of senior leaders (see Strategy 3-20) about the EBP.

## TIPS: Evaluation Planning

- Acknowledge that evaluation is critical to demonstrate an impact and becomes even more important when robust evidence is not available.

- Take time to collect baseline data prior to piloting the EBP change.

- Include process (i.e., knowledge, attitude, behavior) and outcome indicators to create a comprehensive evaluation plan.

- Measure outcomes to identify impact of a practice change.

- Include balancing measures to identify and manage risks.

- Select project-specific key indicators to avoid collecting unnecessary data.

- Use identical data collection items and tools from pre- and post-pilot for comparable results.

- Use process data to determine next steps if the desired outcomes are not achieved.

- Compare evaluation results with those reported in the literature.

- If using a Likert scale, avoid midpoints (e.g., "uncertain") to help intrepretation of findings.

**Figure 9.1**   Chart Suggestions: A Thought-Starter

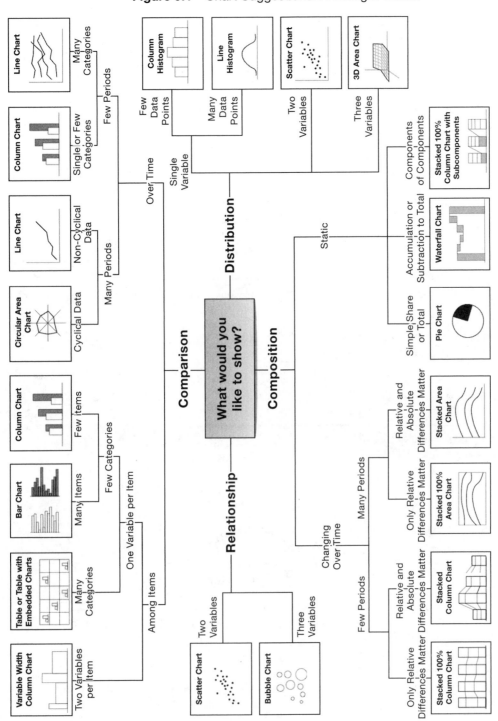

## Example 9.1    Clinician Questionnaire

### Oral Mucositis Clinician Questionnaire Answer Key

**INSTRUCTIONS**: Please take a few minutes to provide valuable feedback to the Oral Mucositis Committee. Your responses are anonymous and will be used to improve care for patients with oral mucositis.

**Area:** _____    **Date:** _____

### SECTION I: Knowledge assessment

**INSTRUCTIONS:** Please select the ONE best answer for each question.

1. Loss of saliva is thought to contribute to increased risk of oral mucositis from which of the following?
   - ☐ a. Increased mucosal trauma and irritation from loss of surface lubrication
   - ☒ b. Increased microbial colonization
   - ☐ c. Dehydration of the mucosal surface
   - ☐ d. a & b
   - ☐ e. All of the above

2. Mouthwashes containing alcohol should be used when a patient has oral mucositis?
   - ☐ a. True
   - ☒ b. False (to avoid further irritation to damaged oral mucosa)

3. Mint or cinnamon flavoring in oral care products can cause pain for patients with oral mucositis.
   - ☒ a. True
   - ☐ b. False

4. Throat pain is often a precursor to oral mucositis in head and neck cancer patients.
   - ☒ a. True
   - ☐ b. False

5. Mild pain from oral mucositis can initially be treated with which of the following?
   - ☒ a. Bland oral rinses (e.g., saline)
   - ☐ b. Topical anesthetics
   - ☐ c. Nonsteroidal anti-inflammatory drugs
   - ☐ d. As-needed (PRN) dosing of systemic analgesic
   - ☐ e. Around-the-clock dosing of systemic analgesic

6. Oral mucositis can contribute to which of the following?
   - ☐ a. Pain
   - ☐ b. Sepsis or infection
   - ☐ c. Dehydration
   - ☐ d. Inability to eat
   - ☒ e. All of the above

7. When teaching patients about oral care, which of the following instructions is incorrect?
   - ☐ a. Brush your teeth at least two times per day.
   - ☐ b. Use a soft or ultra-soft toothbrush.
   - ☐ c. Biotene toothpaste is recommended during treatment.
   - ☐ d. Brush for 2 minutes and hold the toothbrush at a 45-degree angle.
   - ☒ e. Cap the head of the toothbrush between use.

| 8. How much toothpaste should be used each time teeth are brushed? | ☐ a. Enough to cover the top of the bristles<br>☒ b. Pea size or less<br>☐ c. Enough to create foam<br>☐ d. None of the above |
|---|---|
| 9. What is the proper oral care instruction for patients without teeth? | ☒ a. Clean gums two or three times per day with gauze or with a washcloth or paper towel that is wet with tap water.<br>☐ b. Patients without teeth do not need oral care instruction.<br>☐ c. Brush two times per day with a soft toothbrush.<br>☐ d. None of the above. |
| 10. What are the proper oral care instructions for flossing? | ☐ a. Floss once per day<br>☐ b. Unwaxed floss<br>☐ c. Waxed floss<br>☐ d. a & b<br>☒ e. a & c<br>☐ f. None of the above |
| 11. Oral rinses are used to do which of the following? | ☐ a. Promote cleaning and plaque removal.<br>☐ b. Prevent infections.<br>☐ c. Reduce the risk of long-term cavity development.<br>☐ d. Promote comfort.<br>☒ e. All of the above. |
| 12. Which of the following oral rinses are appropriate for oncology patients? | ☐ a. Plain water<br>☐ b. Salt and baking soda<br>☐ c. Biotene Dry Mouth Mouthwash<br>☒ d. All of the above |
| 13. Which of the following is true about nutritional intake in patients experiencing oral mucositis? | ☐ a. They should eat anything possible as their calorie needs are greater.<br>☐ b. They should use a soft or liquid diet to ease swallowing discomfort.<br>☒ c. They should avoid foods that would potentially injure oral tissue.<br>☐ d. They will need central venous nutrition (CVN) so there are no additional nutrition considerations. |

*continues*

**Example 9.1    Clinician Questionnaire (Continued)**

### SECTION I: Knowledge assessment (Continued)

14. Which product is recommended for lip care?

☒ a. Lanolin
☐ b. Carmex
☐ c. Chapstick
☐ d. Vaseline

15. When educating caregivers in the care of oral mucositis, which of the following instructions should be included?

☐ a. Explain how to revise brushing when oral mucositis is present.
☐ b. Demonstrate how to monitor the appearance of the oral cavity each day.
☐ c. Explain the importance of seeking medical assistance if mouth sores or oral pain interfere with dietary intake.
☐ d. Explain foods to avoid if mouth sores or soreness develops.
☒ e. All of the above.

### SECTION II: Perception or attitude assessment

**INSTRUCTIONS:** Please indicate the number that best describes your perception or attitude about oral mucositis in oncology patients.

| | Strongly Disagree | Disagree | Agree | Strongly Agree |
|---|---|---|---|---|
| 1.  Our patients receive oral care at least twice per day. | 1 | 2 | 3 | 4 |
| 2.  I am able to identify which patients need to have oral mucositis prevention. | 1 | 2 | 3 | 4 |
| 3.  Using oral care products for oral mucositis enhances the quality of nursing care in the clinic or unit. | 1 | 2 | 3 | 4 |
| 4.  I feel knowledgeable about carrying out oral mucositis prevention. | 1 | 2 | 3 | 4 |
| 5.  Completing oral care enables me to meet the oral health needs of most oncology patients. | 1 | 2 | 3 | 4 |
| 6.  Oral health influences general health in both children and adults. | 1 | 2 | 3 | 4 |

| | Strongly Disagree | Disagree | Agree | Strongly Agree |
|---|---|---|---|---|
| 7. Completing oral care is important for my patients. | 1 | 2 | 3 | 4 |
| 8. Informing patients and families about the importance of oral care is essential for prevention and to reduce severity of oral mucositis. | 1 | 2 | 3 | 4 |
| 9. Available patient education materials are helpful in reducing severity of oral mucositis. | 1 | 2 | 3 | 4 |
| 10. Having cancer patients see a dentist before starting treatment reduces the severity of oral mucositis. | 1 | 2 | 3 | 4 |
| 11. I have easy access to oral rinses for patients with mouth or throat soreness. | 1 | 2 | 3 | 4 |
| 12. I feel support to provide oral care for cancer patients at risk for oral mucositis. | 1 | 2 | 3 | 4 |

Bensinger et al., 2008

EXAMPLES

TOOLS

## Example 9.2   Clinician Questionnaire and Answer Key

### SECTION I: Perception assessment

| INSTRUCTIONS: Please indicate the number that best communicates your perception of pain assessment for older adults. | Strongly Disagree | Disagree | Agree | Strongly Agree |
|---|---|---|---|---|
| 1.  I feel well prepared to carry out pain assessment for older adults. | 1 | 2 | 3 | 4 |
| 2.  I am able to access tools that support pain assessment for older adults. | 1 | 2 | 3 | 4 |
| 3.  Documentation of pain assessment findings is easy to complete. | 1 | 2 | 3 | 4 |
| 4.  I have enough time to complete pain assessment for older adults. | 1 | 2 | 3 | 4 |
| 5.  I am able to use the patient-preferred pain assessment scale for older adults. | 1 | 2 | 3 | 4 |
| 6.  I feel supported in my efforts to complete pain assessment for older adults. | 1 | 2 | 3 | 4 |
| 7.  Pain assessment for older adults is difficult because of problems with cognition (e.g., delirium). | 1 | 2 | 3 | 4 |
| 8.  Older adults have difficulty using the 0–10 numeric rating scale. | 1 | 2 | 3 | 4 |
| 9.  Pain assessment for older adults is managed with the use of reliable pain assessment methods. | 1 | 2 | 3 | 4 |
| 10. Pain assessment is important for quality care for older adult patients. | 1 | 2 | 3 | 4 |

### SECTION II: Knowledge assessment (with answer key)

INSTRUCTIONS: Please select the ONE best answer for each question.

|  | True | False |
|---|---|---|
| 1.  Observable changes in vital signs must be relied on to verify a patient's statement that he or she has severe pain. | ☐ | ☒ |
| 2.  Patients can sleep in spite of moderate or severe pain. | ☒ | ☐ |

| SECTION II: Knowledge assessment (with answer key) | True | False |
|---|---|---|
| 3.  Older adults with pain should be encouraged to endure as much pain as possible before resorting to a pain relief measure. | ☐ | ☒ |
| 4.  If a patient's pain is relieved by administration of a placebo, the pain is not real. | ☐ | ☒ |
| 5.  Older adults who use opioid medications regularly will eventually become addicted to them. | ☐ | ☒ |
| 6.  Patients with mild to moderate cognitive impairment can provide a self-report of pain intensity. | ☒ | ☐ |
| 7.  Research shows that older adults feel painful sensations less intensely than younger adults. | ☐ | ☒ |
| 8.  Older adults with pain may be at greater risk of falling. | ☐ | ☒ |
| 9.  Older adults with pain may be less able to participate in rehabilitation activities (e.g., ambulating). | ☒ | ☐ |

### SECTION III: Current practice

**INSTRUCTIONS:** Please fill in an answer for each question based on your nursing practice in caring for older adults.

I am able to identify the patient-preferred pain assessment scale _____ % of the time.

I am able to consistently use the patient-preferred pain assessment scale _____ % of the time.

For older adults in pain, I am able to assess pain every 4 hours _____ % of the time.

For older adults in pain, I am able to compare their pain rating with their acceptable level of pain _____ % of the time.

Cullen, 2013; Hamilton & Edgar, 1992; Herr, Bojoro, Steffensmeier, & Rakel, 2006; IOM, 2011c; McCaffery & Ferrell, 1997; McLennon, 2005; Registered Nurses' Association of Ontario, 2007

EXAMPLES

TOOLS

## Example 9.3    Chart Audit Forms

### Inpatient Oral Assessment and Oral Care

| Patient record number: | | Area: | |
|---|---|---|---|
| | Admission<br>Date: _____ | Day 1<br>Date: _____ | Day 4<br>Date: _____ |
| Oral assessment documented: at least once on the day of admission; at least two times on Day 1, if not discharged that day; and at least two times on Day 4, if still hospitalized. | ☐ Yes<br>☐ No | ☐ Yes<br>☐ No | ☐ Yes<br>☐ No |
| Oral assessment total score: | Score: _____ | Score 1: _____<br>Score 2: _____ | Score 1: _____<br>Score 2: _____ |
| Oral care documented: at least once on the day of admission; at least two times on Day 1, if not discharged that day; and at least two times on Day 4, if still hospitalized. | ☐ Yes<br>☐ No | ☐ Yes<br>☐ No | ☐ Yes<br>☐ No |
| Mark interventions: | ☐ Denture care<br>☐ Floss<br>☐ Gauze<br>☐ Gel/Biotene®<br>☐ Gel/fluoride<br>☐ Lip care<br>☐ Lip care/lanolin<br>☐ Rinse<br>☐ Toothbrush<br>☐ Toothbrush, electric<br>☐ Toothbrush, soft<br>☐ Toothpaste<br>☐ Toothpaste/Biotene<br>☐ Troxel syringe<br>☐ Washcloth<br>☐ Gum massage<br>☐ Palate plate care | ☐ Denture care<br>☐ Floss<br>☐ Gauze<br>☐ Gel/Biotene<br>☐ Gel/fluoride<br>☐ Lip care<br>☐ Lip care/lanolin<br>☐ Rinse<br>☐ Toothbrush<br>☐ Toothbrush, electric<br>☐ Toothbrush, soft<br>☐ Toothpaste<br>☐ Toothpaste/Biotene<br>☐ Troxel syringe<br>☐ Washcloth<br>☐ Gum massage<br>☐ Palate plate care | ☐ Denture care<br>☐ Floss<br>☐ Gauze<br>☐ Gel/Biotene<br>☐ Gel/fluoride<br>☐ Lip care<br>☐ Lip care/lanolin<br>☐ Rinse<br>☐ Toothbrush<br>☐ Toothbrush, electric<br>☐ Toothbrush, soft<br>☐ Toothpaste<br>☐ Toothpaste/Biotene<br>☐ Troxel syringe<br>☐ Washcloth<br>☐ Gum massage<br>☐ Palate plate care |

EXAMPLES

TOOLS

| | Admission<br>Date: _____ | Day 1<br>Date: _____ | Day 4<br>Date: _____ |
|---|---|---|---|
| Oral solutions documented: | ☐ Yes<br>☐ No | ☐ Yes<br>☐ No | ☐ Yes<br>☐ No |
| Mark interventions: | ☐ Hydrogen peroxide, half-strength<br>☐ Mouthwash<br>☐ Mouthwash/Biotene<br>☐ Normal saline<br>☐ Baking soda<br>☐ Salt and soda<br>☐ Water<br>☐ Gelclair<br>☐ Salivart | ☐ Hydrogen peroxide, half-strength<br>☐ Mouthwash<br>☐ Mouthwash/Biotene<br>☐ Normal saline<br>☐ Baking soda<br>☐ Salt and soda<br>☐ Water<br>☐ Gelclair<br>☐ Salivart | ☐ Hydrogen peroxide, half-strength<br>☐ Mouthwash<br>☐ Mouthwash/Biotene<br>☐ Normal saline<br>☐ Baking soda<br>☐ Salt and soda<br>☐ Water<br>☐ Gelclair<br>☐ Salivart |

### Ambulatory Oral Assessment and Oral Care

**Patient record number:**                                   **Area:**

| | Visit date:<br>_____ | Visit date:<br>_____ | Visit date:<br>_____ |
|---|---|---|---|
| Oral screening completed by nursing assistant or medical assistant: | ☐ Yes<br>☐ No | ☐ Yes<br>☐ No | ☐ Yes<br>☐ No |
| Changes to mouth or throat: | ☐ Yes<br>☐ No | ☐ Yes<br>☐ No | ☐ Yes<br>☐ No |
| Oral assessment documented by nurse, if applicable: | ☐ Yes<br>☐ No<br>☐ Not applicable | ☐ Yes<br>☐ No<br>☐ Not applicable | ☐ Yes<br>☐ No<br>☐ Not applicable |
| Oral assessment total score: | Score: _____ | Score: _____ | Score: _____ |
| Oral care education documented by nurse: | ☐ Yes<br>☐ No | ☐ Yes<br>☐ No | ☐ Yes<br>☐ No |
| Oral care interventions documented as part of patient education (e.g. Biotene toothpaste, lanolin lip care, salt-and-soda rinses): | | | |

Farrington, Cullen, & Dawson, 2013

EXAMPLES

TOOLS

## Example 9.4    Patient Questionnaire About Oral Care

**INSTRUCTIONS:** The following are situations that patients with your illness have said are important. Please circle the number that shows the extent to which each has been a problem for you during the past week.

1.  How much **mouth and throat soreness** did you have in the past week:

| None | | | | | | | | | | Worst Possible |
|---|---|---|---|---|---|---|---|---|---|---|
| 0 | 1 | 2 | 3 | 4 | 5 | 6 | 7 | 8 | 9 | 10 |

2.  How much did **mouth and throat soreness** affect you during the past week with:
    a.  Difficulty sleeping:

| No Trouble Sleeping | | | | | | | | | | Unable to Sleep |
|---|---|---|---|---|---|---|---|---|---|---|
| 0 | 1 | 2 | 3 | 4 | 5 | 6 | 7 | 8 | 9 | 10 |

    b.  Difficulty eating:

| No Trouble Eating | | | | | | | | | | Unable to Eat |
|---|---|---|---|---|---|---|---|---|---|---|
| 0 | 1 | 2 | 3 | 4 | 5 | 6 | 7 | 8 | 9 | 10 |

    c.  Difficulty brushing your teeth:

| No Trouble Brushing Teeth | | | | | | | | | | Unable to Brush Teeth |
|---|---|---|---|---|---|---|---|---|---|---|
| 0 | 1 | 2 | 3 | 4 | 5 | 6 | 7 | 8 | 9 | 10 |

    d.  Difficult because of a dry mouth:

| No Trouble with Dry Mouth | | | | | | | | | | Worst Possible Dry Mouth |
|---|---|---|---|---|---|---|---|---|---|---|
| 0 | 1 | 2 | 3 | 4 | 5 | 6 | 7 | 8 | 9 | 10 |

**INSTRUCTIONS:** Please answer the questions below. These questions will ask you about oral care and how you clean your mouth. Please circle the answer that best describes what you have done the past week.

| | Seldom/ Never | Once a Week | Once a Day | Twice a Day | More than Twice a Day |
|---|---|---|---|---|---|
| 3. How often do you brush your teeth? | 1 | 2 | 3 | 4 | 5 |

4. Which toothpaste do you use?
   - ☐ a. Aquafresh
   - ☐ b. Biotene
   - ☐ c. Colgate
   - ☐ d. Crest
   - ☐ e. Other (please specify): _____

| | Seldom/ Never | Once a Week | Once a Day | Two or Three Times a Day | Four or More Times a Day |
|---|---|---|---|---|---|
| 5. How often do you use salt & soda mouth rinses? | 1 | 2 | 3 | 4 | 5 |

6. Do you use lip balm?
   - ☐ a. Yes, which brand _____
   - ☐ b. No

**INSTRUCTIONS:** Please circle the number that best communicates your perception about your mouth and oral care during your cancer treatment.

| | Strongly Disagree | Disagree | Agree | Strongly Agree |
|---|---|---|---|---|
| 7. I feel I know what to do to prevent mouth sores during my cancer treatment. | 1 | 2 | 3 | 4 |
| 8. The materials I received were helpful. | 1 | 2 | 3 | 4 |
| 9. I feel well prepared for good oral care during my cancer treatment. | 1 | 2 | 3 | 4 |
| 10. Special toothpaste is helping me manage my mouth sores better. | 1 | 2 | 3 | 4 |
| 11. Special oral rinses are helping me manage my mouth sores better. | 1 | 2 | 3 | 4 |

Other comments:

_____

_____

*Thank you for participating in this project and for your comments.*

Please return your completed form to _____

(Gussgard, Jokstad, Hope, Wood, & Tenenbaum, 2015; Kartin et al., 2014; Kushner et al., 2008; Rosenthal et al., 2008)

## Example 9.5 EBP Project Report to Quality Improvement Program

### Performance Improvement Program: Quarterly Report

| | |
|---|---|
| Center/department/division/unit: | 3West |
| Submitted by: | |
| Project title: | Oral Mucositis Assessment |
| Project team members: | |
| Date issue identified: | |
| Status: | ☒ Complete ☐ In progress |
| Safety project: | ☐ Yes ☒ No |

### Project source:

| | | |
|---|---|---|
| ☒ Core data, unit, audit | ☐ Patient satisfaction | ☒ Interprofessional project |
| ☐ Benchmarking | ☐ Sentinel/adverse event | ☒ Evidence-based practice |
| ☐ Other data source | | |

### Area of improvement (Check all that apply):

| | | |
|---|---|---|
| ☒ Quality (clinical outcomes) | ☐ Cost | ☐ People (clinician/credentialing) |
| ☐ Service (efficiency—internal process) | ☐ Growth (new or expanding service) | |

| | |
|---|---|
| Define: Project purpose | Implement a standardized, evidence-based oral assessment scale to address oral mucositis for both ambulatory and inpatient adult and pediatric oncology patients. |
| Measure: Data/information about current situation | Current documentation related to oral assessment does not adequately capture oral mucosa changes for adult or pediatric oncology patients experiencing oral mucositis. Incomplete documentation of changes in the oral mucosa prohibits timely implementation of prevention and treatment strategies. |
| Analyze: Root cause and data | Oral assessment documentation meets the needs of the majority of patients within the institution. Nursing documentation of oral assessment for oncology patients needs to improve. |
| Improve: Implementation strategies | Education (online and live inservices); slogan and logo; creative prompts (wind-up teeth). |
| Control: Maintain gains and integrate into workflow | Policy; process evaluation (clinician questionnaire); integrate new tool into documentation; chart audits of documentation in the patient health record to evaluate compliance; report into quality improvement system. |

## Tool 9.1    Selecting Process and Outcome Indicators

**INSTRUCTIONS:** Identify key indicators for each of the evaluation components (knowledge, attitude, behavior, outcome, balancing measures). Data collection may be automated if the data are available electronically or may require manual collection.

| KNOWLEDGE | |
|---|---|
| **Indicator** | **Information to Consider** |
| Extent of the clinical issue (e.g., incidence, prevalence, rate) | ■ Incidence of the problem in the country<br>■ Rate of an adverse outcome reported in the literature |
| Gap in local outcome compared to higher performers or in evidence reports | ■ Rate of an adverse outcome in the organization, unit, clinic, or setting<br>■ Rate for higher performers |
| How to assess the clinical issue | ■ Components of an evidence-based assessment<br>■ Frequency of assessment<br>■ Tool for assessment and scoring<br>■ Link between assessment and interventions |
| Interventions for prevention or treatment | ■ Key interventions<br>■ Location of supplies and how to obtain supplies<br>■ How to use equipment<br>■ Precautions for interventions (e.g., patients to exclude, patient risk, how to minimize risk) |
| Documentation of assessments and interventions | ■ Where documentation is available within the documentation system<br>■ How to differentiate assessment findings for documentation (e.g., pressure injury stages) |

| PERCEPTION or ATTITUDE | |
|---|---|
| **Indicator** | **Example of Wording** |
| Importance of clinical topic | <Insert clinical topic> is an important clinical issue for patients on my unit. |
| Relevance of topic to quality and safety | Addressing <insert clinical topic> is a priority for high-quality, safe patient care. |
| Feeling knowledgeable | I feel knowledgeable in <insert clinical topic>. |
| Feeling supported | I feel supported in completing <insert clinical topic>. |

*continues*

EXAMPLES

TOOLS

## Tool 9.1   Selecting Process and Outcome Indicators (Continued)

### PERCEPTION or ATTITUDE

| Indicator | Example of Wording |
| --- | --- |
| Sufficient time to learn | I have had sufficient time to learn how to complete <insert clinical topic>. |
| Resources available | <insert clinical topic> resources are readily available for use with patients. |
| Helpfulness of resource materials | <insert clinical topic> resources are helpful. |
| Know who can assist | I know who can assist me with <insert clinical topic> care. |
| Access to an expert | I have ready access to an expert to help troubleshoot the <insert clinical topic> protocol. |
| Ability to carry out protocol | I am able to carry out the <insert clinical topic> protocol. |
| Ability to carry out key steps | I am able to carry out key steps in the <insert clinical topic> protocol. |
| Ease of documentation | Documentation of <insert clinical topic> is easy. |

### BEHAVIOR or PRACTICE

| Indicator | Information to Consider | Data Collection Method |
| --- | --- | --- |
| When to evaluate documentation | ■ First expected documentation (e.g., within 24 hours of admission)<br><br>■ When to evaluate repeated documentation, based on documentation frequency and expected length of stay | ■ Chart audit or patient health record report |
| Documentation by which clinicians | ■ Registered nurse<br><br>■ Nursing assistant<br><br>■ Medical assistant<br><br>■ Physician<br><br>■ Pharmacist<br><br>■ Therapist<br><br>■ Nurse practitioner/physician assistant<br><br>■ Hospitalist<br><br>■ Other | ■ Chart audit or patient health record report |

| Indicator | Information to Consider | Data Collection Method |
|---|---|---|
| Key documentation components | ■ Completion of critical variables within \<insert clinical topic\><br><br>■ Scoring of variables within \<insert clinical topic\><br><br>■ Frequency of each variable within \<insert clinical topic\><br><br>■ Completion of patient education<br><br>■ Distribution of patient education materials<br><br>■ Complete key steps within interventions<br><br>■ Frequency of completing key steps within interventions | ■ Chart audit or patient health record report |
| Current practices | ■ Correct identification of patients for EBP change<br><br>■ Frequency, timing, or completeness of key steps within interventions | ■ Observation<br><br>■ Interview<br><br>■ Self-report |
| Patient volume or cost | ■ Number of patients who could benefit from the EBP change<br><br>■ Length of stay<br><br>■ Discharge disposition (e.g., improve rate of patients returning home) | ■ Report from billing or EHR |

## OUTCOMES

Determine where to identify reported outcomes to consider including in the evaluation plan for the EBP change:

■ Clinical practice guidelines

■ Research reports

■ Quality improvement data

■ Reportable measures

■ Benchmarks

■ Organizational data (e.g., length of stay, cost)

## BALANCING MEASURES

Determine where to identify outcomes that may conflict with desired outcomes for use in the evaluation plan for the EBP change:

■ Conflicting research findings

■ Monitor incident reports of associated risks

■ Competing practice recommendations

■ Quality improvement data

■ Organizational data (e.g., length of stay, cost)

## Tool 9.2    Developing Topic-Specific Process and Outcome Indicators

**INSTRUCTIONS:** Identify key indicators for each of the evaluation components (knowledge, attitude, behavior, outcome, balancing measures). Develop or adapt wording to match topic-specific elements to include in the EBP evaluation.

| KNOWLEDGE | | |
|---|---|---|
| **Indicator** | **Project-Specific** | **Items to Include** |
| Extent of the clinical issue (e.g., incidence, prevalence, rate) | | ☐ |
| Gap in local outcome compared to higher performers or in evidence reports | | ☐ |
| How to assess the clinical issue | | ☐ |
| Interventions for prevention or treatment | | ☐ |
| Where to document assessments and interventions | | ☐ |

| PERCEPTION or ATTITUDE | | |
|---|---|---|
| **Indicator** | **Project-Specific** | **Items to Include** |
| Importance of clinical topic | | ☐ |
| Relevance of topic to quality and safety | | ☐ |
| Feeling knowledgeable | | ☐ |
| Feeling supported | | ☐ |
| Sufficient time to learn | | ☐ |
| Resource materials available | | ☐ |
| Helpfulness of resource materials | | ☐ |
| Know who can assist | | ☐ |
| Access to an expert | | ☐ |
| Ability to carry out protocol | | ☐ |
| Ability to carry out key steps | | ☐ |
| Ease of documentation | | ☐ |

| BEHAVIOR OR PRACTICE | | | |
|---|---|---|---|
| **Indicator** | **Project-Specific** | **Data Collection Method** | **Items to Include** |
| When to evaluate documentation | | ☐ Patient chart audit<br>☐ Patient health record report | ☐ |
| Documentation by which clinician(s) | ☐ Registered nurse<br>☐ Nursing assistant<br>☐ Medical assistant<br>☐ Physician<br>☐ Pharmacist<br>☐ Therapist<br>☐ Nurse practitioner/ physician assistant<br>☐ Other | ☐ Chart audit<br>☐ Patient health record report | ☐ |
| Key documentation components | | ☐ Chart audit<br>☐ Patient health record report | ☐ |
| Key components of practice | | ☐ Observation<br>☐ Interview<br>☐ Self-report<br>☐ Chart audit<br>☐ Patient health record report | ☐ |
| Patient volume or cost | | ☐ Report from billing<br>☐ Patient health record report | ☐ |

| OUTCOMES | | | | |
|---|---|---|---|---|
| **Sources** | **Reported Outcomes** | **Project Data to Obtain** | **Who Can Provide the Data?** | **Items to Include** |
| Clinical practice guidelines | | | | ☐ |
| Research reports | | | | ☐ |
| Quality improvement data | | | | ☐ |
| Reportable measures | | | | ☐ |
| Benchmarks | | | | ☐ |
| Organizational data (e.g., length of stay, cost) | | | | ☐ |

*continues*

**Tool 9.2   Developing Topic-Specific Process and Outcome Indicators (Continued)**

| | BALANCING MEASURES | | | |
|---|---|---|---|---|
| Sources | Outcomes to Monitor | Project Data to Obtain | Who Can Provide the Data? | Items to Include |
| Conflicting research findings | | | | ☐ |
| Monitor incident reports of associated risks | | | | ☐ |
| Competing practice recommendations | | | | ☐ |
| Quality improvement data | | | | ☐ |
| Organizational data (e.g., length of stay, cost) | | | | ☐ |

**NOTE:** Select project-specific key indicators for each evaluative component. You must be selective in order to collect relevant data and avoid unnecessary data collection. Select indicators that will help you understand problems and measure changes.

## Tool 9.3    Audit Form

**INSTRUCTIONS:** This tool is designed to audit practice for <topic>. Insert the patient record number and answer each element. Take notes on a separate paper for challenges with identifying data.

**Patient record number:** _____    **Area:** _____

| | Admission/Visit date: | Day1/Visit date: | Day 2/Visit date: |
|---|---|---|---|
| <Insert topic> screening completed by nursing assistant or medical assistant | ☐ Yes<br>☐ No | ☐ Yes<br>☐ No | ☐ Yes<br>☐ No |
| Clinical changes for <insert symptom> noted | ☐ Yes<br>☐ No | ☐ Yes<br>☐ No | ☐ Yes<br>☐ No |
| <Insert symptom> documented by nurse, if applicable | ☐ Yes<br>☐ No<br>☐ Not applicable | ☐ Yes<br>☐ No<br>☐ Not applicable | ☐ Yes<br>☐ No<br>☐ Not applicable |
| <Insert topic> total score | Score: _____ | Score: _____ | Score: _____ |
| <Insert topic> education documented by nurse | ☐ Yes<br>☐ No | ☐ Yes<br>☐ No | ☐ Yes<br>☐ No |
| <Insert topic> care interventions documented (or add comment) | ☐ <intervention 1><br>☐ <intervention 2><br>☐ <intervention 3><br>☐ <intervention 4><br>☐ <intervention 5><br>☐ <intervention 6> | ☐ <intervention 1><br>☐ <intervention 2><br>☐ <intervention 3><br>☐ <intervention 4><br>☐ <intervention 5><br>☐ <intervention 6> | ☐ <intervention 1><br>☐ <intervention 2><br>☐ <intervention 3><br>☐ <intervention 4><br>☐ <intervention 5><br>☐ <intervention 6> |

## Tool 9.4    Clinician Questionnaire

**Unit/clinic:** _____    **Date:** _____

**INSTRUCTIONS:** Please take a few minutes to provide valuable feedback related to <topic>. Your responses are anonymous and will be used to improve care for patients with <topic>.

### SECTION I: Knowledge assessment

**INSTRUCTIONS:** Please select the ONE best answer for each question.

| | |
|---|---|
| 1. <insert item> | ☐ a.<br>☐ b.<br>☐ c.<br>☐ d. |
| 2. <insert item> | ☐ a.<br>☐ b.<br>☐ c.<br>☐ d. |
| 3. <insert item> | ☐ a.<br>☐ b.<br>☐ c.<br>☐ d. |
| 4. <insert item> | ☐ True<br>☐ False |
| 5. <insert item> | ☐ True<br>☐ False |
| 6. <insert item> | ☐ True<br>☐ False |

### SECTION II: Perception or attitude assessment

**INSTRUCTIONS:** Please indicate the number that best describes your perception or attitude about <topic>.

| | Strongly Disagree | Disagree | Agree | Strongly Agree |
|---|---|---|---|---|
| 1. All patients in <clinic/unit> receive <insert topic> care at least <frequency>. | 1 | 2 | 3 | 4 |
| 2. I am able to identify which patients need to have <insert topic> prevention. | 1 | 2 | 3 | 4 |
| 3. Using <insert topic or product> enhances the quality of nursing care in the <clinic/unit>. | 1 | 2 | 3 | 4 |
| 4. I feel knowledgeable about carrying out <insert topic>. | 1 | 2 | 3 | 4 |

| SECTION II: Perception or attitude assessment | | | | |
|---|---|---|---|---|
| | Strongly Disagree | Disagree | Agree | Strongly Agree |
| 5. Completing \<insert topic\> enables me to meet the health needs of most patients. | 1 | 2 | 3 | 4 |
| 6. Completing \<insert topic\> care is important for my patients. | 1 | 2 | 3 | 4 |
| 7. Informing patients and families about the importance of \<insert topic\> care is essential for the prevention and reduced severity of \<insert outcome\>. | 1 | 2 | 3 | 4 |
| 8. Available patient education materials are helpful in reducing \<insert outcome\>. | 1 | 2 | 3 | 4 |
| 9. Documentation of \<insert topic\> is easy to complete. | 1 | 2 | 3 | 4 |
| 10. I have easy access to equipment/supplies for providing \<insert topic\> care. | 1 | 2 | 3 | 4 |
| 11. I have ready access to experts for assistance providing \<insert topic or product\> care. | 1 | 2 | 3 | 4 |
| 12. I feel supported to provide \<insert topic\> care. | 1 | 2 | 3 | 4 |

EXAMPLES

TOOLS

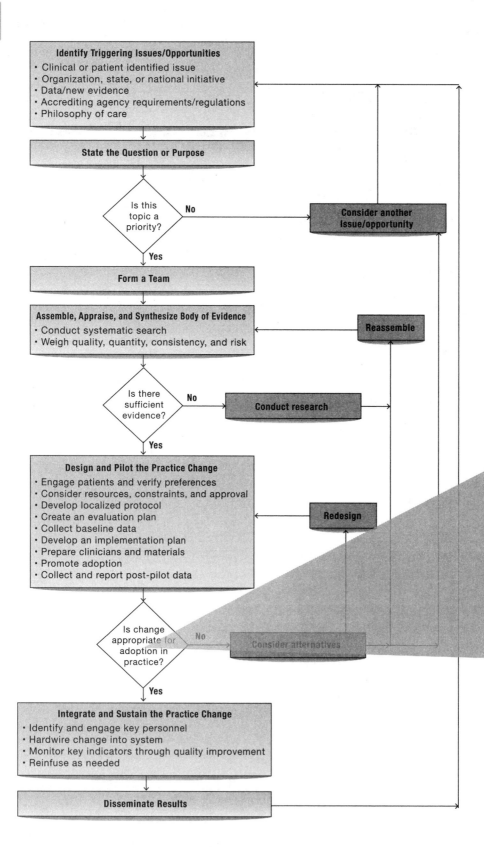

# IS CHANGE APPROPRIATE FOR ADOPTION IN PRACTICE?

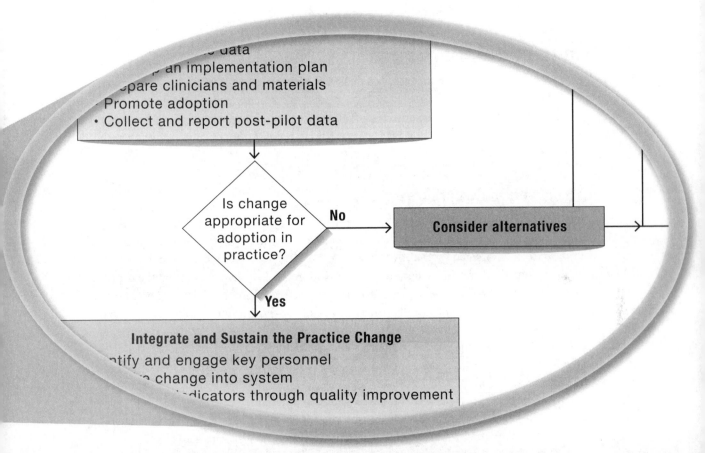

data
an implementation plan
pare clinicians and materials
• Promote adoption
• Collect and report post-pilot data

Is change appropriate for adoption in practice?

**No** → **Consider alternatives**

**Yes**

**Integrate and Sustain the Practice Change**
tify and engage key personnel
change into system
dicators through quality improvement

*"Vitality shows in not only the ability to persist, but in the ability to start over."*

–F. Scott Fitzgerald

A voiding unnecessary changes while integrating evidence-based practice (EBP) innovations to improve care is among the most important challenges in healthcare (Dixon-Woods, Amalberti, Goodman, Bergman, & Glasziou, 2011; IOM, 2015a). Next, the EBP process comes to this decision point: Is the change appropriate for practice? Prior to the decision to adopt a practice change, pilot testing is imperative. Consider use of pilot testing as parallel to a Phase 1 trial in research designed to identify risk or unintended outcomes of the innovation and system effects (Dixon-Woods et al., 2011). The pilot step allows the intervention and implementation plan to be tested and refined in context, addressing potential threats that will increase the chance for successful adoption in practice before full-scale implementation occurs. Implementation success can be measured by assimilation (the process of moving from awareness to adoption, resulting in a practice becoming routine or institutionalized) and fidelity (the extent to which the practice change is carried out as intended) (Panzano, Sweeney, Seffrin, Massatti, & Knudsen, 2012).

# Use Evaluation Data

The team reviews evaluative data from the pilot and decides whether the EBP practice change worked to improve outcomes as the evidence indicated and whether the implementation plan worked to promote adoption. Data from the evaluation are reviewed (see Tool 10.1). Each component of the evaluation informs the decision about effectiveness of the EBP change, use of the EBP protocol in the pilot area, and expanding rollout to other appropriate areas.

## Outcome Data and Balancing Measures

Outcome data and balancing measures provide the team with direction when determining whether the EBP change is appropriate for adoption in practice. Patient and/or organization quality and safety indicators make up the outcomes targeted for improvements (e.g., hospital-acquired infections, clinician retention). Balancing measures monitor for systemic effects and unintended consequences from the practice change (e.g., risk for falls when implementing an early ambulation intervention). Balancing measures are particularly important to consider when the evidence is not clear or risk is evident. Outcome data and balancing measures collected in the pilot should be compared pre- and post-practice change and then benchmarked with outcomes reported in the literature and by other organizations. If the practice change is not carried out as intended (low fidelity), outcomes may fail to improve (e.g., if steps are skipped in an EBP central line dressing change protocol, bloodstream infection rates may not improve and could even increase). If the intervention fails to achieve the expected outcomes, it may be a function of implementation failure rather than the EBP protocol or intervention itself (Panzano et al., 2012). Deciding whether outcomes met the intended goal for improvement is central to making a decision about next steps.

## Process Data

Process data supplement outcome data and may help to define barriers or solutions for the practice change. Process data include components from evaluation: knowledge, attitudes, and behaviors (see Chapter 9). Process data are also helpful in determining areas for improvement and next steps for the team.

## Knowledge

Knowledge of EBP has a direct influence on the adoption of a practice change (Pashaeypoor, Ashktorab, Rassouli, & Alavi-Majd, 2016; Rogers, 2003). Clinician knowledge should improve following implementation, when using strategies to build knowledge and commitment (see Chapter 8). If clinician knowledge does not improve, or remains lower than projected, additional education and outreach are needed (see Strategies 2-1 and 2-9). Target education to the established knowledge gaps identified in the baseline data.

## Attitudes

The attitudes component of evaluation captures clinician and patient/family feedback about both the EBP protocol and implementation. The perceived complexity, observability, and trialability are predictive of EBP adoption (Pashaeypoor et al., 2016). Usually, perceptions improve post-pilot through use of effective implementation strategies (Block, Lilienthal, Cullen, & White, 2012; Dolezal, Cullen, Harp, & Mueller, 2011). However, on certain projects, clinician perceptions may not improve, such as when the practice is difficult to use (e.g., nasogastric tube placement verification requiring sampling gastric aspirates) (Farrington, Lang, Cullen, & Stewart, 2009; Gilbertson, Rogers, & Ukoumunne, 2011; Peter & Gill, 2009) or when the clinician has gained new insights into the complexity of a practice that was previously viewed as routine (e.g., blood pressure measurement) (Cullen, Dawson, & Williams, 2010; Dole, 2009; Dole et al., 2011). If clinician perceptions are more positive post-pilot and do not indicate a need to revise the EBP protocol, the clinician is ready for adoption of the intervention. If clinician perceptions are rated lower than expected post-pilot, consider protocol revisions and/or expanding implementation strategies that build the practice change into the system (e.g., checklist, documentation, standing orders, patient reminders), making adoption easier. Choose specific implementation strategies that address items rated below the goal. For example, if clinicians rate "ease of documentation" low, adapt the documentation format.

## Behaviors

The practices or behaviors component of evaluation is also useful in determining next steps. This evaluation is often completed through a chart audit to capture use of the EBP protocol. Increased use of the electronic health record promises better access to process data. Critical indicators identified in the evidence and included in the EBP protocol will be captured in the behaviors component of evaluation. If clinicians are not completing key steps in the process (low intervention fidelity), consider the feasibility and the need to adapt the EBP protocol and/or implementation plan. Often, using one of two strategies may help: 1) troubleshoot use for complex patients (see Strategy 2-19) or 2) integrate practice change into the workflow (see Strategy 3-2). Patient health behaviors are also key to determining whether the practice change worked. If patient health behaviors don't change, the outcome is unlikely to improve. Determine the need to adapt patient/family involvement and decision aids (see Strategy 3-18) and revise the protocol and/or implementation.

## The Decision Point

When both process and outcome data are positive, as the body of evidence predicted, the decision to adopt and integrate is straightforward. In the real world, the data are less likely to be clear, and in most cases there continues to be opportunity to improve processes. Yet clinical decisions need to be made. Patients/families and clinicians often do not have the luxury of waiting for research to provide a definitive direction for practice. Clinicians must decide to move forward with adopting the EBP practice changes or consider other alternatives (see Figure 10.1). An EBP framework for making a decision between current practice and a practice innovation includes three sequential questions to guide teams through this decision point (see Tool 10.2):

1. Do the data suggest that the practice change is better than current practice?

2. Is the collection of more information worthwhile?

3. Should we wait for more evidence?

Tools may also help teams make the decision to implement (Johnson, Tuzzio, Renz, Baldwin, & Parchman, 2016) (see Tool 10.3).

**Figure 10.1**   Indications for Deciding: Is the Change Appropriate for Adoption in Practice?

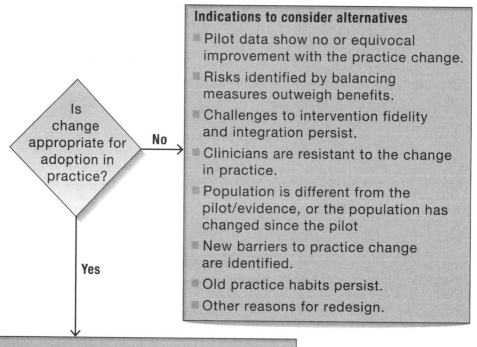

## Change Is Appropriate for Adoption in Practice

Planning for expanding the practice change beyond the pilot unit begins with creating awareness and interest through implementation and collecting baseline data for evaluation. In some cases, it may be appropriate to roll out an intervention to similar populations (e.g., adult medical surgical) first while repeating pilot testing only in high-risk populations with unique needs (e.g., pediatric oncology). Making the decision to roll out to other areas will be facilitated by involvement of representatives from that area. As with pilot testing, consider timing of implementation, capitalizing on times of increased awareness and interest but avoiding times where other changes compete for time and attention. Consider staggering the rollout or coordinating with information technology updates (Sparger et al., 2012).

When the decision is made to adopt a practice change, also consider eliminating old practices, which are often firmly entrenched in the clinical workflow. New practices cannot be fully adopted if old approaches, which lack evidence, persist. Old practice habits that are particularly resistant to change have been called "sacred cow" practices (Hanrahan et al., 2015; Makic, Rauen, Watson, & Poteet, 2014). The process of removing these practices, or eliminating sacred cows, is also described as de-implementation, de-innovation, or de-adoption, and is not simply the reverse of implementing an innovation. The challenges are different and may be even more difficult (Ubel & Asch, 2015). See Chapter 11 for more details about integrating the EBP practice change.

## Change Is Not Appropriate for Adoption in Practice

If the change is not ready for adoption in practice, consider these alternatives: Redesign and repilot the practice change, reassemble the evidence, or consider another issue/opportunity to address.

### Redesign and Repilot

Sometimes, failure of an innovation is not caused by failure of the EBP protocol itself, but rather by the complexity of the change or an inability to let go of the old practice (Sparger et al., 2012). In this case, it is appropriate to loop back, redesign the practice change based on evaluation data, and then repilot. For de-implementation, see Chapter 11.

### Reassemble

If redesign is indicated but options are not clear, it can be useful to reassemble the evidence. Reexamine the evidence for solutions to the problems you have identified (e.g., mismatch between practice recommendation and patient resources). It is appropriate to continue following the literature. If new research in the topic area emerges, loop back to assemble, appraise, and synthesize it with the evidence you have already reviewed.

## Consider Another Issue/Opportunity

Occasionally, it may be determined that the EBP change is not appropriate for adoption in practice—for example, the intervention is too costly, risks outweigh the benefits, organizational priorities change, or new literature provides significant contradiction. In this case, it may be appropriate to abandon the current EBP change and loop back to consider other issues and opportunities, essentially beginning the EBP process again. If the decision is made to abandon the practice change, the rationale and any data should be clearly communicated to stakeholders.

### TIPS: Making the Decision to Adopt

- Use outcome data to determine whether the practice change was beneficial.
- Use process evaluation data to determine whether the protocol needs to be revised.
- Use process data to identify implementation strategies that were effective during the pilot.
- Use process data to identify additional tools or resources needed to integrate the practice change into workflow.
- Stagger the rollout of practice changes to avoid overloading clinicians and to ensure adequate time for implementation.
- Plan for information technology changes that could delay rollout.
- Consider use of pilot testing as parallel to a Phase 1 trial in research designed to identify risk or unintended outcomes of the innovation and system effects.
- Remember that a delay in making the decision has associated risk.

## Tool 10.1   Decision to Adopt an EBP

**INSTRUCTIONS:** Insert evaluative data from the pilot. Review results as a team to determine whether evidence-based practice should be adopted as piloted.

### KNOWLEDGE

☐ Knowledge pre-data (i.e., total mean percent correct): _____

☐ Knowledge post-data (i.e., total mean percent correct): _____

☐ Knowledge improvement (comparing pre-data to post-data): _____

| Sufficient improvement? | ☐ Yes ☐ No |
|---|---|

If no, describe action needed:

| Is mean score > 80%? | ☐ Yes ☐ No |
|---|---|
| Specific items of concern? | ☐ Yes ☐ No |

If yes, describe problem and solution:

### ATTITUDE

| Key Indicator/Item | Pre-Data Mean | Post-Data Mean | Change | Threshold Achieved |
|---|---|---|---|---|
| | | | | ☐ Yes ☐ No |
| | | | | ☐ Yes ☐ No |
| | | | | ☐ Yes ☐ No |
| | | | | ☐ Yes ☐ No |

*Sample threshold = post-data mean > 3.25; 1–4 scale using Tool 9.4.

### BEHAVIOR

| Key Indicator/Item | Pre-Data Frequency/Mean | Post-Data Frequency/Mean | Change | Threshold Achieved |
|---|---|---|---|---|
| | | | | ☐ Yes ☐ No |
| | | | | ☐ Yes ☐ No |
| | | | | ☐ Yes ☐ No |

*Sample threshold = post-data percent improvement

*continues*

## Tool 10.1    Decision to Adopt an EBP (Continued)

### OUTCOMES

| **Anticipated Outcome #1:** | |
|---|---|
| ☐ Outcome pre-data | |
| ☐ Outcome post-data | |
| Improvement in outcome: | ☐ Yes<br>☐ Not sufficient |

If not, describe problem and solution:

| **Anticipated Outcome #2:** | |
|---|---|
| ☐ Outcome pre-data | |
| ☐ Outcome post-data | |
| Improvement in outcome: | ☐ Yes<br>☐ Not sufficient |

If not, describe problem and solution:

| **Anticipated Outcome #3:** | |
|---|---|
| ☐ Outcome pre-data | |
| ☐ Outcome post-data | |
| Improvement in outcome: | ☐ Yes<br>☐ Not sufficient |

If not, describe problem and solution:

| **Balancing Measure #1:** | |
|---|---|
| ☐ Outcome pre-data | |
| ☐ Outcome post-data | |
| Change in outcome: | ☐ Yes<br>☐ No |

If yes, describe problem and solution:

### CORRECTIVE ACTION NEEDED

## Tool 10.2 EBP Framework for Making Decisions About Adoption of EBP in Practice

**INSTRUCTIONS:** Read each section and answer questions sequentially. Discuss as a group to determine if the EBP change is appropriate.

### 1. Do the data suggest that the practice change is better than current practice?

Outcomes and balancing measures data should be used to determine the extent of the benefit (net benefit minus net risk or cost). Decision theory suggests that practice changes resulting in a net benefit should be implemented and that the strength and quality of evidence are irrelevant. However, in real-world clinical settings, the risk of making a wrong decision should be considered.

☐ Yes, change is appropriate                    ☐ No, consider next question

### 2. Is the collection of more information worthwhile?

Consider whether the benefit of getting more information outweighs the costs (including time) of collecting it. The value of added information can be determined by these questions:

a. How certain are we of the benefit of the practice change? _____

b. What is the potential impact of a wrong decision? _____

c. Would additional information significantly improve uncertainty? _____

d. What is the cost (including time and lost opportunity for improved outcomes) of collecting more data?
_____

If the value of the information exceeds the costs, it may be worthwhile to consider further pilot testing or research.

☐ No, change is appropriate                    ☐ Yes, consider next question

### 3. Should we wait for more evidence?

Consider the risk of implementing now versus waiting, with these questions:

a. How long will it take? _____

b. How likely is it that further evidence will change the practice recommendation? _____

c. What is the cost (e.g., risk) of delaying? _____

d. What would the cost be if the change were implemented and then found to be inferior?
_____

e. Would implementing prevent ongoing testing and future research, or could it be done concurrently?
_____

☐ No, change is appropriate                    ☐ Yes, consider further pilot testing or research (see Chapter 6)

(Chalkidou, Lord, Fischer, & Littlejohns, 2008)

## Tool 10.3    Decision to Implement

**INSTRUCTIONS**: Determine whether a new clinical tool or process is relevant and worth implementing or adapting for your practice. Use it individually or as a point for team discussion.

| 1. To what extent do you agree that this intervention: | Strongly Agree | Agree | Disagree | Strongly Disagree |
|---|---|---|---|---|
| a) Addresses a common or high-priority problem in our practice | 1 | 2 | 3 | 4 |
| b) Could be modified to meet the needs of our practice | 1 | 2 | 3 | 4 |
| c) Would be simple to implement in our practice | 1 | 2 | 3 | 4 |
| d) Is likely to improve processes or patient outcomes in our practice | 1 | 2 | 3 | 4 |
| e) Could be pilot tested in our practice prior to fully implementing | 1 | 2 | 3 | 4 |
| f) Is relevant to our patient population (from the patient or provider perspective) | 1 | 2 | 3 | 4 |
| g) Would work for our patient population | 1 | 2 | 3 | 4 |

| 2. Consider how you would adopt or adapt this intervention in your practice. What level of resources would you need in the following areas? | Low | | | High | Don't Know |
|---|---|---|---|---|---|
| a) Extent of training for clinicians | 1 | 2 | 3 | 4 | |
| b) Changes to workflow, roles, and tasks among team members | 1 | 2 | 3 | 4 | |
| c) Technical assistance to modify the patient health record or data systems | 1 | 2 | 3 | 4 | |
| d) New and/or additional financial investment/support | 1 | 2 | 3 | 4 | |
| e) Support from local practice/clinic leader | 1 | 2 | 3 | 4 | |
| 3. What is the likelihood that you will adopt or adapt this intervention in your practice in the next year? | 1 | 2 | 3 | 4 | |

4. If you were going to adapt this intervention to your practice, note your ideas about what you would change.

(Research Toolkit, 2013)

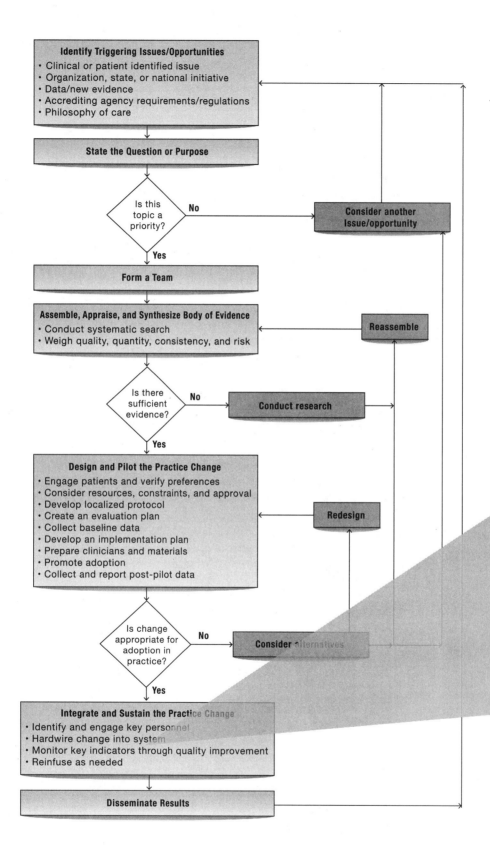

**Identify Triggering Issues/Opportunities**
- Clinical or patient identified issue
- Organization, state, or national initiative
- Data/new evidence
- Accrediting agency requirements/regulations
- Philosophy of care

**State the Question or Purpose**

Is this topic a priority?

No → **Consider another Issue/opportunity**

Yes

**Form a Team**

**Assemble, Appraise, and Synthesize Body of Evidence**
- Conduct systematic search
- Weigh quality, quantity, consistency, and risk

**Reassemble**

Is there sufficient evidence?

No → **Conduct research**

Yes

**Design and Pilot the Practice Change**
- Engage patients and verify preferences
- Consider resources, constraints, and approval
- Develop localized protocol
- Create an evaluation plan
- Collect baseline data
- Develop an implementation plan
- Prepare clinicians and materials
- Promote adoption
- Collect and report post-pilot data

**Redesign**

Is change appropriate for adoption in practice?

No → **Consider alternatives**

Yes

**Integrate and Sustain the Practice Change**
- Identify and engage key personnel
- Hardwire change into system
- Monitor key indicators through quality improvement
- Reinfuse as needed

**Disseminate Results**

# INTEGRATE AND SUSTAIN THE PRACTICE CHANGE

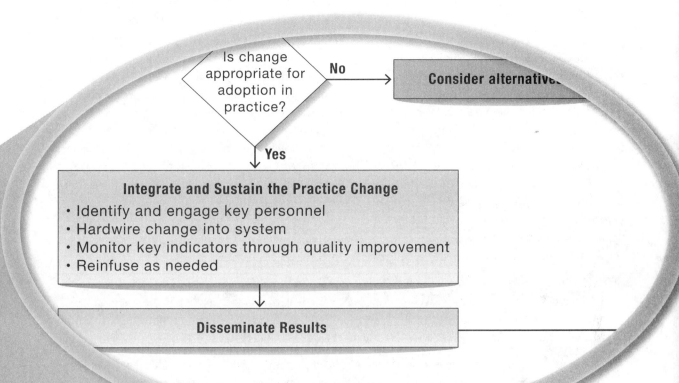

*"If you don't know where you are going, you'll end up somewhere else."*

–Yogi Berra

After the pilot and decision to integrate the practice change in the pilot area, additional work is needed to move from adoption to sustained use of the evidence-based practice (EBP) protocol. When instituting the practice change, the focus on implementation strategies shifts to pursuing integration and sustained use of the EBP change (see Figure 11.1) and learning from evaluative data (Cullen & Adams, 2012; Fleiszer, Semenic, Ritchie, Richer, & Denis, 2016a; Fleuren, van Dommelen, & Dunnink, 2015).

**Figure 11.1** Implementation Phases

A number of implementation strategies will need to continue from earlier phases of implementation. The project team should review the clinician feedback about implementation strategies used during the pilot for this planning. Some strategies may be abandoned, some continued, and others added. Evidence to guide how to sustain practice change is still developing. However, a number of strategies have some evidence supporting continued use for sustainability (see Figure 11.2). This phase of implementation continues to require local leadership to coordinate practice improvements (Fleiszer et al., 2016a; Fleuren et al., 2015; Lowson et al., 2015; Nordqvist, Timpka, & Lindqvist, 2009) and continued participation by champions and point-of-care clinicians (Doyle et al., 2013; Fleiszer et al., 2016a; Ford, Krahn, Wise, & Oliver, 2011; Lowson et al., 2015; Wiltsey, Stirman et al., 2012). This is a time to promote peer influence (Hoke & Guarracino, 2016; Smith & Korenstein, 2015) but also continue to celebrate and recognize completed work (see Strategy 4-1). Progress toward this goal will be neither rapid nor smooth. Senior leaders need to provide visible support that acknowledges the value of the improvement to patient care (Fleiszer et al., 2016a; Ford et al., 2011) and sets the standard for using the EBP process.

Strategies for implementing practice innovations may need to be paired with strategies for removing old habits, including building teams with competing biases, emphasizing evidence over opinion, resisting extending evidence-based changes to unproven areas or populations, and encouraging clinicians to examine biases in their interpretation of evidence (Hanrahan et al., 2015; Ubel & Asch, 2015).

Resistance to change or psychological biases make it difficult for clinicians to let go of outdated practices. Work on implementation continues, and now is an important time to consider de-implementation. Often new EBP practices being implemented will change practice procedures. Sometimes science updates indicate practices need to be abandoned altogether (Nevin et al., 2015; Prasad & Ioannidis, 2014). Implementation and sustainment for practice recommendation reversal or abandonment may create new challenges for de-implementation of old practices (Hanrahan et al., 2015). Eliminating costly, ineffective, or low-value practices remains a national and international priority (van Bodegom-Vos, Davidoff, & Marang-van de Mheen, 2016). More research is needed to provide guidance for de-implementation. Current strategies for de-implementation are to update local policies, integrate EBP into the patient health record, substitute old practices with new ones, and maintain a clear focus on improving outcomes (Montini & Graham, 2015; Nevin et al., 2015; van Bodegom-Vos et al., 2016). Monitor for practice variation, updates to Choosing Wisely®, and professional organization recommendations to stay abreast of practices requiring de-implementation (American Board of Internal Medicine Foundation, 2017; Nevin et al., 2015).

**Figure 11.2**    Evidence-Based Implementation Strategies for Sustainability

| Create Awareness & Interest | Build Knowledge & Commitment | Promote Action & Adoption | Pursue Integration & Sustained Use |
|---|---|---|---|
| **Connecting with Clinicians, Organizational Leaders, and Key Stakeholders** | | | |
| ▪ Highlight advantages* or anticipated impact*<br>▪ Highlight compatibility*<br>▪ Continuing education programs*<br>▪ Sound bites*<br>▪ Journal club*<br>▪ Slogans & logos<br>▪ Staff meetings<br>▪ Unit newsletter<br>▪ Unit inservices<br>▪ Distribute key evidence<br>▪ Posters and postings/fliers<br>▪ Mobile 'show on the road'<br>▪ Announcements & broadcasts | ▪ Education (e.g., live, virtual, or computer-based)*<br>▪ Pocket guides<br>▪ Link practice change & power holder/stakeholder priorities*<br>▪ Change agents (e.g., change champion*, core group*, opinion leader*, thought leader, etc.)<br>▪ Educational outreach or academic detailing*<br>▪ Integrate practice change with other EBP protocols*<br>▪ Disseminate credible evidence with clear implications for practice*<br>▪ Make impact observable*<br>▪ Gap assessment/gap analysis*<br>▪ Clinician input*<br>▪ Local adaptation* & simplify*<br>▪ Focus groups for planning change*<br>▪ Match practice change with resources & equipment<br>▪ Resource manual or materials (i.e., electronic or hard copy)<br>▪ Case studies | ▪ Educational outreach/academic detailing*<br>▪ Reminders or practice prompts*<br>▪ Demonstrate workflow or decision algorithm<br>▪ Resource materials and quick reference guides<br>▪ Skill competence*<br>▪ Give evaluation results to colleagues*<br>▪ Incentives*<br>▪ Try the practice change*<br>▪ Multidisciplinary discussion & troubleshooting<br>▪ "Elevator speech"<br>▪ Data collection by clinicians<br>▪ Report progress & updates<br>▪ Change agents (e.g., change champion*, core group*, opinion leader*, thought leader, etc.)<br>▪ Role model*<br>▪ Troubleshooting at the point of care/bedside<br>▪ Provide recognition at the point of care* | ▪ Celebrate local unit progress*<br>▪ Individualize data feedback*<br>▪ Public recognition*<br>▪ Personalize the messages to staff (e.g., reduces work, reduces infection exposure, etc.) based on actual improvement data<br>▪ Share protocol revisions with clinician that are based on feedback from clinicians, patient, or family<br>▪ Peer influence<br>▪ Update practice reminders |
| **Building Organizational System Support** | | | |
| ▪ Knowledge broker(s)<br>▪ Senior executives announcements<br>▪ Publicize new equipment | ▪ Teamwork*<br>▪ Troubleshoot use/application*<br>▪ Benchmark data*<br>▪ Inform organizational leaders*<br>▪ Report within organizational infrastructure*<br>▪ Action plan*<br>▪ Report to senior leaders | ▪ Audit key indicators*<br>▪ Actionable and timely data feedback*<br>▪ Non-punitive discussion of results*<br>▪ Checklist*<br>▪ Documentation*<br>▪ Standing orders*<br>▪ Patient reminders*<br>▪ Patient decision aids*<br>▪ Rounding by unit & organizational leadership*<br>▪ Report into quality improvement program*<br>▪ Report to senior leaders<br>▪ Action plan*<br>▪ Link to patient/family needs & organizational priorities<br>▪ Unit orientation<br>▪ Individual performance evaluation | ▪ Audit and feedback*<br>▪ Report to senior leaders*<br>▪ Report into quality improvement program*<br>▪ Revise policy, procedure, or protocol*<br>▪ Competency metric for discontinuing training<br>▪ Project responsibility in unit or organizational committee<br>▪ Strategic plan*<br>▪ Trend results*<br>▪ Present in educational programs<br>▪ Annual report<br>▪ Financial incentives*<br>▪ Individual performance evaluation |

* Implementation strategy is supported by at least some empirical evidence in healthcare.
For permission to use, go to https://uihc.org/implementation-strategies-evidence-based-practice-evidence-based-practice-implementation-guide
© Copyright of the Implementation Strategies for Evidence-Based Practice is retained by Laura Cullen, MA, RN, FAAN, and the University of Iowa Hospitals and Clinics.
Cullen, L., & Adams, S. L. (2012). Planning for implementation of evidence-based practice. *Journal of Nursing Administration, 42*(4), 222–230. doi:10.1097/NNA.0B013E31824CCD0A

# Identify and Engage Key Personnel

The team involved in instituting the practice change may be different from the pilot team. This team is now responsible for sustaining the practice in the pilot area, rolling out and standardizing the practice within the institution, and providing ongoing evaluation to determine the need for reinfusion. Action planning is an approach to build EBP work into the system, and it may be beneficial when redesigning team membership (see Tool 11.1) and planning for sustainability. Sequential reporting within shared governance committees (see Figure 11.3) and the quality improvement program ensures that the message reaches stakeholders (see Strategy 3-20). The integration team may now include, as key stakeholders, experts from quality or performance improvement, clinician education or orientation, policy, and documentation committees.

# Hardwire Change Into the System

Creating a practice routine hardwires the behavior change as the routine workflow (Innis & Berta, 2016; Spyridonidis & Calnan, 2011). The practice change should become the new norm. No clear formula exists for hard-wiring the practice into the clinicians' workflow. Strategies described in this phase will facilitate sustained use of EBP. Some early implementation strategies need to continue across later implementation phases to promote sustainability. Practice changes with continued commitment from change agents and senior leaders to maintain attention and resources may be helpful. Clinicians are busy and can easily revert to old habits, so active implementation strategies are still needed to maintain or build ownership from the clinicians involved (Davies, Tremblay, & Edwards, 2010; Spyridonidis & Calnan, 2011; Stenberg & Wann-Hansson, 2011; Tucker, Bieber, Attlesey-Pries, Olson, & Dierkhising, 2012).

# Monitor Key Indicators Through Quality Improvement (QI)

Continued evaluation is needed to track integration and identify any need for reinfusion. Linking back to the quality improvement (QI) cycle to monitor key indicators will be helpful (Gruen et al., 2008; Hulscher, Schouten, Grol, & Buchan, 2013; Lindamer et al., 2009; Maher, Gustafson, & Evans, 2010). Long-term evaluation monitors and analyzes structure, process, and outcome data (see Chapter 9). Process and outcome indicators are essential to monitor. Indicators are narrowed from those used in the pilot to those deemed critical to follow (i.e., to maintain fidelity) or those still showing an opportunity for improvement. No more than three to five process indicators and two outcome indicators should be collected long term, to keep resources focused on integration without exhausting them on evaluation (Fleiszer et al., 2016a; Fleuren et al., 2015). Structure indicators may be appropriate to consider monitoring in some EBP changes. In some cases, the structure evaluation refers to the physical environment supporting and sustaining the EBP (e.g., airflow in the operating room, milieu in a behavioral unit, environmental hazards for falling). Clinician expertise or training may also be an important structure indicator to track (e.g., pain certification in the Post Anesthesia Care Unit). The infrastructure supporting the EBP change will be important to identify now as well. An organizational, departmental, or unit committee may be charged with maintaining or continuously improving practices based on the EBP pilot (Lowson et al., 2015). Review and consideration of the structure supporting the EBP are valuable for ensuring that the institution can support sustaining the change. Some flexibility is needed. Indicators to track during this phase may change as the needs evolve.

**Figure 11.3**   Reporting in Shared Governance Structure Supporting Integration of EBP

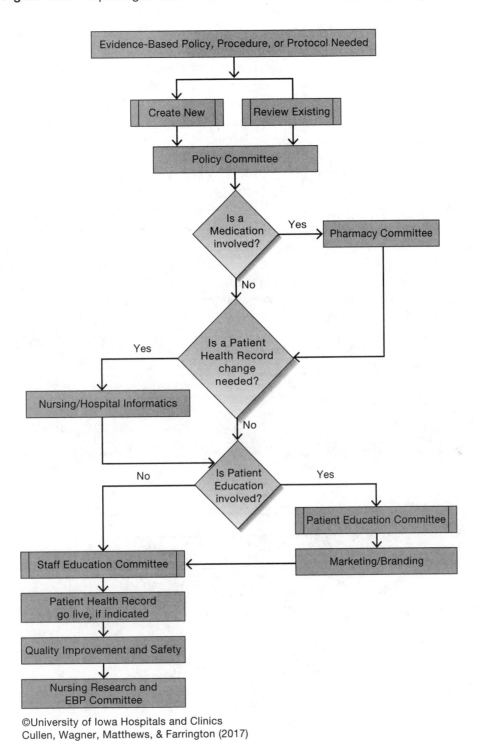

©University of Iowa Hospitals and Clinics
Cullen, Wagner, Matthews, & Farrington (2017)

Data are collected and shared using audit and feedback techniques (see Strategies 3-12, 3-13, and 4-6). Think carefully about how to present data to stakeholders. Select a graph for reporting pilot results to make interpretation easy (see Figure 9.1) (Abela, 2013; Carey & Lloyd, 2001), or consider using an online or software application (e.g., http://labs.juiceanalytics.com/chartchooser/index.html). Data are collected and tracked to demonstrate sustained gains, continued incremental improvements, or need for reinfusion (see Figure 11.4) (Benneyan, Lloyd, & Plsek, 2003; Carey & Lloyd, 2001; Mohammed, Worthington, & Woodall, 2008). Data can be displayed using a histogram, run chart, or statistical process control chart. Each type of graph can demonstrate clinically important improvements for interpretation by clinical experts. A histogram can be used early in the integration process, when fewer data points are available (see Tool 11.2). As data are tracked over time and additional data points are available, a more robust graphical display is possible. A run chart is an option that is easy to develop and interpret (see Tool 11.3). A run chart may be used with at least 10 to 12 data points (NHSScotland Quality Improvement Hub, 2016; Perla, Provost, & Murray, 2011). Run charts are more powerful than histograms by providing a mechanism to identify statistically significant changes in practices or outcomes. Statistical process control charts are the most robust way to report evaluative data that display practice patterns over time (see Tool 11.4). Statistical process control charts require a minimum of 15 data points. A run chart or statistical process control chart can be used to identify statistically significant trends caused by specific intervention or environmental factors, known as "special cause variation" (Benneyan, 1998a, 1998b; Carey & Lloyd, 2001). EBP improvements seek to generate positive special cause variation.

**Figure 11.4**   Trended Outcome Data

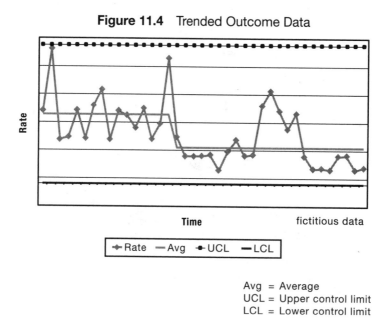

Avg = Average
UCL = Upper control limit
LCL = Lower control limit

# Reinfuse as Needed

A need for reinfusion can be identified from the data. Proactive planning for reinfusion and adaptation is also needed to sustain the gains achieved through the pilot (Gruen et al., 2008; Lindamer et al., 2009). Often, practices tend to slip back in the 3- to 6-month period after the pilot, if strategies for pursuing integration and sustained use are not sufficient. Plan periodic data feedback to keep busy clinicians focused (see Strategies 4-2 and 4-6) (Fleiszer et al., 2016a; Fleuren et al., 2015; Lowson et al., 2015). Part of reinfusion is building ongoing training into orientation and educational programs (Doyle et al., 2013; Fleiszer et al., 2016a; Hulscher et al., 2013; Lowson et al., 2015). More research is needed on sustainability of EBP protocols to determine exact timing for reinfusion. In the early phases of project integration, a minimum of quarterly reinfusion may be helpful.

The post-pilot period was also used to collate data for internal reporting (Innis & Berta, 2016). Internal and external dissemination can occur during the integration phase (see Chapter 12). Presentation and/or publication may be appropriate and can require an additional investment from the team. Dissemination should not divert attention and resources from integration efforts to avoid creating the need to repeat work on implementation because practice reverted to old habits. Keep the team focused to attain sustained change. Be flexible with selecting and timing of continued implementation strategies, using audit and actionable data feedback (see Strategy 4-6) to achieve the goal. Each project will follow its own timeline and path to integration (Rogers, 2003).

## TIPS: Integrate and Sustain the Practice Change

- Build on action planning from implementation to reinvigorate the team.

- Add key stakeholders as needed.

- Review post-pilot data to determine key implementation strategies to continue or modify.

- Review post-pilot data to determine key indicators to trend integration and sustainability or to stimulate reinfusion.

- Determine whether a phased approach would help with rollout or scaling up in other areas.

- Keep senior leaders informed to guide their continued active discussion, planning, and facilitation of the EBP improvement.

- Integrate project work into existing committee responsibilities.

## Tool 11.1   Action Plan for Sustaining EBP

**INSTRUCTIONS:** This tool is designed with key steps for integrating and sustaining an EBP change. Review the outlined steps and identify any steps to remove and delete that row. Fill in remaining cells to develop a comprehensive integration plan. Include the key step, specific actions for each step, individuals by name, materials or resources needed, anticipated date for completion, metric to demonstrate completion of the activity, and mark done. Discuss as a team and update regularly.

| Project Director Name: | Team: | |
|---|---|---|
| Project Purpose: To integrate the _____ EBP practice change into routine workflow as standard practice on _____ (Unit/clinic) | | |
| **Key Step or Objective** | **Specific Activities to Meet Objective** | **Person Responsible** |
| Review team membership to focus on integration | Review team membership and determine need to link within shared governance | |
| | Reconfigure team: Add strategic members | |
| Internal strategic reporting | Practice/policy committee name: _____ | |
| | Informatics/electronic health record representative _____ (name) | |
| | Patient education committee _____ (name) | |
| | Staff education committee _____ (name) | |
| | Quality/performance improvement committee _____ (name) | |
| | EBP committee _____ (name) | |
| Identify key data to trend | Identify process indicators with opportunity for improvement | |
| | Narrow to key process indicators with greatest impact on outcome | |
| | Identify key outcome indicators | |
| | Identify balancing measure required to reduced undesired effect, needing ongoing monitoring | |
| Mobilize QI methods | Generate report within QI/PI system | |
| | Select appropriate graph to display data trends (e.g., run or statistical process control chart) | |

| | Materials or Resources Needed | Due Date | Evaluation | Done Date |
|---|---|---|---|---|
| | Team plan/charter with membership outlined | | Updated team membership list | |
| | Project summary to share | | Email and meet/invite | |
| | Flowchart of committees within shared governance structure | | Report project update with proposed policy update | |
| | | | Report project update with proposed changes in order sets, documentation, etc. | |
| | | | Report project update with proposed patient educational materials with reading level assessment | |
| | | | Report project update with proposed plan | |
| | | | Report project update with integration plan | |
| | | | Report project findings with integration plan | |
| | Data management resources | | Considered knowledge, attitude, and practices/behaviors for clinicians and patients | |
| | | | Created list of < 10 indicators for each: knowledge, attitude, and practices/behaviors (see Tools 9.1 and 9.2) | |
| | | | Top 2: _____ _____ | |
| | | | Determined unintended consequence to monitor: _____ | |
| | | Quarterly | Example 9.5 | |
| | | | Histogram for immediate post-pilot (see Tool 11.2) | |

*continues*

EXAMPLES

TOOLS

## Tool 11.1   Action Plan for Sustaining EBP (Continued)

| Key Step or Objective | Specific Activities to Meet Objective | Person Responsible |
|---|---|---|
| | Monitor data using audit, and report using actionable feedback | |
| | Identify interprofessional champions for QI cycle | |
| Select integration strategies | Review Implementation Strategies for EBP | |
| | Select strategies to continue and to add | |
| | Determine timing for proactive and regular reinfusion | |
| | Identify local champion with responsibility to lead through integration | |
| Set goal | Establish target for integration that indicates change is hardwired | |
| | Determine when goal is met to remove from future training programs or competency training, if appropriate | |
| External reporting of lessons learned | Select a venue reaching target audience | |
| | Choose conference abstract (paper or poster) and/or manuscript | |
| | Develop and submit an abstract following author guidelines | |
| Garner continued senior leadership support | Send notification of team success to assist team leaders in recognizing team | |
| | Report through QI system to senior leaders and board | |
| | Acknowledge leadership support in success | |
| Monitor for need to reinvigorate team | Follow trended data for deterioration | |
| Determine need to cycle back to top of Iowa Model | Identify whether topic work was divided into pieces (e.g., assessment completed first, intervention next) | |
| | Evidence changes practice recommendation | |
| | Data indicate deterioration in practice | |

| Materials or Resources Needed | Timeline | Evaluation | Done Date |
|---|---|---|---|
| | | | |
| | | Discipline specific champions: _____ | |
| See Figure 11.2 | | Team discussion using 15% solutions activity (Lipmanowicz & McCandless, 2014) | |
| | | List strategies with responsibility for follow-up | |
| | Begin 3 months after pilot evaluation | Quarterly until target reached and sustained for 1 year | |
| | | Clinician champion: _____ _____ | |
| Review pilot evaluation data | | Key data meet or exceed goal for 1 year | |
| | | Evaluate quarterly | |
| | | Abstract submission <organization> | |
| | | ☐ Paper/oral <br> ☐ Poster | |
| Expert review before submission | | Due <date> | |
| | | Email summary of success | |
| Brief project/executive summary (see Examples 6.4 and 12.1) | | Report project summary | |
| Example 9.5 | | Public recognition or send a thank-you note | |
| | | Monitor quarterly | |
| | | Next round will address: <topic> | |
| | | Librarian-assisted search | |
| | | Monitor quarterly | |

EXAMPLES

TOOLS

## Tool 11.2   Histograms

**INSTRUCTIONS:** The procedures for developing, displaying, and interpreting a histogram are outlined as a checklist. Complete each step and mark as each step is done.

## Benefits and Limitations

- Easy to understand
- Demonstrates progress toward goal
- Provides an easy-to-identify improvement or need for reinfusion
- Does not indicate if change is normal variation or special cause
- Does not indicate statistical or clinical significance
- Demonstrates static, not dynamic data

## Procedure

- ☐ Obtain data software with graphical capability
- ☐ Determine indicators to graph
- ☐ Select frequency of data reporting (e.g., monthly)
  - ○ Determine number of available data points for $x$-axis
- ☐ Select graph: histogram versus run chart or statistical process control chart
  - ○ Consider audience: expertise and preference for data display
  - ○ Use most robust data display option
- ☐ Retrieve or enter data into a spreadsheet or statistical software
- ☐ Plot, arrange, connect data points, and then format data display
  - ○ Maintain full display of $y$-axis end points (e.g., 0–100%)
- ☐ Determine whether a benchmark is available and beneficial to include, add if available
- ☐ Label axis and legends clearly
- ☐ Determine stability or variation in data that indicates whether performance improvement was achieved or intervention is needed
- ☐ Distribute data display with next steps to keep data actionable
- ☐ Consider strategic internal dissemination to executives

## Interpreting Histograms

- ☐ Locate the operational definition of the indicator being displayed
- ☐ Consider which measure of central tendency is being displayed (e.g. mean, median)
- ☐ Look for variation
  - ○ Identify the baseline data point
  - ○ Identify the most recent data point

☐ Determine the change from baseline

☐ Determine if improvement is demonstrated in the data (i.e., change in the desired direction)

☐ Determine if goal was achieved and maintained (e.g., more than one post-pilot data point)

☐ Ask questions to expand the understanding of the data

☐ Describe what the data mean, as a story

## Example

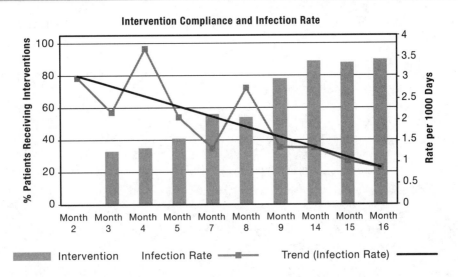

**Intervention Compliance and Infection Rate**

fictitious data

Books and software are listed that provide direction for creating and using histograms.

■ Carey, R. G., & Lloyd, R. C. (2001). *Measuring quality improvement in healthcare: A guide to statistical process control applications.* Milwaukee, WI: ASQ Quality Press.

■ KhanAcademy. (2016). Creating a histogram [Video file]. Retrieved from https://www.khanacademy.org/math/cc-sixth-grade-math/cc-6th-data-statistics/histograms/v/histograms-intro

■ Microsoft. (n.d.). Create a histogram. Retrieved from https://support.office.com/en-us/article/Create-a-histogram-B6814E9E-5860-4113-BA51-E3A1B9EE1BBE

■ MySecretMathTutor. (2011, September 1). Statistics–how to make a histogram [Video file]. Retrieved from https://www.youtube.com/watch?v=KCH_ZDygrm4

■ Smith, J. M. (2014). *Meaningful graphs: Converting data into informative Excel® charts.* United States of America: Author.

■ Statistics How To. (2013). Make a histogram in easy steps. Retrieved from http://www.statisticshowto.com/make-histogram

## Tool 11.3   Run Charts

**INSTRUCTIONS:** The procedures for developing, displaying, and interpreting a run chart are outlined as a checklist. Complete each step and mark as each step is done. Use the examples as a visual tool.

## Benefits and Limitations

- Demonstrates progress toward goal and sustained use of practice improvement
- Easy to identify random vs. non-random change/variation
- Provides an easy-to-identify need for reinfusion
- Improves strength of interpretation by using robust analysis that may demonstrate a clinically significant or statistically significant impact
- Control charts without limits
- Require no statistical calculations
- Easy to understand
- Will not detect all special cause variation
- Require a minimum of 10 data points (although some rules have been extended for use when at least 5 data points are available)

## Procedure

- [ ] Obtain data software with graphical capability
- [ ] Determine indicators to graph
- [ ] Select frequency of data reporting (e.g., monthly)
  - ○ Consider audience: expertise and preference for data display
  - ○ Use most robust data display option
- [ ] Select graph: run chart versus histogram, or statistical process control chart
- [ ] Determine number of available data points for *x*-axis
- [ ] Retrieve or enter data into a spreadsheet or statistical software
- [ ] Plot, arrange, connect data points, and then format data display
  - ○ Maintain full display of *y*-axis end points (e.g., 0–100%)
- [ ] Include a median—indicated by a line through the data points
- [ ] Determine whether a benchmark is available and beneficial to include, add if available
- [ ] Label axis and legends clearly
- [ ] Determine stability or variation in data that indicates whether performance improvement was achieved or intervention is needed

☐ Distribute data display with next steps to keep data actionable

☐ Consider strategic internal dissemination to executives

☐ Determine when to freeze the median/mean or limits to demonstrate improvement and/or establish a new goal

## Interpreting Run Charts

Use these rules to determine if there is special cause (statistically significant and non-random) as compared to common cause variation (what is usually expected in healthcare data). Data that break these rules indicate special cause variation that requires further investigation.

**Rule 1: Identify a shift:** six or more consecutive data points above or below the median (ignore the values that fall on the median and continue the count)

☐ If the graph includes fewer than 20 data points (not on the median) then 7 or more equals a shift

☐ If 20 or more data points (not on the median) then 8 or more equals a shift

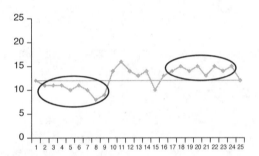

**Rule 2: Identify a trend:** number of consecutive ascending or descending points; dependent on number of data points. Ignore one of two consecutive data points that are identical.

☐ If there are 5–8 total data points then 5 or more consecutive ascending or descending indicate special cause

☐ If there are 9–20 total data points then 6 or more indicate special cause

☐ If there are 21–100 total data points then 7 or more indicate special cause

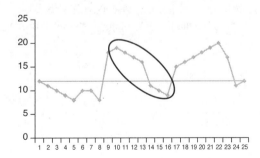

*continues*

EXAMPLES

TOOLS

## Tool 11.3　Run Charts (Continued)

### Interpreting Run Charts (Continued)

<u>**Rule 3**</u>: **Identify a run:** consecutive data points on the same side of the median. Count number of times the data line crosses the median line AND add one.

☐ Use an established probability to determine whether there are more or fewer than the expected number. (http://www.qihub.scot.nhs.uk/media/529936/run%20chart%20rules.pdf or  http://sixsigmastudyguide. com/run-chart)

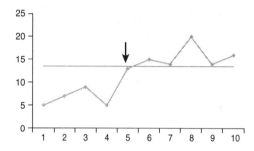

<u>**Rule 4**</u>: **Identify an astronomical point:** data points that are different from all or a majority of other values as well as being different from the highest and lowest values usually seen

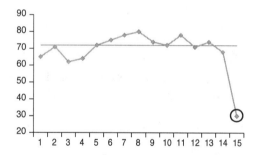

## Example

Avdić, A., Tucker, S., Evans, R., Smith, A., & Zimmerman, M. B. (2016). Comparing the ratio of mean red blood cell transfusion episode rate of 1 unit versus 2 units in hematopoietic stem cell transplant patients. *Transfusion, 56*(9), 2346–2351. doi:10.1111/trf.13708

## Resources

Books and software are listed that provide direction for creating and using run charts.

- Berardinelli, C., & Yerian, L. (n.d.). Run charts: A simple and powerful tool for process improvement [Web log post]. Retrieved from https://www.isixsigma.com/tools-templates/control-charts/run-charts-a-simple-and-powerful-tool-for-process-improvement

- Blossom, P. (2013, April 1). Create a run chart [Video file]. Retrieved from https://www.youtube.com/watch?v=0FNzoB19G4A

- Carey, R. G., & Lloyd, R. C. (2001). *Measuring quality improvement in healthcare: A guide to statistical process control applications.* Milwaukee, WI: ASQ Quality Press.

- Institute for Healthcare Improvement. (n.d.-a). Run chart tool. Retrieved from http://www.ihi.org/resources/pages/tools/runchart.aspx

- Institute for Healthcare Improvement. (n.d.-b). Whiteboard: Run chart [Video file]. Retrieved from http://www.ihi.org/education/IHIOpenSchool/resources/Pages/AudioandVideo/Whiteboard7.aspx

- National Health Service. (n.d.-c). Run chart rules for interpretation. Retrieved from http://www.qihub.scot.nhs.uk/media/529936/run%20chart%20rules.pdf

- Perla, R. J., Provost, L. P., & Murray, S. K. (2011). The run chart: A simple analytical tool for learning from variation in healthcare processes. *BMJ Quality & Safety, 20*(1), 46–51. doi:10.1136/bmjqs.2009.037895.

- Six Sigma study guide. ((2014, January 20). Run chart: Creation, analysis, & rules. Retrieved from http://sixsigmastudyguide.com/run-chart

- Smith, J. M. (2014). *Meaningful graphs: Converting data into informative Excel® charts.* United States of America: Author.

EXAMPLES

TOOLS

## Tool 11.4    Statistical Process Control Charts

**INSTRUCTIONS:** The procedures for developing, displaying, and interpreting a statistical process control chart are outlined as a checklist. Complete each step and mark as each step is done. Use the examples as a visual tool.

## Benefits and Limitations

▪ Demonstrates progress toward goal and sustained use of practice improvement

▪ Easy to identify random vs. non-random change/variation

▪ Provides an easy-to-identify need for reinfusion

▪ Improves strength of interpretation by using robust analysis that may demonstrate a clinically significant or statistically significant impact

▪ Will not detect all special cause variation

▪ Requires a minimum of 15 data points

## Procedure

☐ Obtain data software with graphical capability

☐ Determine indicators to graph

☐ Select frequency of data reporting (e.g., monthly)

   ○ Consider audience: expertise and preference for data display

   ○ Use most robust data display option

☐ Select graph: statistical process control chart versus histogram or run chart

☐ Determine number of available data points for *x*-axis

☐ Determine whether displaying continuous or discrete data and select the type of chart to use

☐ Retrieve or enter data into a spreadsheet or statistical software

☐ Plot, arrange, connect data points, and then format data display

   ○ Maintain full display of *y*-axis end points (e.g., 0–100%)

☐ Include a mean—indicated by a line through the data points

☐ Determine whether a benchmark is available and beneficial to include, add if available

☐ Label axis and legends clearly

☐ Determine stability or variation in data that indicates whether performance improvement was achieved or intervention is needed

   ○ Mark the time points on the graph when interventions occurred.

○ Look for common cause and special cause variation. Common cause variation is expected and is the usual variation seen in real life (e.g., time needed to go from home to work varies). Special cause variation is a statistically significant change in trended data (e.g., construction or an accident significantly interfering with your travel time between home and work). Identify special cause variation by using the seven rules outlined in the section that follows.

○ Note that an improvement from an EBP change in practice procedures may shift the mean or create a positive special cause variation that is in the desired direction (e.g., significantly fewer hospital-acquired events).

☐ Identify key components of the graph:

○ Find the mean, indicated by a line through the center of the data points on the graph.

○ Identify Zone C:  First locate the mean. Then locate the first line on either side of the mean. Zone C is one sigma or approximately one standard deviation away from the mean. Sigma is used to indicate data spread. If the data are normally distributed (i.e., bell-shaped curve), Zone C will contain about 68% of the data points.

○ Next identify Zone B: This is approximately two standard deviations on either side of the mean. If the data are normally distributed, Zone B will contain about 95% of the data points.

○ Lastly identify Zone A: This is approximately three standard deviations on either side of the mean. Zone A will contain 99% of the data, if data are normally distributed.

○ Upper control limit (UCL) is three sigmas (or standard deviations) above the mean. The UCL may be displayed with a static or roving line on the upper edge of Zone A.

○ Lower control limit (LCL) is three sigmas below the mean. The LCL will be displayed with a static or roving line, matching the UCL, and is located on the lower edge of Zone A. In healthcare the LCL may be zero and not included on the graph.

○ In some cases, only the three sigmas or UCL and LCL will be displayed because they are fairly easily applied in practice.

☐ Distribute data display with next steps to keep data actionable

☐ Consider strategic internal dissemination to executives

☐ Determine when to freeze the mean or limits to demonstrate improvement and/or establish a new goal

*continues*

**Tool 11.4    Statistical Process Control Charts (Continued)**

**Interpreting Statistical Process Control Charts**

**INSTRUCTIONS:** Use these rules to determine if there is special cause (statistically significant and non-random) as compared to common cause variation (what is usually expected in healthcare data). Data that break these rules indicate special cause variation that requires further investigation.

■ **Rule 1: Beyond Limits:** Any point beyond Zone A

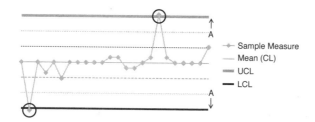

■ **Rule 2: Zone A:** Two of three consecutive points in Zone A or beyond

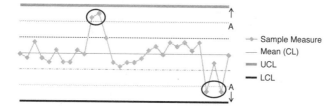

■ **Rule 3: Zone B:** Four of five data points in Zone B or beyond on the same side of the center line

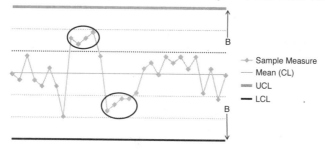

■ **Rule 4: Zone C:** Eight consecutive data points on either side of the center line in Zone C or beyond

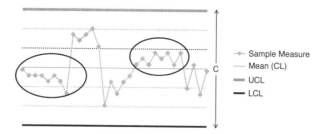

■ **Rule 5: Trend:** Six or more data points steadily increasing or decreasing

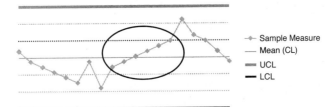

■ **Rule 6: Over-Control:** Fourteen consecutive data points alternating up and down (sawtooth pattern)

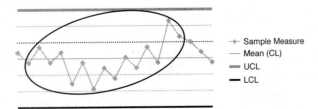

■ **Rule 7: Stratification:** Fifteen consecutive data points within Zone C

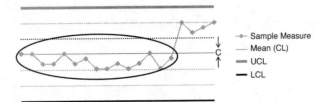

## Example

Fisher, D., Cochran, K., Provost, L., Patterson, J., Bristol, T., Metzguer, K., ... McCaffrey, M. (2013). Reducing central line-associated bloodstream infections in North Carolina NICUs. *Pediatrics, 132*(6), 1–8. doi:10.1542/peds.2013-2000

*continues*

EXAMPLES

TOOLS

## Tool 11.4   Statistical Process Control Charts (Continued)

## Resources

Articles, books, and online resources are listed that provide direction for creating and using statistical process control charts.

- Benneyan, J. C., Lloyd, R. C., & Plsek, P. E. (2003). Statistical process control as a tool for research and healthcare improvement. *Quality & Safety in Health Care, 12*(6), 458–464.

- Carey, R. G., & Lloyd, R. C. (2001). *Measuring quality improvement in healthcare: A guide to statistical process control applications.* Milwaukee, WI: ASQ Quality Press.

- Institute for Health Improvement [IHI Open School]. (2014a, May 5). Whiteboard: Control charts [Video file]. Retrieved from https://www.youtube.com/watch?v=9kmblj5zRtA

- Institute for Health Improvement [IHI Open School]. (2014b, May 5). Whiteboard: Static vs. dynamic data [Video file]. Retrieved from https://www.youtube.com/watch?v=UJqvC_uo63M

- Mohammed, M. A., Worthington, P., & Woodall, W. H. (2008). Plotting basic control charts: Tutorial notes for healthcare practitioners. *Quality & Safety in Health Care, 17*(2), 137–145. doi:10.1136/qshc.2004.012047

- National Health Service. (n.d.-a). Quality and service improvement tools: Statistical process control (SPC). Retrieved from http://webarchive.nationalarchives.gov.uk/20121108103848/http://www.institute.nhs.uk/quality_and_service_improvement_tools/quality_and_service_improvement_tools/statistical_process_control.html

- National Health Service. (n.d.-b). Quality and service improvement tools: Variation—an overview. Retrieved from http://webarchive.nationalarchives.gov.uk/20121108105624/http://www.institute.nhs.uk/quality_and_service_improvement_tools/quality_and_service_improvement_tools/variation_-_an_overview.html

- National Health Service. (2010). Explanation of statistical process control charts: Changes to the presentation of information in the *Staphylococcus aureus* bacteremia quarterly reports. Retrieved from http://www.wales.nhs.uk/sites3/page.cfm?orgid=379&pid=13438

- Schmaltz, S. (2011). A selection of statistical process control tools used in monitoring health care performance. Rockville, MD: Agency for Healthcare Research and Quality. Retrieved from http://qualitymeasures.ahrq.gov/expert/expert-commentary.aspx?id=16454

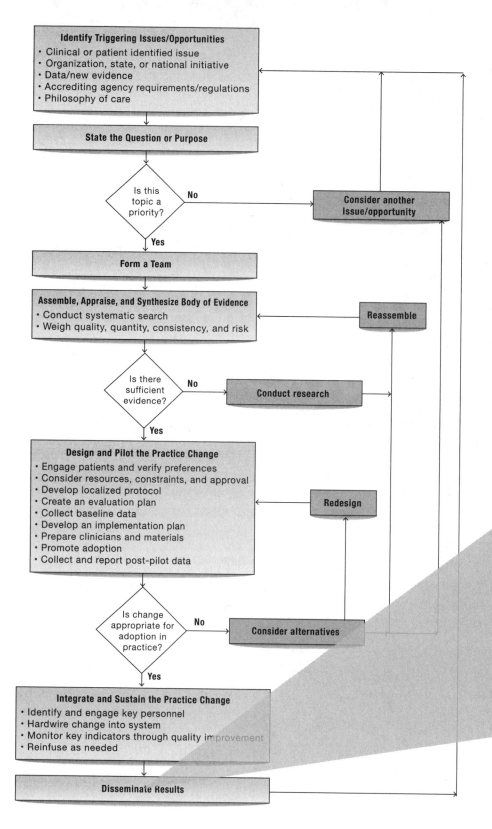

# DISSEMINATE RESULTS

**Yes**

**Integrate and Sustain the Practice Change**
- Identify and engage key personnel
- Hardwire change into system
- Monitor key indicators through quality improvement
- Reinfuse as needed

**Disseminate Results**

*"If opportunity doesn't knock, build a door."*

–Milton Berle

**D**issemination should occur within the organization and externally to the greater nursing and health-care communities. Formal and informal internal dissemination of results begins shortly after the pilot evaluation is complete (Lipman, Lange, Cohen, & Peterson, 2014). Reporting pilot results is an important step toward integration of the practice change.

## Internal Dissemination

Internal dissemination should include reporting within the organization's shared governance and quality improvement (QI) structures. Figure 11.3 is an example of a flowchart for reporting in a shared governance structure to support integration of evidence-based practice (EBP) changes. Reporting through the QI program or directly to senior leaders (see Strategy 2-23) is strategic for demonstrating the direct link among the practice change, the EBP infrastructure, and organizational priorities (see Strategy 3-20). Senior leadership support grows if the return on investment from the EBP change is demonstrated and clearly articulated.

Reporting pilot results to areas subsequently rolling out the practice change will help garner interest. When disseminating internally, include a brief project summary in newsletters, blogs, or on intranet sites where clinicians are accustomed to looking for updates and announcements (see Example 12.1 and Strategy 3-8). These summaries should include the project title; project director and interprofessional team member names and credentials; purpose and rationale; brief synthesis of evidence; practice change; implementation strategies; and evaluation results. Be creative but brief, and tailor the information to the audience (e.g., nurse, medical assistant, pharmacy).

Consider developing a project poster to rotate between the appropriate clinical areas (see Example 12.2 and Tool 12.1) (Williams & Cullen, 2016). You can use this same poster for orientation of new clinicians to emphasize the expectation for continuous improvement through EBP.

## External Dissemination

A decision to disseminate externally cannot be made until after evaluative findings are analyzed. Dissemination outside of the organization expands nursing knowledge and encourages similar EBP changes in other organizations. External dissemination of results from EBP projects may be accomplished through oral presentations, poster presentations, or peer-reviewed publications.

## Approval Process

Prior to external dissemination of EBP, institutional approval may be required (see Example 12.3). Simple notification of the EBP, Research, and/or QI office or a senior nurse administrator may be sufficient. If Institutional Review Board (IRB) review and approval is expected prior to dissemination of EBP work, consider either submitting a Human Subjects Research Determination (HSRD) form or filing for an exemption with the human subjects review committee (see Tool 12.2) (Adams, Farrington, & Cullen, 2012; Fineout-Overholt, Gallagher-Ford, Mazurek Melnyk, & Stillwell, 2011; Forsyth, Wright, Scherb, & Gaspar, 2010; Lekan, Hendrix, McConnell, & White, 2010; Wood & Morrison, 2011).

If your institution does not require IRB approval for QI and EBP work but it is required externally (e.g., by a journal), you may need to retrospectively submit the QI or EBP project to the IRB to provide documentation of the determination that the work is not human-subjects research. Check with your institution's IRB for the best approach.

## Conference Abstracts

Consider submitting an EBP abstract for presentation at a local, national, or international research, EBP, QI, or nursing specialty conference (see Example 12.4 and Tool 12.3). Most conferences post a call for abstracts several months before the conference. The abstract submission process typically allows you to specify whether you are interested in a poster presentation and/or an oral presentation. Pilot or preliminary data are more suitable for a poster versus an oral presentation. Carefully follow the abstract submission guidelines. You will be notified if your abstract is accepted and will receive further instructions and deadlines at that time. Tool 12.3 is a template that can be used to write an EBP abstract, and Example 12.4 is an example of an EBP abstract.

## Presentation Preparation

External presentations make the EBP work visible beyond the organization. Proactive planning must occur in order to be prepared for either an oral presentation or a poster presentation.

# Publication

Publishing is an additional opportunity for dissemination of project results outside the organization (see Example 12.6 and Tool 12.5). Publication can be a lengthy but rewarding process. Several decisions need to be made early in the process:

- **Authorship:** Whom to include, the order in which authors' names will appear, contributions, and commitment to publish (International Committee of Medical Journal Editors, 2017)

- **Journal selection:** Determining the target audience, deciding on primary and secondary journal choices, impact factor, access, and cost to publish

- **Timeline:** Deadlines for submission and turnaround time

The first author listed is responsible for coordinating manuscript completion for submission. Include clinicians on the team, as they can describe the practice change among other sections. Refer to the journal's author guidelines early in the writing process to determine the type of submission (e.g., review, brief, report), formatting requirements, and publication style. Be prepared to write and rewrite several times before submission. Consider SQUIRE 2.0 criteria to include when outlining key sections and content (SQUIRE, 2015). Invite an experienced author to help guide the process and provide a final round of edits before submission.

Submit a well-written and edited manuscript to increase the potential for being accepted. Manuscripts that are poorly written or have punctuation and spelling errors will detract from the message and are more likely to be rejected (Adams et al., 2012; Fineout-Overholt et al., 2011; Veness, 2010; Wenzel, Dünser, & Lindner, 2011). Journals may offer editorial assistance for new authors. Some journals invite potential authors to send a query letter, with or without an abstract, to the editor regarding the match between the manuscript and journal. Appendix C includes publications by EBP staff nurse interns.

## TIPS: EBP Dissemination

- Disseminate internally and externally.

- Report project purpose, synthesis of the evidence, practice change, implementation, and evaluation results.

- Determine early in the process how to reflect authorship and acknowledgment that reflect both project work and writing.

- Get help reviewing and editing presentations and publications.

- Develop the manuscript, poster presentation, or oral presentation targeting the audience.

- Use an Internet search engine to locate author guidelines for manuscript preparation and formatting. If you cannot find the author guidelines on the journal's home page, you can easily locate them by combining the journal name and the term *author guidelines*.

- Determine the institution's policy regarding publication of QI data.

- Treat EBP projects as QI for external reporting and follow institutional policies regarding notification or approvals required before external dissemination of EBP project results.

- If IRB approval is required for dissemination, consider requesting a letter from the IRB that the project is not human-subjects research.

- Think positive. Give it a try—you are now an expert on your project and the topic.

- Consider elements from SQUIRE 2.0 for content to report.

## Example 12.1   EBP Project Summary

### Project Title

Nasogastric Tube Placement in Pediatric and Neonatal Patients

### Project Director and Team

Michele Farrington, BSN, RN, CPHON, staff nurse, University of Iowa Hospitals and Clinics, 3JCP (project director); Sheryl Lang, MA, RN, CPNP, CNA-BC, nurse manager, University of Iowa Hospitals and Clinics, 3JCP; Laura Cullen, DNP, RN, FAAN, EBP scientist, University of Iowa Hospitals and Clinics, Office of Nursing Research, EBP and Quality; Stephanie Stewart, MSN, RNC-NIC, advanced practice nurse, University of Iowa Hospitals and Clinics, NICU

### Project Summary

Nasogastric (NG) tube placement is a common procedure used for pediatric and neonatal patients. However, there is little research regarding the use of NG tubes in children and neonates. Placement of an NG tube is indicated in order to aspirate stomach contents for diagnostic or therapeutic reasons or to provide a route for feedings or administration of medications. NG tube placement needs to be checked frequently and can best be monitored in the following ways: aspiration of gastrointestinal (GI) contents, testing aspirate pH, measuring the external length of the tube to ensure that it matches the length documented after insertion, and diagnostic imaging or X-ray. X-ray remains the only certain way to document tube placement. Bedside methods used to check enteral tube placement are less accurate, so aspiration and at least one other verification method should be used every time confirmation of tube placement is indicated. If there is doubt about where the tube is placed, the licensed independent practitioner should be consulted about the need to obtain an X-ray.

Nurses throughout the University of Iowa Children's Hospital were asked to complete a survey related to NG tube practices before receiving education related to the practice change, and then again after the standard of practice had been updated, based on information from an extensive literature search. These are some of the more interesting survey results. Measuring insertion length for an NG tube is done by measuring from the nare to the earlobe to midway between the xiphoid process and umbilicus; 46.6% of nurses reported using this process on the pre-implementation questionnaire, whereas 87.5% reported using this process post-implementation. A large number of nurses (95.5%) responded on the pre-implementation questionnaire that they check NG tube placement by auscultation of air over the abdomen, whereas the post-implementation results showed an increase in the number of nurses checking tube placement by verifying that the measured mark is aligned at the nare, aspirating fluid of a specific color, and measuring the pH of the aspirate using evidence-based approaches. On both the pre- and post-implementation questionnaires, most nurses reported never taking care of a patient who had a misplaced NG tube (79.5% and 83.3%, respectively). Feeding tube misplacements are not a common occurrence and are reported in the literature to occur approximately 4% of the time.

Standardization of NG tube practices throughout the pediatric and neonatal units at the University of Iowa Children's Hospital will potentially decrease tube misplacement rates, which will ultimately lead to increased patient comfort and decreased potential complications. Avoided complications will then lead to a decreased length of stay and hospital costs.

**Example 12.2   EBP Poster**

## Low-Dose Ketamine Infusions for Post-Operative Pain in Opioid-Tolerant Orthopedic Spine Patients: An Evidence-Based Practice Project

Allison Hanson, BSN, RN; Michele Farrington, BSN, RN, CPHON; Trudy Laffoon, MA, RN-BC; Cindy Dawson, MSN, RN, CORLN; Mary Nace, BSN, RN, ONC; Carol Strabala, BSN, RN, ONC; Judy Swafford, BS, RN, ONC; Megan Farnsworth, MNHP, RN, ONC; Gloria Dorr, MA, RN-BC; Denise Litwiller, MSN, RN-BC; Megan Davis-DeGeus, ARNP, MSN; Anne Smith, MSN, RN-BC; Sharon Baumler, MSN, RN, CORLN, OCN; Laura Cullen, DNP, RN, FAAN; Nicole Ramney, BSN, RN-BC; Lee Kral, PharmD, BCPS, RPh, BS; Timothy Brennan, MD, PhD; and Sergio Mendoza-Lattes, MD
University of Iowa Hospitals and Clinics, Iowa City, IA

### Purpose
To determine if low-dose ketamine infusions can lower post-operative pain for opioid-tolerant orthopedic spine surgery patients

### Process
Iowa Model of Evidence-Based Practice to Promote Quality Care (Titler, et al., 2001)

### Synthesis of Evidence
- Opioid-tolerant patients have complex pain management needs (Dykstra, 2012)
- Untreated acute pain may lead to development of persistent pain (Dunwoody, et al. 2008)
  - Cost of chronic pain estimated at $635 billion/year in the United States (Dykstra, 2012)
    - Medical treatment
    - Lost worker productivity
- Low-dose ketamine infusions may provide analgesia for opioid-tolerant patients undergoing surgery (Loftus, et al., 2010)
  - Resets opioid receptors
  - Less opioid given post-operatively
  - Decreased opioid side effects
- Ketamine side effects warrant special attention and patients need frequent monitoring (Abrishankar, et al. 2012)
- Patients receiving intra-operative ketamine used about 30% less morphine in the first 24 hours and 37% less morphine in the first 48 hours after surgery (Loftus, et al. 2010)
  - Opioid-tolerant patients
  - Lumbar spine surgery
- Lower morphine consumption rates post-operatively if received IV ketamine bolus at end of surgery (Bilgin, et al. 2005)

### Practice Change
- Best Practice Advisory:
  - Opioid-tolerant orthopedic spine patients
    - Based on pre-operative medication history
      - Opioid use for ≥ 3 months
    - Expected post-operative length of stay >24 hours
  - Encourage consistent, timely referrals for pre-operative evaluation by pharmacist or staff physician from acute pain service
  - Develop a surgical pain treatment plan collaboratively with patient
  - Distribute ketamine patient education handout
- Updated:
  - Nursing ketamine policy
  - IV ketamine medication administration guideline
  - Ketamine order set
  - Ketamine medication administration record

### Evaluation
**Staff Questionnaires**
- Nurses and licensed independent practitioners (pain clinic and orthopedic clinic & unit)
  - Pre-Implementation: n=50/77 (65% response rate)
  - Post-Implementation: n=22/88 (25% response rate)
- Staff knowledge results
  - 72% correct (pre) improved to 77% correct (post)

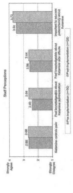

**Patient Questionnaires**
- Distributed pre- and post-implementation to spine surgery patients who received a ketamine infusion post-operatively
- Key concepts – ketamine contributes to pain management

### Implementation Strategies

Cullen, L. & Adams, S. (2012). Planning for implementation of evidence-based practice. *Journal of Nursing Administration*, 42(4), 222-230.

### Conclusions and Next Steps
**Conclusions**
- Staff knowledge improved regarding ketamine for pain
- Opioid-tolerant patients having orthopedic spine surgery were identified proactively before surgery and pain treatment plans were developed
- Interprofessional communication and collaboration were instrumental to project success

**Next Steps**
- Re-infusion of staff education for all inpatient areas caring for patients with ketamine infusions
- Integrate Best Practice Advisory into electronic record to identify all opioid-tolerant patients pre-operatively and consider development of pain treatment plans

### Acknowledgment
Partial funding provided by the Center for Pain Medicine and Regional Anesthesia, UI Health Care.

(Farrington, Hanson, Laffoon, & Cullen, 2015)

## Example 12.3   Institutional EBP Policy

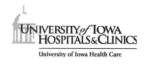

# Policy and Procedure Manual

**Evidence Based Practice Projects: Initiation,**        **N-A-12.003**
**Implementation, Reporting and Dissemination**

## POLICY

1.  Support for exploration and/or development of evidence-based practice (EBP) projects is available through the Nursing Research, Evidence-Based Practice, and Quality (NREQ) Office by calling 384-9098 or from a divisional representative.

2.  Resources available on the nursing research and EBP intranet sites, or by contacting the NREQ Office, include: a) *The Iowa Model Revised: Evidence-Based Practice to Promote Excellence in Health Care©*, b) *Implementation Strategies for Evidence-Based Practice©*, c) *EBP building Blocks: Comprehensive Strategies, Tools, and Tips* book, and d) an article on planning for implementation of EBP. [1, 2, 3]

3.  EBP project directors are responsible for recommending evidence-based revisions of policies, procedures, protocols, standards, and guidelines to appropriate Department of Nursing Services and Patient Care committees, as needed (e.g., PNP, NIS, QIS).

4.  EBP project directors are responsible for reporting practice recommendations and project findings within the shared governance structure. A flowchart outlining the order for committee reporting is available on the nursing shared governance intranet site.

5.  EBP project results are reported following the pilot and periodically (e.g., quarterly, every 6 weeks) until the project goal is obtained using the Performance Improvement Program – Quarterly Report form which is located on the CQSPI website. This report is submitted to the divisional and departmental Quality Improvement and Safety Committees.

6.  External dissemination is encouraged. Consultation regarding external dissemination and approval is available by calling the NREQ Office at 384-9098.

## RELATED STANDARDS AND LINKS

- N-A-12.001      Approval to do Research within the Department of Nursing Services and Patient Care

- N-A-12.002      Funding of Nursing Research Proposals

- N-A-12.004      Approval for Students to do Course Projects

- N-A-13.003      References: Guidelines for Documenting

**Example 12.3    Institutional EBP Policy**

**REFERENCES**

[1]    Iowa Model Collaborative. (2017). Iowa Model of Evidence-Based Practice: Revisions and validation. *Worldviews on Evidence-Based Nursing,14*(3), 175–182. doi:10.1111/wvn.12223

[2]    Cullen, L., & Adams, S. (2012). Planning for implementation of evidence-based practice. *Journal of Nursing Administration, 42*(4), 222–230. doi:10.1097/NNA.0b013e31824ccd0a

[3]    Cullen, L., Hanrahan, K., Tucker, S., Rempel, G., & Jordan, K. (2012). *Evidence-based practice building blocks: Comprehensive strategies, tools, and tips.* Iowa City, IA: Office of Nursing Research, Evidence-Based Practice and Quality, Department of Nursing Services and Patient Care, University of Iowa Hospitals and Clinics.

Last Revised:       10/15

**EXAMPLES**

**TOOLS**

**EXAMPLES**

**TOOLS**

## Example 12.4   EBP Abstract

### Project Title

Low-Dose Ketamine Infusions for Post-Operative Pain in Opioid-Tolerant Orthopedic Spine Patients: An Evidence-Based Practice Project

### Team Members

Allison Hanson, BSN, RN; Michele Farrington, BSN, RN, CPHON; Trudy Laffoon, MA, RN-BC; Cindy Dawson, MSN, RN, CORLN; Mary Nace, BSN, RN, ONC; Carol Strabala, BSN, RN, ONC; Judy Swafford, BS, RN, ONC; Megan Farnsworth, RN, MNHP; Gloria Dorr, MA, RN-BC; Denise Litwiller, MSN, RN-BC; Megan Davis-DeGeus, ARNP, MSN; Anne Smith, MSN, RN-BC; Sharon Baumler, MSN, RN, CORLN, OCN; Laura Cullen, DNP, RN, FAAN; Nicole Ranney, BSN, RN-BC; Lee Kral, PharmD, BCPS, RPh, BS; Timothy Brennan, MD, PhD; and Sergio Mendoza-Lattes, MD

### Purpose and Rationale

The purpose of this evidence-based practice project was to determine whether low-dose ketamine infusions can lower post-operative pain for opioid-tolerant orthopedic spine surgery patients. Opioid-tolerant patients have complex pain management needs (Dykstra, 2012), and untreated acute pain may lead to the development of persistent pain (Dunwoody et al., 2008). Benefits of ketamine for opioid-tolerant patients have been shown, but ketamine side effects warrant special attention (Abrishamkar et al., 2012). The Iowa Model of Evidence-Based Practice to Promote Quality Care (Titler et al., 2001) guided the process.

### Synthesis of Evidence

The cost of chronic pain (related to medical treatment and lost worker productivity) is estimated at $635 billion per year in the United States (Dykstra, 2012). Ketamine, used as an analgesic in low doses, may be beneficial for opioid-tolerant patients undergoing surgery (Loftus et al., 2010). Potential benefits include resetting opioid receptors, the need for less opioid post-operatively, and decreased opioid side effects (Loftus et al., 2010). In a randomized, double-blind study of opioid-tolerant patients undergoing lumbar spine surgery, patients receiving intraoperative ketamine used approximately 30% less morphine in the first 24 hours and 37% less morphine in the first 48 hours after surgery (Loftus et al., 2010). A double-blind study comparing ketamine administration, different durations, and timing related to the operative procedure demonstrated lower morphine consumption rates post-operatively for patients who received an intravenous ketamine bolus at the end of surgery (Bilgin et al., 2005). Patients receiving ketamine infusions need frequent monitoring for side effects (Abrishamkar et al., 2012).

## Practice Change

The acute pain service created a consistent referral process for opioid-tolerant patients undergoing spine surgery to determine whether ketamine infusions would be appropriate. The pharmacist meets pre-operatively with the patient to collaboratively develop a surgical pain treatment plan based on current medications, dosages, duration of use, etc. and provides a ketamine patient education handout, if appropriate. The pain treatment plan provided guidance for intraoperative and post-operative pain management using ketamine.

## Implementation Strategies

The Implementation Guide (Cullen & Adams, 2012), divided into four phases, was used to guide implementation. To create awareness and interest, a slogan and logo were developed, and a change champion presented information to clinicians. To build knowledge and commitment, an action plan was created, education was provided, and a report was given to senior leaders. To promote action and adoption, resource materials (e.g., pocket cards); a patient education brochure; and progress reports and updates were created and shared. To pursue integration and sustained use, the nursing ketamine policy and medication administration guideline were revised and approved. The ketamine order set and medication administration record were also updated.

## Evaluation

Patient questionnaires were distributed pre-implementation regarding ketamine and pain management. Clinicians (nurses and licensed independent practitioners) questionnaires assessing knowledge and attitudes related to ketamine were also distributed pre-implementation. Pre-implementation clinicians perceptions (n=50) demonstrated the following: ketamine controls pain (2.6; 1–4 Likert scale), feel knowledgeable about ketamine administration (2.3), feel knowledgeable about ketamine side effects (2.4), and potential patients who may benefit from ketamine are easy to identify (2.3). The clinician questionnaire stimulated interest in ongoing education related to ketamine and pain management. Patient and clinician questionnaires will also be distributed post-implementation.

## Example 12.5    EBP Presentation

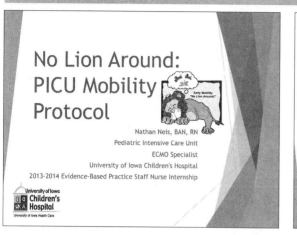

# No Lion Around: PICU Mobility Protocol

Nathan Neis, BAN, RN
Pediatric Intensive Care Unit
ECMO Specialist
University of Iowa Children's Hospital
2013-2014 Evidence-Based Practice Staff Nurse Internship

University of Iowa Children's Hospital
University of Iowa Health Care

---

## Purpose Statement

▶ The purpose of this evidence-based practice project was to initiate an early mobilization program in the PICU to safely improve pediatric patient outcomes.

University of Iowa Children's Hospital
University of Iowa Health Care

---

## Team Members

▶ Sameer Kamath, MD, MS
▶ Kayla Krueger, PT
▶ Brianna Clarahan, PT
▶ Michele Farrington, BSN, RN, CPHON
▶ Angela Otto, BSN, RN, CNML
▶ Mandi Houston, BSN, RN, CCRN
▶ Jennifer Erdahl, BSN, RN, CCRN

▶ Laura Cullen, DNP, RN, FAAN
▶ Paula Levett, MS, RN, CCRN
▶ Kristen Rempel
▶ Kimberly Jordan
▶ Matthew Reed, RRT
▶ Melissa Smith, OT

University of Iowa Children's Hospital
University of Iowa Health Care

---

## Synthesis of Evidence

▶ Early mobilization: Initiate a patient mobilization protocol within the first few hours of admission to the PICU:

   ▶ PICU culture shift toward mobility as a **required** component of quality daily patient care
   ▶ Change practice patterns by using teamwork to help achieve mobilization of patients
   ▶ Optimize the ICU environment and equipment to allow for proper patient mobilization

University of Iowa Children's Hospital
University of Iowa Health Care

---

## Synthesis of Evidence (cont.)

▶ Mobility decreases:
   ▶ Pressure ulcers
   ▶ Ventilator time/pneumonia
   ▶ UTIs
   ▶ Hospital length of stay
   ▶ Sedation
   ▶ Morbidity/mortality
   ▶ Healthcare costs
▶ Mobility improves:
   ▶ Patient outcomes

University of Iowa Children's Hospital
University of Iowa Health Care

---

## Any evidence that early mobility works?

▶ Majority of the evidence focuses on adult patients

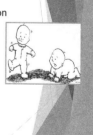

   ▶ University of Iowa Children's Hospital PICU — one of the first to systematically initiate this innovative practice change

▶ Early mobility is shown to be feasible and safe in ICU patients

University of Iowa Children's Hospital
University of Iowa Health Care

## Practice Change

- **ALL** PICU patients except:
  - Elevated ICP
  - Traumatic brain injury
  - Physician discretion
- Providers order following admission:
  - Mobility level
  - Physical therapy and occupational therapy consults
- Providers order patient-specific HR, RR, BP, and O2 sat ranges (Recommended 25% variation from baseline)

## Practice Change (cont.)

- Providers order pre-medications for pain to be given before mobility
- Nursing staff provides Family Guide once readiness for mobility is determined
- During daily rounds, interdisciplinary team assesses readiness to progress to the next mobility level

## Practice Change (cont.)

- Changes made to the pediatric admission order set
- Changes made to nursing documentation regarding mobility level, patient tolerance, and equipment used

## Implementation Strategies

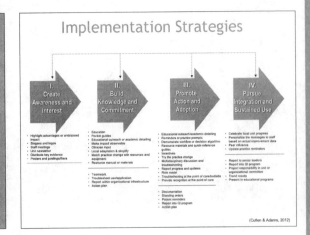

(Cullen & Adams, 2012)

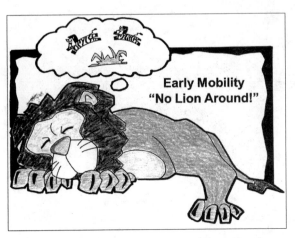

Early Mobility
"No Lion Around!"

## The Algorithm: Nurses and Providers!

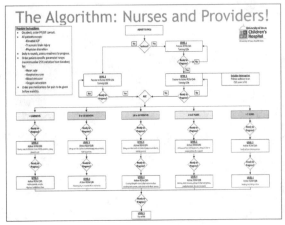

*continues*

EXAMPLES

TOOLS

## Example 12.5    EBP Presentation (Continued)

### The Algorithm – Families!

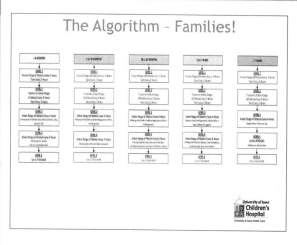

### Handout: Patient and Family Education

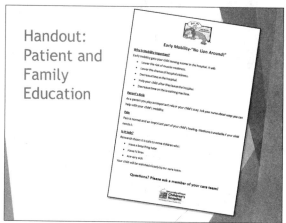

### Evaluation: Clinician Participants

| Sample | Pre (n=58) | Post (n=95) |
|---|---|---|
| Staff Nurses | 43 | 68 |
| Respiratory Therapists | 9 | 13 |
| Physicians (Attending) | 3 | 6 |
| Nurse Practitioners | 1 | 5 |
| Physician (Fellow) | 2 | 3 |

### Evaluation: Clinician Knowledge

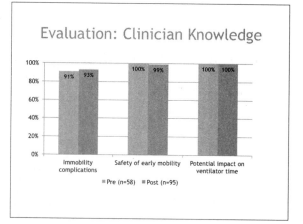

### Evaluation: Clinician Perceptions

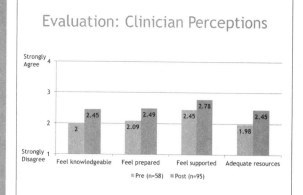

### Evaluation: Clinician Perceptions (cont.)

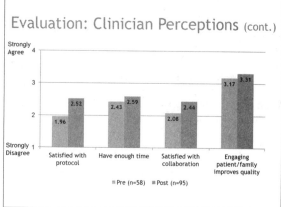

**EXAMPLES**

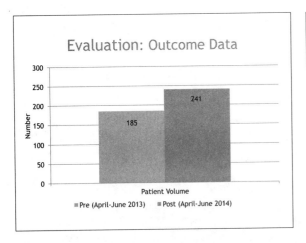

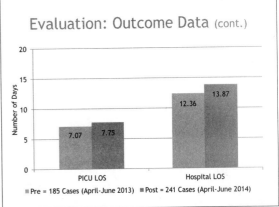

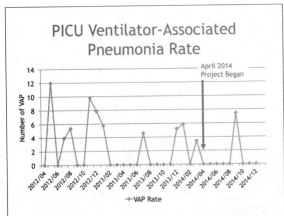

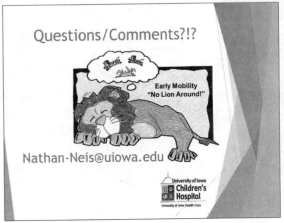

**TOOLS**

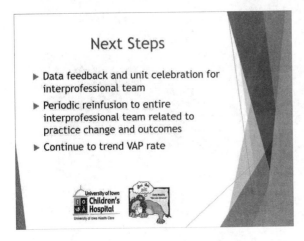

(Cullen, Hanrahan, et al., in press; Neis, 2015)

EXAMPLES

TOOLS

**Example 12.6    EBP Publication**

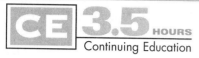

CE **3.5** HOURS
Continuing Education

By Diane Madsen, BSN, RN, Tamara Sebolt, BSN, RN, Laura Cullen, MA, RN,
Beverly Folkedahl, BSN, RN, COCN, CWCN, Toni Mueller, MSN, RN, CCRN,
Corinne Richardson, BSN, RN, and Marita Titler, PhD, RN, FAAN

# Listening to Bowel Sounds:
## An Evidence-Based Practice Project

*Nurses find that a traditional practice isn't the best indicator of returning gastrointestinal motility in patients who've undergone abdominal surgery.*

**Overview:** Nurses' practice of listening to bowel sounds was first proposed in 1905 and continues today, largely unquestioned. The authors developed a project to determine whether any compelling evidence exists for using this method to assess for the return of gastrointestinal (GI) motility following abdominal surgery. Literature on the subject was evaluated and an assessment of nursing practice was conducted. Based on the literature review and the assessment, a nursing practice guideline was developed, implemented, and evaluated. (Note that the nursing practice guideline outlined in this article was evaluated for use with abdominal surgery patients only and hasn't been evaluated in and may not be appropriate for other patient populations). The results were positive and indicate that clinical parameters other than bowel sounds, such as the return of flatus and the first postoperative bowel movement, are appropriate in assessing for the return of GI motility after abdominal surgery. Bowel sound assessment was discontinued and patient outcomes were evaluated to make sure that the practice change had no adverse effect on patients' recovery.

*Diane Madsen is a staff nurse; Tamara Sebolt is a nurse manager; Laura Cullen is an advanced practice nurse and evidence-based practice coordinator; Beverly Folkedahl is an advanced practice nurse; Toni Mueller is associate director of perioperative nursing; Corinne Richardson is a staff nurse; and Marita Titler is director of research, quality, and outcomes management, all in the Department of Nursing at the University of Iowa Hospitals and Clinics, Iowa City. The project was supported by the Evidence-Based Practice Staff Nurse Internship at the University of Iowa Hospitals and Clinics. The authors wish to thank Joseph J. Cullen, MD, professor of surgery at the University of Iowa College of Medicine and chief of the surgical service at the Veterans Affairs Medical Center, Iowa City, for his assistance. Contact author: laura-cullen@uiowa.edu. The authors of this article have no other significant ties, financial or otherwise, to any company that might have an interest in the publication of this educational activity.*

**Example 12.6    EBP Publication (Continued)**

What's the best indication of returning gastrointestinal (GI) motility in patients who've undergone abdominal surgery? A century ago, nurses first began listening for bowel sounds as a sign of such recovery. Since then, the practice has persisted largely unquestioned and is supported more by tradition than by evidence.

It has become apparent, as nursing practice has evolved, that this is the case with many nursing activities. In order to improve the quality of care, it's vital that nurses question their current practices to determine whether they're based on evidence or merely on tradition.

The Iowa Model of Evidence-Based Practice to Promote Quality Care successfully promotes the integration of evidence into practice.[1] The model outlines the implementation of an evidence-based practice project (see Figure 1, page 42). Identifying a practice problem or new knowledge triggers the evidence-based practice process. Leaders in the health care facility and on the nursing unit then review the proposal to determine what priority it should be given, and they assemble a team to carry it out.

The team selects, reviews, critiques, and synthesizes the evidence in the literature. If the research evidence is sufficient, the team initiates change. If the evidence is insufficient, the team reviews other evidence or suggests more research. The team then pilots and evaluates the practice change to determine whether revisions are needed before integrating and applying the change in other clinically appropriate areas. More evaluation and dissemination of results is essential to integrate the practice into daily care.

This article describes the results of an evidence-based practice project that began when one of us (DM), a staff nurse on a GI surgery unit, questioned the practice of listening to bowel sounds to assess for gastric motility. We followed the Iowa Model described above.

### CLINICAL ISSUE

Our evidence-based practice project began with the identification of a clinical problem, which we framed in a series of questions that hadn't been sufficiently addressed in the nursing literature:

- Why do we listen to bowel sounds?
- What evidence supports listening to bowel sounds?
- Are bowel sounds a valuable tool for determining the return of GI motility after abdominal surgery?
- Does bowel sound assessment promote early intervention, such as feeding, or recovery in abdominal surgery patients?

Alteration in GI motility following abdominal surgery was first documented with the introduction of X-rays in the 1890s, and in 1905 (as reported by Nachlas and colleagues) Cannon first proposed auscultation of bowel sounds to determine whether GI motility had returned after abdominal surgery.[2] Nursing students are taught to listen for as long as five minutes in each of the four quadrants of the abdomen to determine whether bowel sounds are present; nurses may therefore spend up to 20 minutes per patient on one component of the nursing assessment.[3-5] Given the imperative to improve patient outcomes and the pressure to use nursing time more efficiently, it's necessary to question the validity of this traditional nursing practice.

### SYNTHESIS OF THE EVIDENCE

Locating research evidence was a challenge. Literature searches were attempted with the help of other nurses and librarians, but with few results. The basic research in this area is old and in some cases wasn't listed in Medline when this project began. To find the literature, we used a "snowball" method[6] (meaning that an initial information source referred us to other sources); in this case, a surgical motility researcher shared his collection of articles and provided leads, resulting in a more effective literature retrieval.

> There are no nursing interventions associated with the presence or absence of bowel sounds.

Published research on the correlation between bowel sounds and GI motility is sparse and dates to the 1960s. Recent research has focused on using pacemakers or drugs to speed recovery, with inconsistent findings that aren't clinically useful. We looked for studies that involved the return of GI motility after abdominal surgery as well as the use of assessment for bowel sounds in abdominal surgery patients. Critique and synthesis of the evidence included primary findings from clinical research describing the pattern of returning GI motility, as well as secondary findings from research that

*continues*

**Example 12.6   EBP Publication (Continued)**

**Figure 1.** The Iowa Model of Evidence-Based Practice to Promote Quality Care

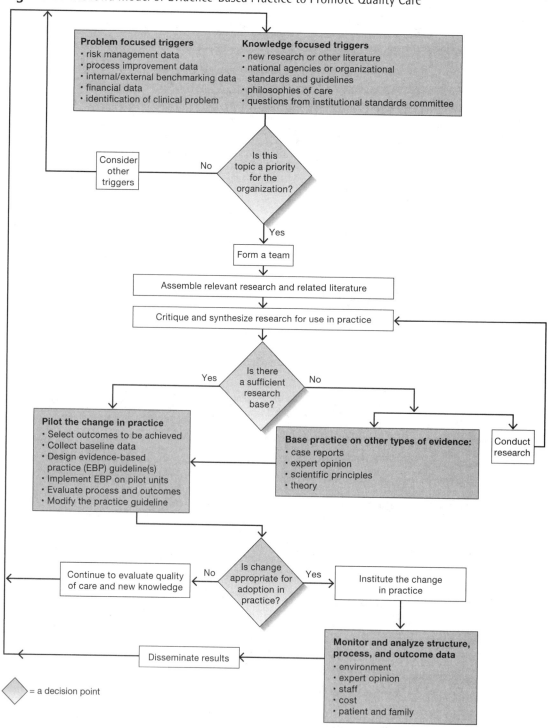

## Example 12.6    EBP Publication (Continued)

addressed other questions. Several randomized, controlled trials; 15 experimental studies; and three systematic reviews were included in the evidence synthesis (see Table 1, page 46). More evidence from available research, expert opinion, and case studies report the practice of listening to bowel sounds to determine motility only as a matter of tradition.

The return of GI motility after abdominal surgery follows a predictable pattern, beginning with random electrical impulses, then random muscle contractions, eventually becoming coordinated myoelectrical activity, and then propulsion.[7] The return of GI motility begins in the small intestine; it is then seen in the stomach and, finally, the colon (first on the right side, then on the left).[7-10] The timing of the return of postoperative GI motility varies according to the surgical procedure[11] and other clinical variables, but motility is usually seen in the small intestine in four to 24 hours, the stomach in two to four days, and the colon in three to seven days postoperatively (see Figure 2, at right).

Early postoperative bowel sounds probably don't represent the return of normal GI motility[2, 12, 13]; rather, they most likely represent uncoordinated early contraction in the small intestine.[14-16] Therefore, auscultation of the abdomen during the early recovery phase after abdominal surgery isn't a good assessment of the recovery of postoperative motility.[15]

Preventing oral intake in the first days after abdominal surgery has been standard practice because of concern that complications such as anastomotic leakage, dehiscence, wound disruption, vomiting, and aspiration might arise,[17, 18] but recent research has questioned this tradition.[19-21] Bufo and colleagues speculate that the tradition of prohibiting early feeding may be a holdover from a time when now-outdated anesthetics that were associated with more nausea and vomiting were in use.[22] Recent research suggests that early feeding is, in fact, safe for patients, and bowel sounds do not indicate feeding tolerance.[17, 22-26] Patient outcomes of early feeding include tolerance of oral intake and improved patient comfort; early feeding may also reduce length of hospital stay and stimulate recovery of motility.[17-19, 22] The recent work on early feeding and other research on reducing the routine use of nasogastric tubes are additional contributions to the growing body of evidence on recovery of postoperative motility.

The primary markers for returning GI motility after abdominal surgery are the return of flatus and bowel movement, indicating recovery of the colon.[27-30] Additional indications of recovery from postoperative ileus are the patient's ability to tolerate oral intake without nausea or vomiting, the return of appetite, and an absence of other symp-

**Figure 2.** Timing of Return of Postperative GI Motility

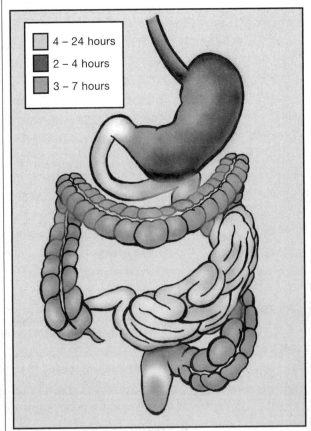

□ 4 – 24 hours
■ 2 – 4 hours
□ 3 – 7 hours

Motility is usually seen in the small intestine in four to 24 hours, the stomach in two to four days, and the colon in three to seven days.

toms of ileus, such as distension, feeling bloated, and cramps.[17, 22-26, 31] In addition to monitoring for returning GI motility, postoperative assessment should include pain assessment and the monitoring of vital signs and intake and output.

Interviewing patients can help reveal some of the important signs of returning GI motility. Instead of approaching patients with a stethoscope in hand, nurses can ask how they feel and whether flatus, bowel movements, and appetite have returned. There are additional benefits to this approach. Spending time with patients and listening to their needs—as well as allowing more time to answer questions—helps establish rapport and educate patients on postoperative preventive management.

### CURRENT PRACTICE

We created questionnaires for practitioners that were designed to identify their understanding of GI

*continues*

## Example 12.6   EBP Publication (Continued)

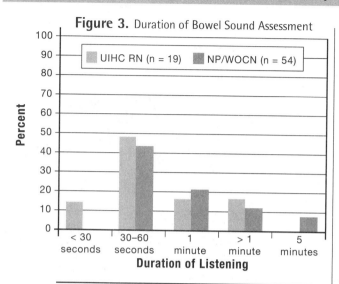

**Figure 3.** Duration of Bowel Sound Assessment

UIHC = University of Iowa Hospitals and clinics staff nurses; NP/WOCN = nurse practitioners with wound, ostomy, and continence certification.

motility and their current assessment practices after abdominal surgery (sample questionnaires are available from the authors). We solicited nurse practitioners (NPs) with wound, ostomy, and continence certification (n = 206) and selected nurse experts (who may not have had such certification) from our organization (n = 25). We also sent questionnaires on current practice to surgeons within our organization (n = 15). Return of the survey was considered an indication of consent to participate. Sixty-eight NPs (33%) and 19 staff nurse experts (76%) returned questionnaires. Of the 68 questionnaires from the NP group, only 54 (26%) were useable, because several respondents indicated that their clinical practice area didn't include abdominal surgery. Nine (60%) of the 15 general surgeons responded.

The nursing questionnaires included six multiple choice questions, one item asking practitioners to rank the importance of clinical parameters, and two short answer items. The results showed that all nurses who responded to the questionnaire continued to listen to bowel sounds following abdominal surgery. Nearly 60% of NPs and 90% of the nurses at our organization auscultate in four quadrants every four to eight hours. Despite the fact that most nursing textbooks advise listening for up to five minutes in each of the four quadrants to determine whether bowel sounds are present, the majority of nurses actually listen for less time (see Figure 3, above). Nurses monitor a number of other clinical indicators of GI motility when caring for the patient who has undergone abdominal surgery. The indicators most often ranked as important were pain, distension, firmness, vomiting, and bowel sounds (see Figure 4, page 45). The nurse experts also listed the clinical parameters they used to monitor changes in the patient's clinical condition and that would prompt notification of the surgeon (see Figure 5, page 45). Parameters listed most often were vomiting, distension, pain, wound drainage, and firmness.

The surgeon questionnaire included seven short-answer items on the physiology of bowel recovery, practice preferences, and key clinical parameters. The physicians reported that the three most important clinical parameters that indicate the return of GI motility are return of flatus (89%), bowel movement (44%), and appetite (44%). The majority of the surgeons (78%) reported that the monitoring of bowel sounds by nurses is not helpful to them in patient management. The five nursing assessments most valued by surgeons were the return of flatus (78%) and bowel movement (67%) (both of which are indicators of recovery), and distension (44%), nausea (44%), and vomiting (44%) (all three of which are negative indicators). Of interest are the differences between nurses and surgeons in their rankings of parameters indicating a need to notify surgeons.

There are no nursing interventions associated with the presence or absence of bowel sounds. Other assessments will reveal the absence of bowel motility and suggest appropriate interventions. For example, the nurse can ask the patient if he's nauseated and, if so, treat the nausea. Similarly, the nurse may treat abdominal distension by inserting a nasogastric tube. If distension is present in a patient who already has a nasogastric tube, the nurse should check the tube's placement and patency.

### CHANGING PRACTICE

Based on our review of the growing body of evidence in the literature and the questionnaire results discussed here, we decided that a change in care was needed. We instituted a practice change in our organization, eliminating the practice of listening for bowel sounds after abdominal surgery. Prior to making the change, several things needed to happen. One step was to work with the nursing informatics group to change the online documentation system to allow the documentation of useful assessments rather than just listening for bowel sounds. Next, we developed a program on the practice change, to be led by two staff nurses who understood the evidence for not listening to bowel sounds, as well as the new documentation standards and who led change on the surgical unit.

Prior to the staff education from nurse leaders, we conducted a pretest to assess knowledge among surgical unit nurses. A poster displayed in the unit report room reviewed the literature on the history and physiology of bowel sound assessment and the

**Example 12.6    EBP Publication (Continued)**

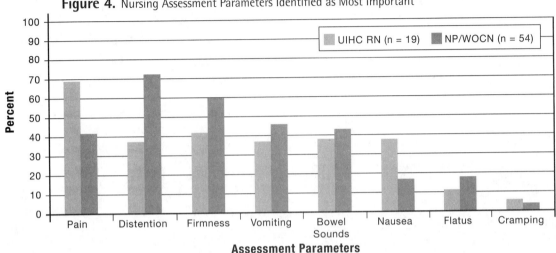

**Figure 4.** Nursing Assessment Parameters Identified as Most Important

UIHC = University of Iowa Hospitals and Clinics staff nurses; NP/WOCN = nurse practitioners with wound, ostomy, and continence certification.

**Figure 5.** Clinical Parameters for Notification of Surgeon

UIHC = University of Iowa Hospitals and Clinics staff nurses; NP/WOCN = nurse practitioners with wound, ostomy, and continence certification.

return of GI motility, as well as results from the questionnaires, which described the current practice patterns and preferences among the NP, staff nurse, and surgeon groups.

Using evidence helped us promote acceptance of the new protocol. Several nurses were selected to facilitate the change by training the trainers—working with small groups of nurses on the same shifts who would then educate other nurses. This arrangement allowed questions to be answered as nurses piloted the new guidelines and acted as role models and troubleshooters at the bedside. Another poster in the unit report room helped nurses use the revised online documentation. Additional assessment guides were placed at computers where nurses and other care providers document. Also, a pocket assessment guide was made available to each nurse to use when assessing patients. The guide included 10 assessment items written on one side and, on the reverse, questions to ask the patient. These tools helped remind nurses to comprehensively document each of the relevant assessment parameters.

*continues*

## Example 12.6    EBP Publication (Continued)

Table 1. Selected Studies Used in the Development of Guidelines for Nurse Monitoring of Patients

| Subjects and Procedure | Study Description and Relevant Findings |
|---|---|
| **Benson MJ, et al. *Gastroenterology* 1994;106(4):924-36.** | |
| 29 consecutive patients (23 patients were in sample) undergoing intra-abdominal surgery for sigmoid carci-noma; compared rectal cisapride with placebo on proximal small bowel migrating myoelectric complex (MMC), monitored with manometer | Randomized, placebo-controlled, double-blind study<br>• Bowel sounds and flatus were compared as indicators of motility, but flatus was the primary clinical indicator; both are insensitive and indirect indicators of motility.<br>• Clinical resolution of ileus (passage of flatus) preceded the complete recovery of small bowel motility (bowel sounds occurred even earlier).<br>• "Bowel sounds are thought to arise from the movement of an air–water interface in the upper gastrointestinal (GI) tract. Their return in the post-op state does not, judging from our data, correlate with the complete recovery of proximal small bowel motility." (Bowel sounds returning before motility may allow a change in treatment or feeding.)[page 935] |
| **Boghaert A, et al. *Acta Anaesthesiol Belg* 1987;38(3):195-9.** | |
| 53 adult patients undergoing any type of surgery; monitored cisapride effect on return of postoperative motility in patients with ileus | Randomized, double-blind trial<br>• Recovery of the left colon may take up to 7 days and coincides with the end of postoperative ileus.<br>• Bowel sounds may be present even though propulsive motility hasn't yet returned.<br>• Passage of flatus, unlike the presence of bowel sounds, may be considered a direct indicator of colonic peri-stalsis, the start of which marks the end of postoperative ileus. |
| **Bohm B, et al. *Arch Surg* 1995;130(4):415-9.** | |
| 12 canines underwent laparoscopic placement or conventional laparotomy for electrode placement. Myoelectric activity was monitored during laparo-scopic right colectomy, conventional right colectomy, or anesthesia alone; measuring median time to return of nor-mal myoelectrical activity | Prospective randomized, controlled study in the canine model<br>• Postoperative motility, indicated by 1st bowel movement, returned faster after laparoscopic procedures than with "open" procedures.<br>• Motility returned 1st to the small intestine, then to the stomach. |
| **Bufo AJ, et al. *Dis Colon Rectum* 1994;37(12):1260-5.** | |
| 38 consecutive patients (36 in sample) undergoing colorectal operations | Nonrandomized prospective study<br>• 31 of 36 patients tolerated early feeding and had shorter mean length of hospital stay (5.7 days); patients with traditional, conservative treatment had, on average, an 8-day stay; patients with ileus had a 10.6-day stay.<br>• Most patients had return of flatus and bowel movement within 3 to 5 days (mean = 4.2 days).<br>• Neither bowel sounds nor flatus determined patients' tolerance of oral intake or was a good indicator of when to resume feeding. |
| **Condon RE, et al. *Am J Physiol* 1995;269(3 Pt 1):G408-17.** | |
| 48 patients undergoing elective major abdominal surgery (1984 to 1994) had colonic smooth muscle electrical activity recorded | Experimental design with convenience sample<br>• Ileus resolved 3.8 days postoperatively (range, 2 to 6 days) as indicated by flatus and bowel movement (bowel sounds were not used as an indicator).<br>• Right colon returned before left colon.<br>• Ileus recovery was also indicated by flatus, defecation, and the ability to consume solids without nausea or vomiting.<br>• Normal colonic activity was seen after the seventh postoperative day. |

And finally, a resource manual helped orient new nurses. The manual is updated periodically and includes research articles, computer documentation guides, survey results, and project evaluation data.

### PROTOCOL LIMITATIONS

The practice protocol was implemented and evalu-ated on a general surgery unit with abdominal surgery patients. The new protocol was limited to abdominal surgery patients, because the research in the literature review did not include other surgical procedures or patient populations. The protocol may not be appro-priate for medical patients, because their impaired motility would probably not follow the same pattern seen with postoperative paralytic ileus, as described in the abdominal surgery research literature.

In the new protocol, assessing the unconscious patient for clinical indicators of GI motility is simi-lar to assessing the conscious one. Regardless of the patient's level of awareness, the return of bowel sounds after abdominal surgery represents the return of uncoordinated contractions in the small intestine, not propulsive contractions in the colon. The presence or absence of abdominal distension or firmness, vomiting, and bowel movements should be assessed to determine the status of GI motility in the unconscious patient. The signs that should trig-ger notification of the surgeon are nearly the same: vomiting, abdominal distension or firmness, and increased wound drainage.

Pain is an additional indicator to monitor in postoperative patients and may indicate impaired recovery of GI motility. The use of epidural anal-gesia has led to better pain management but requires pain assessment that's tailored to the patient's condition.

## Example 12.6    EBP Publication (Continued)

### After Abdominal Surgery

| Subjects and Procedure | Study Description and Relevant Findings |
|---|---|
| **Ducerf C, et al. *Ann Surg* 1992;215(3):237-43.** | |
| 10 patients following cholecystectomy, underwent 4 days of monitoring by electromyographic recordings | Experimental design with convenience sample<br>• Defined normal postsurgical recovery as "absence of abnormal clinical signs and the presence of gas expulsion between 2nd and 3rd day after surgery." [page 238]<br>• 3 hours after surgery, phase III of MMC was present in short duration and shorter intervals; duration of MMC increased progressively from the 1st to the 4th postoperative day.<br>• A circadian pattern emerged on the 2nd day and became normal on the 4th postoperative days. |
| **Graber JN, et al. *Surgery* 1982;92(1):87-92.** | |
| 6 monkeys undergoing three surgical procedures | Experimental design, random order of procedure with each monkey serving as its own control<br>• Subjects exhibited the following pattern of return of motility: antrum at 3.4 hours; small bowel at 6.5 hours; right colon at 45 hours; sigmoid colon at 55 hours.<br>• Contractile activity may not be equivalent to coordinated gut propulsion.<br>• Colonic ileus lasted up to 48 hours, regardless of the degree of bowel handling.<br>• A delay in gastric emptying was seen as long as 48 hours after operation.<br>• Bowel movement occurred by 2nd postoperative day. |
| **Hotokezaka M, et al. *Dig Dis Sci* 1996;41(5):864-9.** | |
| 11 patients undergoing colon surgery; recorded gastric myoelectric activity | Prospective experimental design<br>• Patients were given a clear liquid diet after passage of flatus or feces, followed by a regular diet when liquids were tolerated 24 to 48 hours after surgery.<br>• There was no correlation between presence of gastric dysrhythmias and clinical recovery of gastrointestinal function; rapid recovery of gastric myoelectrical activity did not correspond with clinical course of the patient following surgery.<br>• The stomach recovered more slowly than the small intestine and more rapidly than the colon. |
| **Huge A, et al. *Dis Colon Rectum* 2000;43(7):932-9.** | |
| 19 patients undergoing left hemicolectomy, sigmoid resection, or primary anastomosis; monitored postoperative colonic tone barostat and manometry | Experimental design with convenience sample<br>• 18 of 19 patients had their 1st stool on postoperative day 3; 1 on postoperative day 4.<br>• 7 of 19 patients had propagating contractile events on postoperative day 2 and 8 had them on postoperative day 3.<br>• There was no relationship between propagating contractions and flatus or 1st bowel movement. Bowel sounds were present in 2/3 of patients on postoperative day 1 and in all by day 3. "Consequently, auscultation of bowel sounds and recording of colonic motility did not correlate well. We suspect that the bowel sounds originated mainly in the small bowel, which has been shown to resume its motility before the colon." [page 937] |
| **Schippers E, et al. *Dig Dis Sci* 1991;36(5):621-6.** | |
| 13 patients undergoing different surgical procedures; measured mechanical activity in the jejunum and compared patients' mechanical return of motility by procedure and early feeding | Prospective, convenience sample<br>• Return of motility in small intestine did not coincide with clinical recovery from postoperative ileus.<br>• 1st flatus occurred on 3rd postoperative day in cholecystectomy patients and on 4th day in those who underwent large bowel resection.<br>• Myoelectrical activity began on the day of the procedure in cholecystectomy patients (4.5 hours after procedure) and later in those who underwent large bowel resection (56.4 hours after the procedure).<br>• Small intestine motility returned first and colon motility returned last.<br>• Feeding changed the interdigestive pattern in the small intestine within minutes of ingestion.<br>• Return of initial electrical and motor activity is *not* associated with clinical recovery from postoperative ileus (clinical recovery was indicated by 1st flatus and 1st stool). |

### EVALUATION OF OUTCOMES

The evaluation of evidence-based practice includes three components: nursing knowledge, the process of implementation, and patient outcomes.

**Nursing knowledge.** The pretest and posttest instruments were identical 10-item questionnaires that addressed those items of postoperative nursing knowledge deemed most critical in the literature we reviewed. We surveyed only nurses working on the general surgery pilot unit. Sixty-three percent of the preeducation group and 83% of the posteducation group responded to the questionnaires. Respondents showed improvement after the educational poster sessions: the pretest and posttest mean scores were 53% and 94% correct, respectively. One item on the questionnaire accounted for all but one of the wrong answers, indicating that the item probably should have been revised.

**Implementation process.** We evaluated the implementation process in two ways: at the time of the posttest, we asked the nurses to complete an additional questionnaire on the implementation process to find out whether facilitation of the new guideline was adequate, and we also audited the nursing charts to assess nurses' compliance with the new guideline. The rate of response to the implementation process questionnaire was 42%. Eighty-five percent of RN respondents agreed or strongly agreed (on a four-point Likert scale) that they felt prepared to implement the practice change. All of the RNs agreed or strongly agreed that they felt knowledgeable enough to carry out the new guideline. The majority of respondents (85%) agreed or strongly agreed that they were able to identify the postoperative signs of returning gastrointestinal motility. In addition, 85% of nurses reported using the guideline.

*continues*

## Example 12.6    EBP Publication (Continued)

### A New Practice Guideline

*The following guideline on gastrointestinal (GI) assessment after abdominal surgery was developed as a result of the evidence-based practice project conducted by the authors.*

#### Policy

After abdominal surgery, abdominal assessment is completed at least every eight hours until the patient experiences first flatus and first bowel movement, and then twice daily and as needed until discharge.

#### Procedure

1. **Explain** the procedure to the patient.
2. **Interview** the patient regarding the presence or absence of the following subjective symptoms indicative of postoperative ileus or return of GI motility:
   - abdominal pain, discomfort
   - flatus within the previous 8 hours
   - bowel movement within the previous 12 to 24 hours, stool
   - nausea, vomiting, or both
   - feeling bloated
   - return of appetite, feeling hungry
   - abdominal cramps
   - referred pain (for example, shoulder pain)
3. **Place** the patient in the supine position for assessment, and ensure comfort (for example, raise the head of the bed slightly).
4. **Inspect** the patient's abdomen, including assessment of presence or absence of
   - distention.
   - drainage from the wound.
5. **Palpate** the patient's abdomen, if it's distended, in a systematic fashion, taking care not to cause discomfort. Palpation includes assessment of presence or absence of
   - abdominal firmness.
   - abdominal tenderness.

We evaluated nurses' use of the new guideline by auditing the charts of consecutive admissions before and after implementation, with a preimplementation group of 32 patients and a postimplementation group of 49. The results indicated that nurses assessed for nausea, vomiting, and abdominal distension before and after the new guideline was implemented, and also assessed for flatus, bowel movement, and appetite. Nurses documented bowel movements before and after the new protocol was implemented as part of standard intake–output monitoring. But documentation of flatus (50% before implementation; 67% after implementation) and appetite (3% before implementation and 57% after implementation) both increased with use of the new practice protocol.

**Patient outcomes.** Monitoring of patient outcomes is essential when evaluating evidence-based practice. We monitored patient outcomes to determine whether discontinuing the monitoring of bowel sounds was detrimental to patients. The patient outcomes in the abdominal surgery population that are most relevant to the return of GI motility are paralytic ileus, bowel obstruction, and early feeding. Comparing the preimplementation and postimplementation patient groups revealed a higher rate of paralytic ileus in the preimplementation group (13%) than in the postimplementation group (4%). No bowel obstructions were documented in either of the two groups. We don't attribute the lower rate of paralytic ileus in the postimplementation group to the introduction of the new practice guideline; rather, the lower rate demonstrates that eliminating the monitoring of bowel sounds wasn't detrimental to patients and probably reflects other patient characteristics. Early feeding of abdominal surgery patients was not evaluated, but that may be the next project for the team.

#### NURSING IMPLICATIONS

This evidence-based practice project has significant implications for nursing. The first and most obvious implication concerns nurses' time. Depending on how closely a nurse follows the textbook recommendations on assessing bowel sounds in postoperative abdominal surgery patients—for up to five minutes per quadrant—nurses could save as much as 20 minutes of nursing care time per patient and have time for more useful patient care activities.

This project also illuminated the importance of questioning traditions. Staff nurses can improve the quality of care by identifying important practice issues that can be addressed by examining the evidence. Evidence may be scarce, but being persistent and employing different strategies to locate it can be effective. For example, overcoming a dearth of available evidence may be possible by collaborating, as we did, with a researcher who knows about the issue and can identify or provide relevant articles to get the team started. As we learned from our experience, overcoming the initial difficulties and completing a project can be rewarding. Implementing evidence-based practice in our organization improved nursing knowledge, nursing process, and patient outcomes. ▼

#### REFERENCES

1. Titler MG, et al. The Iowa Model of Evidence-Based Practice to Promote Quality Care. *Crit Care Nurs Clin North Am* 2001;13(4):497-509.
2. Nachlas MM, et al. Gastrointestinal motility studies as a guide to postoperative management. *Ann Surg* 1972; 175(4):510-22.
3. Interpreting abnormal abdominal sounds. *Nursing* 2000; 30(6):28.
4. Kirton CA. Assessing bowel sounds. *Nursing* 1997; 27(3):64.

## Example 12.6 EBP Publication (Continued)

5. Mehta M. Assessing the abdomen. *Nursing* 2003;33(5):54-5.

6. Greenhalgh T, et al. Diffusion of innovations in service organizations: systematic review and recommendations. *Milbank Q* 2004;82(4):581-629.

7. Livingston EH, Passaro EP, Jr. Postoperative ileus. *Dig Dis Sci* 1990;35(1):121-32.

8. Graber JN, et al. Relationship of duration of postoperative ileus to extent and site of operative dissection. *Surgery* 1982;92(1):87-92.

9. Hotokezaka M, et al. Gastric myoelectric activity changes following open abdominal surgery in humans. *Dig Dis Sci* 1996;41(5):864-9.

10. Schippers E, et al. Return of interdigestive motor complex after abdominal surgery. End of postoperative ileus? *Dig Dis Sci* 1991;36(5):621-6.

11. Bohm B, et al. Postoperative intestinal motility following conventional and laparoscopic intestinal surgery. *Arch Surg* 1995;130(4):415-9.

12. Boghaert A, et al. Placebo-controlled trial of cisapride in postoperative ileus. *Acta Anaesthesiol Belg* 1987;38(3):195-9.

13. Rothnie NG, et al. Early postoperative gastrointestinal activity. *Lancet* 1963;2:64-7.

14. Benson MJ, et al. Small bowel motility following major intra-abdominal surgery: the effects of opiates and rectal cisapride. *Gastroenterology* 1994;106(4):924-36.

15. Huge A, et al. Postoperative colonic motility and tone in patients after colorectal surgery. *Dis Colon Rectum* 2000;43(7):932-9.

16. Morris IR, et al. Changes in small bowel myoelectrical activity following laparotomy. *Br J Surg* 1983;70(9):547-8.

17. Behrns KE, et al. Prospective randomized trial of early initiation and hospital discharge on a liquid diet following elective intestinal surgery. *J Gastrointest Surg* 2000;4(2):217-21.

18. Lewis SJ, et al. Early enteral feeding versus "nil by mouth" after gastrointestinal surgery: systematic review and meta-analysis of controlled trials. *BMJ* 2001;323(7316):773-6.

19. Fearon KC, Luff R. The nutritional management of surgical patients: enhanced recovery after surgery. *Proc Nutr Soc* 2003;62(4):807-11.

20. Holte K, Kehlet H. Prevention of postoperative ileus. *Minerva Anestesiol* 2002;68(4):152-6.

21. Nygren J, et al. New developments facilitating nutritional intake after gastrointestinal surgery. *Curr Opin Clin Nutr Metab Care* 2003;6(5):593-7.

22. Bufo AJ, et al. Early postoperative feeding. *Dis Colon Rectum* 1994;37(12):1260-5.

23. Feo CV, et al. Early oral feeding after colorectal resection: a randomized controlled study. *ANZ J Surg* 2004;74(5):298-301.

24. Gocmen A, et al. Early post-operative feeding after caesarean delivery. *J Int Med Res* 2002;30(5):506-11.

25. Mangesi L, Hofmeyr GJ. Early compared with delayed oral fluids and food after caesarean section. *Cochrane Database Syst Rev* 2002(3):CD003516.

26. Seven H, et al. A randomized controlled trial of early oral feeding in laryngectomized patients. *Laryngoscope* 2003;113(6):1076-9.

27. Bauer JJ, et al. Is routine postoperative nasogastric decompression really necessary? *Ann Surg* 1985;201(2):233-6.

28. Ducerf C, et al. Postoperative electromyographic profile in human jejunum. *Ann Surg* 1992;215(3):237-43.

29. Thoren T, et al. Effects of epidural bupivacaine and epidural morphine on bowel function and pain after hysterectomy. *Acta Anaesthesiol Scand* 1989;33(2):181-5.

30. Tollesson PO, et al. A radiologic method for the study of postoperative colonic motility in humans. *Scand J Gastroenterol* 1991;26(8):887-96.

31. Condon RE, et al. Human colonic smooth muscle electrical activity during and after recovery from postoperative ileus. *Am J Physiol* 1995;269(3 Pt 1):G408-17.

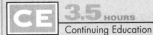

**CE 3.5 HOURS Continuing Education**

**EARN CE CREDIT ONLINE**
Go to www.nursingcenter.com/CE/ajn and receive a certificate within minutes.

**GENERAL PURPOSE:** To give registered professional nurses an opportunity to learn about an evidence-based practice project conducted to see whether any compelling evidence exists for listening to bowel sounds to assess for the return of gastrointestinal (GI) motility after abdominal surgery.

**GENERAL PURPOSE:** After reading this article and taking the test on the next page, you will be able to:

- describe the background information the authors considered in designing their study.
- outline the methodology they used and the factors considered in conducting their study.
- discuss the authors' results and conclusions related to nursing practice guidelines for assessing the return of GI motility.

**TEST INSTRUCTIONS**
**To take the test online, go to our secure Web site at** www.nursingcenter.com/CE/ajn.

**To use the form provided in this issue,**
- record your answers in the test answer section of the CE enrollment form between pages 48 and 49. Each question has only one correct answer. You may make copies of the form. Test code AJN2405.
- complete the registration information and course evaluation. Mail the completed enrollment form and registration fee of $22.75 to **Lippincott Williams and Wilkins CE Group,** 2710 Yorktowne Blvd., Brick, NJ 08723, by December 31, 2007. You will receive your certificate in four to six weeks. For faster service, include a fax number and we will fax your certificate within two business days of receiving your enrollment form. You will receive your CE certificate of earned contact hours and an answer key to review your results. There is no minimum passing grade.

**DISCOUNTS and CUSTOMER SERVICE**
- Send two or more tests in any nursing journal published by Lippincott Williams and Wilkins (LWW) together, and deduct $0.95 from the price of each test.
- We also offer CE accounts for hospitals and other health care facilities online at www.nursingcenter.com. Call **(800) 787-8985** for details.

**PROVIDER ACCREDITATION**
This continuing nursing education (CNE) activity for 3.5 contact hours is provided by LWW, which is accredited as a provider of continuing nursing education by the American Nurses Credentialing Center's Commission on Accreditation and by the American Association of Critical-Care Nurses (AACN 00012278, CERP Category A). This activity is also provider approved by the California Board of Registered Nursing, provider number CEP 11749 for 3.5 contact hours. LWW is also an approved provider of CNE in Alabama, Florida, and Iowa, and holds the following provider numbers: AL #ABNP0114, FL #FBN2454, IA #75. All of its home study activities are classified for Texas nursing continuing education requirements as Type 1. Your certificate is valid in all states. *This means that your certificate of earned contact hours is valid no matter where you live.*

(Madsen et al., 2005)

## Tool 12.1    Creating an EBP Poster

**INSTRUCTIONS:** Creating a poster is an easy way to share information about your EBP project. Refer to the checklist for elements to include in a poster presentation. The poster should be created for readability and focused on key messages.

☐ Use a large font size (> 28).

☐ Be inclusive when listing interprofessional team members of the EBP project.

☐ Consider the following components:

- Project title

- Interprofessional team members' names and credentials

- Purpose statement

- Rationale or background (optional)

- Project framework or EBP process

- Synthesis of evidence

- Practice change

- Implementation strategies

- Evaluation or results

- Next steps

- Conclusions and implications for practice

☐ Place content in columns; readers will read down each column and from left to right.

☐ Credit the funding agency, if applicable.

☐ Use color and images to enhance the story without overdoing it.

☐ Report data in graphs with minimal text for easy interpretation.

☐ Label graphs and legends clearly (e.g., label $x$ and $y$ axes, note sample size).

☐ Provide a link to the program or conference theme, if applicable.

## CITATIONS

American Nurses Association, 2009; Forsyth, Wright, Scherb, & Gaspar, 2010; Hanrahan, Marlow, Aldrich, & Hiatt, 2012; Siedlecki, 2017; Williams & Cullen, 2016.

## Tool 12.2   Institutional Review Board Considerations

**INSTRUCTIONS:** It may be unclear whether EBP work should have Institutional Review Board (IRB) review and approval. This tool provides a checklist of resources and forms to locate within your organization. When questions emerge, seek assistance from an organizational leader and/or EBP expert.

## IRB Review Resources

- ☐ Chair or members of the Nursing Research and EBP Committee
- ☐ Clinical IRB chair (can help differentiate EBP from conduct of research)
- ☐ Organizational policies
- ☐ Office for Human Research Protections: http://www.hhs.gov/ohrp

## IRB Review and Form Completion

- ☐ Always follow institutional policies regarding IRB review for QI.
- ☐ Regular discussions about the approval process between the group responsible for EBP work and the clinical IRB chair may be helpful.
- ☐ Complete a Human Subjects Research Determination request form for review by the institutional IRB clinical chair.
- ☐ When completing the Human Subjects Research Determination request form, use concise QI language instead of research terms:
  - QI/EBP project director (not *principal investigator*)
  - Describe practice change (not *intervention*)
  - Evaluation plan (not *methodological design*)
- ☐ If project results are sensitive, consider reporting in a manner that provides more general outcomes (e.g., a decrease in fall rate by X% instead of a fall rate reduction from X/1000 patient days to Y/1000 patient days).

EXAMPLES

TOOLS

## Tool 12.3    EBP Abstract Template

**INSTRUCTIONS:** Read carefully and follow directions for the conference or program. Include a brief summary of the EBP project-specific information in each section identified. Include all sections in the outline, per call for abstracts directions for specific format and word limits.

**Project Title:**

**Author(s):**

**Purpose and Rationale:** Clearly state the project purpose (include PICO [P = patient population/problem/pilot area, I = intervention, C = comparison, O = outcome] components within the purpose statement) and the rationale for doing the project.

**Synthesis of Evidence:** Provide a synthesis of the available evidence (i.e., not an annotated bibliography).

_____

**Practice Change:** Explain the practice change as a procedure that can be replicated.

_____

**Implementation Strategies:** Describe implementation strategies used to introduce and integrate the change in practice.

_____

**Evaluation:** Describe the evaluation used or planned for the project. Report findings related to both process and outcome indicators.

_____

**Conclusions and Implications for Practice:** Summarize the project findings and how they might be used in practice.

_____

**References:**

_____

**Total Words/Figures Allowed:**

## Tool 12.4   Preparing an EBP Presentation

**INSTRUCTIONS:** Review the checklist and conference directions carefully. Follow each step, checking when complete. Include all elements in the presentation.

- ☐ Carefully read the specifications for the presentation, especially if there is a required or recommended program to use.

- ☐ Know your presentation time limit. A general rule of thumb is to plan to cover one slide in two minutes.

- ☐ Determine what equipment will be provided and notify the sponsoring organization of any special equipment needs, such as access to the Internet or sound.

- ☐ Select a template or design style and use a consistent design style, font style, and font sizes throughout.

- ☐ Create a title slide with byline, institutional logos, and sponsorship (such as grants or other paid endorsements), as appropriate.

- ☐ Report any conflict of interest or intellectual bias.

- ☐ Identify objectives or an outline for the presentation.

- ☐ Identify the key pieces of information you want the audience to learn. Do not bombard the audience with every detail about the project.

- ☐ Use slide titles to inform participants of the pertinence of the content on that slide.

- ☐ Use well-labeled graphs when possible; graphs are easier to read than tables.

- ☐ When adding tables, figures, or images, keep objects proportional (avoid distortion).

- ☐ Include authors' last name and the year of publication for direct citations or specific research studies:

  - ○ Cite directly on the slide in a smaller font size.

  - ○ List complete references for cited materials at the end of the presentation.

- ☐ Use a font size larger than 24 for the slide content and make slide titles slightly larger; references may be in a font that is size 16.

- ☐ Check for consistency in content and formatting.

- ☐ Consider using slide notes as a tool to list additional content to review and cover during an oral presentation.

- ☐ Conclude with implications for practice, research, policy, and future directions.

- ☐ Practice presenting the content for completeness, timing, and flow. Add slides to transition content, if needed.

- ☐ Proofread. Check spelling. Edit. Repeat.

*continues*

## Tool 12.4    Preparing an EBP Presentation (Continued)

☐ Save it! Back it up!

☐ Submit the presentation according to specifications but always take a backup copy on a flash drive when you present.

☐ Consider whether to have handouts or presentation copies available and submit them ahead of time, if applicable.

☐ Allow time for questions.

## CITATIONS

American Nurses Association, 2009; Fineout-Overholt, Gallagher-Ford, Mazurek Melnyk, & Stillwell, 2011; Hanrahan, Marlow, Aldrich, & Hiatt, 2012

## Tool 12.5    Planning for an EBP Publication

**INSTRUCTIONS:** Read author guidelines carefully. Review and discuss the checklist as a team:

- ☐ Determine the target audience.

- ☐ Determine authors to invite to participate in writing (be inclusive). Include clinicians on the team.

- ☐ Determine a primary and secondary choice of journals.

- ☐ Read several issues of potential journals if you are not familiar with the typical content.

- ☐ Send query letters via email, with or without an abstract, to the editor to determine interest in a full manuscript.

- ☐ Read and follow author guidelines closely.

- ☐ Consider SQUIRE 2.0 guidelines.

- ☐ Outline content.

- ☐ Begin writing by capturing ideas and editing later.

- ☐ Plan to rewrite, rewrite, rewrite.

- ☐ Use American Psychological Association (APA) formatting until editing is complete, to avoid confusion with numbering citations during review and edits.

- ☐ Complete final content edits before doing final formatting.

- ☐ Include an acknowledgement of funding sources and individuals providing assistance.

- ☐ Review author guidelines again, prior to submission.

- ☐ After submission, consider reviewers' suggestions carefully and be prepared to edit or address their suggestions.

- ☐ If the manuscript is not accepted, consider resubmitting to another journal.

## CITATIONS

Adams, Farrington, & Cullen, 2012; American Nurses Association, 2009; Fineout-Overholt, Gallagher-Ford, Mazurek Melnyk, & Stillwell, 2011; Hanrahan, Marlow, Aldrich, & Hiatt, 2012; Holland & Watson, 2012; Roush, 2017a, 2017b; Saver, 2014

# REFERENCES

AABB. (2017). Standards portal. Retrieved from http://www.aabb.org/sa/Pages/Standards-Portal.aspx

Aarons, G. A., Ehrhart, M. G., Farahnak, L. R., & Sklar, M. (2014). Aligning leadership across systems and organizations to develop a strategic climate for evidence-based practice implementation. *Annual Review of Public Health, 35,* 255–274. doi:10.1146/annurev-publhealth-032013-182447

Abbott, K. C., & Bakris, G. L. (2004). What have we learned from the current trials? *Medical Clinics of North America, 88*(1), 189–207. doi:10.1016/S0025-7125(03)00129-9

Abbott, L. (2016, April). *Energy Through Motion: An activity intervention for cancer-related fatigue in an ambulatory infusion center.* Paper presented at the 23rd National Evidence-Based Practice Conference, Coralville, IA.

Abbott, L., & Hooke, M. C. (in press). Energy Through Motion: An activity intervention for cancer-related fatigue in an ambulatory infusion center. *Clinical Journal of Oncology Nursing.*

Abdullah, G., Rossy, D., Ploeg, J., Davies, B., Higuchi, K., Sikora, L., & Stacey, D. (2014). Measuring the effectiveness of mentoring as a knowledge translation intervention for implementing empirical evidence: A systematic review. *Worldviews on Evidence-Based Nursing, 11*(5), 284–300. doi:10.1111/wvn.12060

Abela, A. (2013). *Advanced presentations by design: Creating communication that drives action* (2nd ed.). New York, NY: Pfeiffer.

Abraham, A. J., & Roman, P. M. (2010). Early adoption of injectable naltrexone for alcohol-use disorders: Findings in the private-treatment sector. *Journal of Studies on Alcohol and Drugs, 71*(3), 460–466.

Adams, S., & Barron, S. (2009). Use of evidence-based practice in school nursing: Prevalence, associated variables, and perceived needs. *Worldviews on Evidence-Based Nursing, 6*(1), 16–26. doi:10.1111/j.1741-6787.2008.00141.x

Adams, S., Farrington, M., & Cullen, L. (2012). Evidence into practice: Publishing an evidence-based practice project. *Journal of PeriAnesthesia Nursing, 27*(3), 193–202. doi:10.1016/j.jopan.2012.03.004

Aebersold, M. (2011). Using simulation to improve the use of evidence-based practice guidelines. *Western Journal of Nursing Research, 33*(3), 296–305. doi:10.1177/0193945910379791

Agency for Healthcare Research and Quality (AHRQ). (n.d.-a). AHRQuality Indicators. Retrieved from http://www.qualityindicators.ahrq.gov

Agency for Healthcare Research and Quality (AHRQ). (n.d.-b). Assemble the team. Retrieved from https://www.ahrq.gov/professionals/education/curriculum-tools/cusptoolkit/modules/assemble/index.html

Agency for Healthcare Research and Quality (AHRQ). (n.d.-c). Effective health care program: Helping you make better treatment choices: Patient decision aids. Retrieved from https://effectivehealthcare.ahrq.gov/decision-aids/

Agency for Healthcare Research and Quality (AHRQ). (2011a). *Closing the quality gap series: Quality improvement interventions to address health disparities.* Retrieved from http://effectivehealthcare.ahrq.gov/index.cfm/search-for-guides-reviews-and-reports/?pageaction=displayproduct&productid=983

Agency for Healthcare Research and Quality (AHRQ). (2011b). Home. Retrieved from http://www.ahrq.gov

Agency for Healthcare Research and Quality (AHRQ). (2013a). National Guideline Clearinghouse (NGC). Retrieved from https://www.ahrq.gov/cpi/about/otherwebsites/guideline.gov/index.html

Agency for Healthcare Research and Quality (AHRQ). (2013b). Strategy 3: Nurse bedside shift report. Retrieved from http://www.ahrq.gov/professionals/systems/hospital/engagingfamilies/strategy3/index.html

Agency for Healthcare Research and Quality (AHRQ). (2014). Glossary: TeamSTEPPS Long-Term Care instructor guide. Retrieved from http://www.ahrq.gov/teamstepps/longtermcare/references/glossary.html

Agency for Healthcare Research and Quality (AHRQ). (2015a). Explain and motivate use of comparative information. Retrieved from http://www.ahrq.gov/professionals/quality-patient-safety/talkingquality/create/explain/index.html

Agency for Healthcare Research and Quality (AHRQ). (2015b). Tips on designing a quality report. Retrieved from http://www.ahrq.gov/professionals/quality-patient-safety/talkingquality/resources/design/designtips.html

Agency for Healthcare Research and Quality (AHRQ). (2015c). Tips on writing a quality report. Retrieved from http://www.ahrq.gov/professionals/quality-patient-safety/talkingquality/resources/writing/index.html

Agency for Healthcare Research and Quality (AHRQ). (2015d). Your project checklist. Retrieved from http://www.ahrq.gov/professionals/quality-patient-safety/talkingquality/tools/workbook.html

Agency for Healthcare Research and Quality (AHRQ). (2015e). Your project checklist: Translate data into information. Retrieved from http://www.ahrq.gov/professionals/quality-patient-safety/talkingquality/tools/workbook.html

Agency for Healthcare Research and Quality (AHRQ). (2016a). Explain and motivate: Delivering key messages. Retrieved from http://www.ahrq.gov/sites/default/files/wysiwyg/talkingquality/tools/documents/1_explain_and-motivate_delivering_key_messages_final_production.pdf

Agency for Healthcare Research and Quality (AHRQ). (2016b). TeamSTEPPS. Team strategies and tools to enhance performance and patient safety. Retrieved from http://www.ahrq.gov/teamstepps/index.html

Agency for Healthcare Research and Quality (AHRQ). (2017). Engaging patients and families in their health care. Retrieved from https://www.ahrq.gov/professionals/quality-patient-safety/patient-family-engagement/index.html

Aggarwal, M., Singh, S., Sharma, A., Singh, P., & Bansal, P. (2016). Impact of structured verbal feedback module in medical education: A questionnaire- and test score-based analysis. *International Journal of Applied Basic Medical Research, 6*(3), 220–225. doi:10.4103/2229-516X.186968

Agoritsas, T., Heen, A. F., Brandt, L., Alonso-Coello, P., Kristiansen, A., Akl, E. A., . . . Vandvik, P. O. (2015). Decision aids that really promote shared decision making: The pace quickens. *BMJ, 350,* g7624. doi:10.1136/bmj.g7624

Agre, P. E. (2005, October 7). *How to be a leader in your field: A guide for students in professional schools.* Retrieved from http://polaris.gseis.ucla.edu/pagre/leader.html

AGREE Collaboration. (2010). Appraisal of guidelines for research and evaluation. Retrieved from http://www.agreetrust.org/

Aitken, L. M., Burmeister, E., Clayton, S., Dalais, C., & Gardner, G. (2011). The impact of nursing rounds on the practice environment and nurse satisfaction in intensive care: Pre-test post-test comparative study. *International Journal of Nursing Studies, 48*(8), 918–925. doi:10.1016/j.ijnurstu.2010.10.004

Alanen, S., Välimäki, M., Kaila, M., & ECCE Study Group. (2009). Nurses' experiences of guideline implementation: A focus group study. *Journal of Clinical Nursing, 18*(18), 2613–2621. doi:10.1111/j.1365-2702.2008.02754.x

Al Ayubi, S. U., Pelletier, A., Sunthara, G., Gujral, N., Mittal, V., Bourgeois, F. C. (2016). A mobile app development guideline for hospital settings: Maximizing the use of and minimizing the security risks of "bring your own devices" policies. *JMIR mHealth and uHealth, 4*(2), e50. doi:10.2196/mhealth.4424

Albarracín, D., McNatt, P. S., Klein, C. T. F., Ho, R. M., Mitchell, A. L., & Kumkale, G. T. (2003). Persuasive communications to change actions: An analysis of behavioral and cognitive impact in HIV prevention. *Health Psychology, 22*(2), 166–177. doi:10.1037/0278-6133.22.2.166

Aldeyab, M. A., Kearney, M. P., McElnay, J. C., Magee, F. A., Conlon, G., Gill, D., . . . Scott, M. G. (2011). A point prevalence survey of antibiotic prescriptions: Benchmarking and patterns of use. *British Journal of Clinical Pharmacology, 71*(2), 293–296. doi:10.1111/j.1365-2125.2010.03840.x

Aletraris, L., Edmond, M. B., & Roman, P. M. (2015). Adoption of injectable naltrexone in U.S. substance use disorder treatment programs. *Journal of Studies on Alcohol and Drugs, 76*(1), 143–151. doi:10.15288/jsad.2015.76.143

Alexander, L., & Allen, D. (2011). Establishing an evidence-based practice inpatient medical oncology fluid balance measurement policy. *Clinical Journal of Oncology Nursing, 15*(1), 23–25. doi:10.1188/11.CJON.23-25

Alfonso, E., Blot, K., & Blot, S. (2016). Prevention of hospital-acquired bloodstream infections through chlorhexidine gluconate-impregnated washcloth bathing in intensive care units: A systematic review and meta-analysis of randomised crossover trials. *Eurosurveillance, 21*(46), 1–11. doi:10.2807/1560-7917.ES.2016.21.46.30400

Alkhateeb, F. M., & Doucette, W. R. (2009). Influences on physicians' adoption of electronic detailing (e-detailing). *Informatics for Health and Social Care, 34*(1), 39–52. doi:10.1080/17538150902779402

Allegranzi, B., Conway, L., Larson, E., & Pittet, D. (2014). Status of the implementation of the World Health Organization multimodal hand hygiene strategy in United States of America health care facilities. *American Journal of Infection Control, 42*(3), 224–230.

Alleyne, J., & Jumaa, M. O. (2007). Building the capacity for evidence-based clinical nursing leadership: The role of executive co-coaching and group clinical supervision for quality patient services. *Journal of Nursing Management, 15*(2), 230–243. doi:10.1111/j.1365-2834.2007.00750.x

Al Saif, N., Hammodi, A., Al-Azem, M. A., & Al-Hubail, R. (2015). Tension pneumothorax and subcutaneous emphysema complicating insertion of nasogastric tube. *Case Reports in Critical Care, 2015,* Article ID 690742, 1–4. doi:10.1155/2015/690742

Al-Tawfiq, J. A., Abed, M. S., Al-Yami, N., & Birrer, R. B. (2013). Promoting and sustaining a hospital-wide, multifaceted hand hygiene program resulted in significant reduction in health care-associated infections. *American Journal of Infection Control, 41*(6), 482–486. doi:10.1016/j.ajic.2012.08.009

Ambroggio, L., Thomson, J., Murtagh Kurowski, E., Courter, J., Statile, A., Graham, C., . . . White, C. M. (2013). Quality improvement methods increase appropriate antibiotic prescribing for childhood pneumonia. *Pediatrics, 131*(5), e1623–e1631. doi:10.1542/peds.2012-2635

American Academy of Nursing. (2015). Twenty things nurses and patients should question. Retrieved from http://www.aannet.org/choosing-wisely

American Board of Internal Medicine Foundation. (2017). Choosing wisely. Retrieved from http://www.choosingwisely.org/

American Evaluation Association. (2012). American Evaluation Association guiding principles for evaluators. Retrieved from http://www.eval.org/p/cm/ld/fid=51

American Institutes for Research. (2017). Health systems improvement. Retrieved from http://www.air.org/topic/health/health-systems-improvement

American Nurses Association. (2009). *Determining a standard order of credentials for the professional nurse* [Position statement: Credentials for the professional nurse]. Retrieved from http://nursingworld.org/MainMenuCategories/Policy-Advocacy/Positions-and-Resolutions/ANAPositionStatements/Position-Statements-Alphabetically/Credentials-for-the-Professional-Nurse-Determining-a-Standard-Order-of-Credentials-for-the-Professi.html

American Nurses Credentialing Center. (2017). ANCC Magnet Recognition Program. Retrieved from http://www.nursecredentialing.org/Magnet

Anas, R., & Brunet, F. (2009). Overcoming barriers when implementing evidence at the bedside. *Healthcare Quarterly, 12*(4), 72–78. doi:10.12927/hcq.2013.21129

Anderson, C. A., & Titler, M. G. (2014). Development and verification of an agent-based model of opinion leadership. *Implementation Science, 9*(136), 1–13. doi:10.1186/s13012-014-0136-6

Anderson, R., Kleiber, C., Greiner, J., Comried, L., & Zimmerman, M. (2016). Interface pressure redistribution on skin during continuous lateral rotation therapy: A feasibility study. *Heart & Lung, 45*(3), 237–243. doi:10.1016/j.hrtlng.2016.02.003

Anderson-Carpenter, K. D., Watson-Thompson, J., Jones, M., & Chaney, L. (2014). Using communities of practice to support implementation of evidence-based prevention strategies. *Journal of Community Practice, 22*(1–2), 176–188. doi:10.1080/10705422.2014.901268

Andrews, J., Guyatt, G., Oxman, A. D., Alderson, P., Dahm, P., Falck-Ytter, Y., . . . Schünemann, H. J. (2013). GRADE guidelines: 14. Going from evidence to recommendations: The significance and presentation of recommendations. *Journal of Clinical Epidemiology, 66*(7), 719–725. doi:10.1016/j.jclinepi.2012.03.013

Arditi, C., Rège-Walther, M., Wyatt, J. C., Durieux, P., & Burnand, B. (2012). Computer-generated reminders delivered on paper to healthcare professionals; effects on professional practice and health care outcomes. *Cochrane Database of Systematic Reviews, 2012*(12), 1–123. doi:10.1002/14651858.CD001175.pub3

Armellion, D., Trivedi, M., Law, I., Singh, N., Schilling, M. E., Hussain, E., & Farber, B. (2013). Replicating changes in hand hygiene in a surgical intensive care unit with remote video auditing and feedback. *American Journal of Infection Control, 41*(10), 925–927. doi:10.1016/j.ajic.2012.12.011

Arora, S., Miskovic, D., Hull, L., Moorthy, K., Aggarwal, R., Johannsson, H., . . . Sevdalis N. (2011). Self vs expert assessment of technical and non-technical skills in high fidelity simulation. *American Journal of Surgery, 202*(4), 500–506. doi:10.1016/j.amjsurg.2011.01.024

Arslan, D., Koca, T., Tastekin, D., Basaran, H., & Bozcuk, H. (2014). Impact of poster presentations on academic knowledge transfer from the oncologist perspective in Turkey. *Asian Pacific Journal of Cancer Prevention, 15*(18), 7707–7711. doi:10.7314/APJCP.2014.15.18.7707

Ashida, S., Heaney, C. A., Kmet, J. M., & Wilkins, J. R., III. (2011). Using protection motivation theory and formative research to guide an injury prevention intervention: Increasing adherence to the North American Guidelines for Children's Agricultural Tasks. *Health Promotion Practice, 12*(3), 396–405. doi:10.1177/1524839910362034

Aslam, S., Georgiev, H., Mehta, K., & Kumar, A. (2012). Matching research design to clinical research questions. *Indian Journal of Sexually Transmitted Diseases and AIDS, 33*(1), 49–53. doi:10.4103/0253-7184.93829

Assadi, R., Zarghi, N., Shamloo, A. S., & Nikooiyan, Y. (2012). Evidence-based abstracts: What research summaries should contain to support evidence-based medicine. *International Journal of Evidence-Based Healthcare, 10*(2), 154–158. doi:10.1111/j.1744-1609.2012.00266.x

Atkinson, N. L. (2007). Developing a questionnaire to measure perceived attributes of eHealth innovations. *American Journal of Health Behavior, 31*(6), 612–621.

Avdić, A., Tucker, S., Evans, R., Smith, A., & Zimmerman, M. B. (2016). Comparing the ratio of mean red blood cell transfusion episode rate of 1 unit versus 2 units in hematopoietic stem cell transplant patients. *Transfusion, 56*(9), 2346–2351. doi:10.1111/trf.13708

Avery, K. R., O'Brien, M., Pierce, C. D., & Gazarian, P. K. (2015). Use of a nursing checklist to facilitate implementation of therapeutic hypothermia after cardiac arrest. *Critical Care Nurse, 35*(1), 29–37. doi:10.4037/ccn2015937

Aveyard, P., & Bauld, L. (2011). Incentives for promoting smoking cessation: What we still do not know. [Editorial]. *Cochrane Database of Systematic Reviews, 8*(ED000027). doi:10.1002/14651858.ED000027

Badger, J. M., & Cullen, L. (2015, November). *The mentorship experience.* Presented at the Advanced Practice Institute: Promoting Adoption of Evidence-Based Practice, Rhode Island Hospital, Providence, RI.

Badran, H., Pluye, P., & Grad, R. (2015). Advantages and disadvantages of educational email alerts for family physicians: Viewpoint. *Journal of Medical Internet Research, 17*(2), e49. doi:10.2196/jmir.3773

Bahtsevani, C., Willman, A., Stoltz, P., & Östman, M. (2010). Experiences of the implementation of clinical practice guidelines—Interviews with nurse managers and nurses in hospital care. *Scandinavian Journal of Caring Sciences, 24*(3), 514–522. doi:10.1111/j.1471-6712.2009.00743.x

Bailyn, E. (2015, February 6). The 7 defining traits of thought leaders [Web log post]. Retrieved from http://www.huffingtonpost.com/evan-bailyn/the-7-defining-traits-of-_b_6624338.html

Baker, A., Young, K., Potter, J., & Madan, I. (2010). A review of grading systems for evidence-based guidelines produced by medical specialties. *Clinical Medicine, 10*(4), 358–363. doi:10.7861/clinmedicine.10-4-358

Balakas, K., & Sparks, L. (2010). Teaching research and evidence-based practice using a service-learning approach. *Journal of Nursing Education, 49*(12), 691–695. doi:20.4938/02585845-30200842-07

Balla, J. I., Heneghan, C., Glasziou, P., Thompson, M., & Balla, M. E. (2009). A model for reflection for good clinical practice. *Journal of Evaluation in Clinical Practice, 15*(6), 964–969. doi:10.1111/j.1365-2753.2009.01243.x

Balshem, H., Helfand, M., Schünemann, H. J., Oxman, A. D., Kunz, R., Brozek, J., . . . Guyatt, G. H. (2011). GRADE guidelines: 3. Rating the quality of evidence. *Journal of Clinical Epidemiology, 64*(4), 401–406. doi:10.1016/j.jclinepi.2010.07.015

Barnes, B., Barnes, M., & Sweeney, C. D. (2016a). Putting the "meaning" in meaningful recognition of nurses: The DAISY Award. *Journal of Nursing Administration, 46*(10), 508–512. doi:10.1097/NNA.0000000000000394

Barnes, B., Barnes, M., & Sweeney, C. D. (2016b). Supporting recognition of clinical nurses with the DAISY Award. *Journal of Nursing Administration, 46*(4), 164–166. doi:10.1097/NNA.0000000000000320

Barnsteiner, J. H., Reeder, V. C., Palma, W. H., Preston, A. M., & Walton, M. K. (2010). Promoting evidence-based practice and translational research. *Nursing Administration Quarterly, 34*(3), 217–225. doi:10.1097/NAQ.0b013e3181e702f4

Baskerville, N. B., Liddy, C., & Hogg, W. (2012). Systematic review and meta-analysis of practice facilitation within primary care settings. *Annals of Family Medicine, 10*(1), 63–74. doi:10.1370/afm.1312

Basol, R., Larsen, R., Simones, J., & Wilson, R. (2017). Evidence into practice: Hospital and academic partnership demonstrating exemplary professional practice in EBP. *Journal of PeriAnesthesia Nursing, 32*(1), 68–71. doi:10.1016/j.jopan.2016.11.002

Bauer, E. (2003, November 10). Be a thought leader! [Web log post]. Retrieved from http://www.elise.com/blog/be_a_thought_leader

Beaty, C. A., Haggerty, K. A., Moser, M. G., George, T. J., Robinson, C. W., Arnaoutakis, G. J., & Whitman, G. J. (2013). Disclosure of physician-specific behavior improves blood utilization protocol adherence in cardiac surgery. *Annals of Thoracic Surgery, 96*(6), 2168–2174. doi:10.1016/j.athoracsur.2013.06.080

Becker, B., Dawson, P., Devine, K., Hannum, C., Hill, S., Leydens, J., . . . Palmquist, M. (1994–2012). Writing@CSU guide: Case studies. Retrieved from http://writing.colostate.edu/guides/research/casestudy/pop2a.cfm

Bedra, M., Golder, S. H., Cha, E., Jeong, I. C., & Finkelstein, J. (2015). Computerized insulin order sets can lead to unanticipated consequences. In J. Mantas, A. Hasman, & M. Househ (Eds.), *Studies in health technology and informatics: Enabling health informatics applications* (pp. 53–56). Burke, VA: IOS Press.

Benishek, L. A., Kirby, K. C., Dugosh, K. L., & Padovano, A. (2010). Beliefs about the empirical support of drug abuse treatment interventions: A survey of outpatient treatment providers. *Drug and Alcohol Dependence, 107*(2–3), 202–208. doi:10.1016/j.drugalcdep.2009.10.013

Bennett, B., & Provost, L. (2015, July). What's your theory? Driver diagram serves as tool for building and testing theories for improvement. *Quality Progress,* 36–43. Retrieved from http://www.ihi.org/resources/Pages/Publications/WhatsYourTheoryDriverDiagrams.aspx

Benneyan, J. C. (1998a). Statistical quality control methods in infection control and hospital epidemiology, Part I: Introduction and basic theory. *Infection Control and Hospital Epidemiology, 19*(3), 194–214. doi:10.2307/30143442

Benneyan, J. C. (1998b). Statistical quality control methods in infection control and hospital epidemiology, Part II: Chart use, statistical properties, and research issues. *Infection Control and Hospital Epidemiology, 19*(4), 265–283.

Benneyan, J. C., Lloyd, R. C., & Plsek, P. E. (2003). Statistical process control as a tool for research and healthcare improvement. *Quality & Safety in Health Care, 12*(6), 458–464. doi:10.1136/qhc.12.6.458

Bensinger, W., Schubert, M., Ang, K. K., Brizel, D., Brown, E., Eilers, J. G., . . . Trotti, A. M., III. (2008). NCCN Task Force report: Prevention and management of mucositis in cancer care. *Journal of the National Comprehensive Cancer Network, 6*(Suppl. 1), S1–S21, quiz S22–S24.

Berardinelli, C., & Yerian, L. (n.d.). Run charts: A simple and powerful tool for process improvement [Web log post]. Retrieved from https://www.isixsigma.com/tools-templates/control-charts/run-charts-a-simple-and-powerful-tool-for-process-improvement

Berenholtz, S. M., Pronovost, P. J., Lipsett, P. A., Hobson, D., Earsing, K., Farley, J. E., . . . Perl, T. M. (2004). Eliminating catheter-related bloodstream infections in the intensive care unit. *Critical Care Medicine, 32*(10), 2014–2020. doi:10.1097/01.CCM.0000142399.70913.2F

Berenson, R. A., & Rice, T. (2016). Beyond measurement and reward: Methods of motivating quality improvement and accountability. *Health Services Research, 50*(Suppl. 2), 2155–2186. doi:10.1111/1475-6773.12413

Berkman, N. D., Lohr, K. N., Ansari, M. T., Balk, E. M., Kane, R., McDonagh, M., . . . Chang, S. (2015). Grading the strength of a body of evidence when assessing health care interventions: An EPC update. *Journal of Clinical Epidemiology, 68*(11), 1312–1324. doi:10.1016/j.jclinepi.2014.11.023

Berkman, N. D., Lohr, K. N., Morgan, L. C., Richmond, E., Kuo, T. M., Morton, S., . . . Tant, E. (2012). Reliability testing of the AHRQ EPC approach to grading the strength of evidence in comparative effectiveness reviews. Methods Research Report (prepared by TRI International–University of North Carolina Evidence-based Practice Center under Contract No. 290-2007-10056-I.) AHRQ Publication No. 12-EHC067-EF. Rockville, MD: Agency for Healthcare Research and Quality.

Berkman, N. D., Lohr, K. N., Morgan, L. C., Kuo, T. M., & Morton, S. C. (2013). Interrater reliability of grading strength of evidence varies with the complexity of the evidence in systematic review. *Journal of Clinical Epidemiology, 66*(10), 1105–1117. doi:10.1016/j.jclinepi.2013.06.002

Bernstein, E., Topp, D., Shaw, E., Girard, C., Pressman, K., Woolcock, E., & Bernstein, J. (2009). A preliminary report of knowledge translation: Lessons from taking screening and brief intervention techniques from the research setting into regional systems of care. *Academic Emergency Medicine, 16*(11), 1225–1233. doi:10.1111/j.1553-2712.2009.00516.x

Berta, W., Ginsburg, L., Gilbart, E., Lemieux-Charles, L., & Davis, D. (2013). What, why, and how care protocols are implemented in Ontario nursing homes. *Canadian Journal on Aging, 32*(1), 73–85. doi:10.1017/S0714980813000081

Bethel, S. A., Seitz, S., Landreth, C. O., Gibson, L., & Whitcomb, J. J. (2012). Energize staff to create a research agenda. *Clinical Nurse Specialist, 26*(5), 272–276. doi:10.1097/NUR.0b013e31825aeb80

Bhatti, N. I., & Ahmed, A. (2015). Improving skills development in residency using a deliberate-practice and learner-centered model. *Laryngoscope, 125*(Suppl. 8), S1–S14. doi:10.1002/lary.25434

Bhogal, S. K., McGillivray, D., Bourbeau, J., Plotnick, L., Bartlett, S., Benedetti, A., & Ducharme, F. M. (2011). Focusing the focus group: Impact of the awareness of major factors contributing to non-adherence to acute paediatric asthma guidelines. *Journal of Evaluation in Clinical Practice, 17*(1), 160–167. doi:10.1111/j.1365-2753.2010.01416.x

Bhogal, S. K., Murray, M. A., McLeod, K. M., Bergen, A., Bath, B., Menon, A., . . . Stacey, D. (2011). Using problem-based case studies to learn about knowledge translation interventions: An inside perspective. *Journal of Continuing Education in Health Professions, 31*(4), 268–275. doi:10.1002/chp.20140

Bick, D., & Graham, I. (Eds.). (2010). *Evaluating the impact of implementing evidence-based practice.* United Kingdom: Wiley-Blackwell Publishing and Sigma Theta Tau International.

Block, J., Lilienthal, M., & Cullen, L. (2015). Thermoregulation for adult trauma patients. In M. Farrington (Series Ed.), *EBP to Go: Accelerating evidence-based practice.* Iowa City, IA: Office of Nursing Research, Evidence-Based Practice and Quality, Department of Nursing Services and Patient Care, University of Iowa Hospitals and Clinics.

Block, J., Lilienthal, M., Cullen, L., & White, A. (2012). Evidence-based thermoregulation for adult trauma patients. *Critical Care Nursing Quarterly, 35*(1), 50–63. doi:10.1097/CNQ.0b013e31823d3e9b

Bloom's taxonomy. (n.d.) Retrieved 2016 from https://en.wikipedia.org/wiki/Bloom%27s_taxonomy

Blossom, P. (2013, April 1). Create a run chart [Video file]. Retrieved from https://www.youtube.com/watch?v=0FNzoB19G4A

Bonomi, M., & Batt, K. (2015). Supportive management of mucositis and metabolic derangements in head and neck cancer patients. *Cancers, 7*(3), 1743–1757. doi:10.3390/cancers7030862

Borchard, A., Schwappach, D. L., Barbir, A., & Bezzola, P. (2012). A systematic review of the effectiveness, compliance, and critical factors for implementation of safety checklists in surgery. *Annals of Surgery, 256*(6), 925–933. doi:10.1097/SLA.0b013e3182682f27

Bornbaum, C. C., Kornas, K., Peirson, L., & Rosella, L. C. (2015). Exploring the function and effectiveness of knowledge brokers as facilitators of knowledge translation in health-related settings: A systematic review and thematic analysis. *Implementation Science, 10*(162), 1–12. doi:10.1186/s13012-015-0351-9

Bosch, M., Faber, M., Cruijsberg, J., Voerman, G. E., Leatherman, S., Grol, R. P., . . . Wensing, M. (2009). Review article: Effectiveness of patient care teams and the role of clinical expertise and coordination: A literature review. *Medical Care Research and Review, 66*(Suppl. 6), 5S–35S. doi:10.1177/1077558709343295

Bosch, M., Tavender, E. J., Brennan, S. E., Knott, J., Gruen, R. L., & Green, S. E. (2016). The many organisational factors relevant to planning change in emergency care departments: A qualitative study to inform a cluster randomised controlled trial aiming to improve the management of patients with mild traumatic brain injuries. *PLoS ONE, 11*(2), e0148091. doi:10.1371/journal.pone.0148091

Bourdeaux, C. P., Davies, K. J., Thomas, M. J., Bewley, J. S., & Gould, T. H. (2014). Using "nudge" principles for order set design: A before-and-after evaluation of an electronic prescribing template in critical care. *BMJ Quality & Safety, 23*(5), 382–388. doi:10.1136/bmjqs-2013-002395

Bowie, P., Bradley, N. A., & Rushmer, R. (2012). Clinical audit and quality improvement—Time for a rethink? *Journal of Evaluation in Clinical Practice, 18*(1), 42–48. doi:10.1111/j.1365-2753.2010.01523.x

Boyal, A., & Hewison, A. (2016). Exploring senior nurses' experiences of leading organizational change. *Leadership in Health Services, 29*(1), 37–51. doi:10.1108/LHS-03-2015-0005

Brackett, T., Comer, L., & Whichello, R. (2013). Do Lean practices lead to more time at the bedside? *Journal for Healthcare Quality, 35*(2), 7–14. doi:10.1111/j.1945-1474.2011.00169.x

Brader, C., & Jaeger, M. (2014). *What makes an interdisciplinary team work? A collection of informed ideas, discussion prompts, and other materials to promote an atmosphere of collaboration, trust, and respect.* Retrieved from http://commons.pacificu.edu/ipp/42

Bradley, E. H., Holmboe, E. S., Mattera, J. A., Roumanis, S. A., Radford, M. J., & Krumholz, H. M. (2004). Data feedback efforts in quality improvement: Lessons learned from US hospitals. *Quality & Safety in Health Care, 13*(1), 26–31. doi:10.1136/qshc.2002.4408

Bragadóttir, H., Kalisch, B. J., & Tryggvadóttir, G. B. (2017). Correlates and predictors of missed nursing care in hospitals. *Journal of Clinical Nursing, 26*(11–12), 1524–1534. doi:10.1111/jocn.13449

Braithwaite, J., Marks, D., & Taylor, N. (2014). Harnessing implementation science to improve care quality and patient safety: A systematic review of targeted literature. *International Journal for Quality in Health Care, 26*(3), 321–329. doi:10.1093/intqhc/mzu047

Brandt, J. A., Edwards, D. R., Sullivan, S. C., Zehler, J. K., Grinder, S., Scott, K. J., . . . Maddox, K. L. (2009). An evidence-based business planning process. *Journal of Nursing Administration, 39*(12), 511–513. doi:10.1097/NNA.0b013e3181c18026

Bray, P., Cummings, D. M., Wolf, M., Massing, M. W., & Reaves, J. (2009). After the collaborative is over: What sustains quality improvement initiatives in primary care practices? *Joint Commission Journal on Quality and Patient Safety, 35*(10), 502–508. Retrieved from http://www.breastfeedingor.org/wp-content/uploads/2012/10/sustaining_qi_in_practices.pdf

Breimaier, H. E., Halfens, R. J. G., & Lohmann, C. (2015). Effectiveness of multifaceted and tailored strategies to implement a fall-prevention guideline into acute care nursing practice: A before-and-after, mixed-method study using a participatory action research approach. *BMC Nursing, 14,* 18. doi:10.1186/s12912-015-0064-z

Breimaier, H. E., Halfens, R. J. G., Wilborn, D., Meesterberends, E., Haase Nielsen, G., & Lohrmann, C. (2013). Implementation interventions used in nursing homes and hospitals: A descriptive, comparative study between Austria, Germany, and the Netherlands. *International Scholarly Research Notices, 2013,* 1–13.

Brenner, M. (2014, March 31). What is thought leadership? Why you need it. And steps to get it right. Retrieved from https://www.linkedin.com/pulse/20140331173356-951391-what-is-thought-leadership-why-you-need-it-and-steps-to-get-t-right

Breslau, E. S., Weiss, E. S., Williams, A., Burness, A., & Kepka, D. (2015). The implementation road: Engaging community partnerships in evidence-based cancer control interventions. *Health Promotion Practice, 16*(1), 46–54. doi:10.1177/1524839914528705

Breslin, M., Mullan, R. J., & Montori, V. (2008). The design of a decision aid about diabetes medications for use during the consultation with Type 2 diabetes. *Patient Education and Counseling,73*(3), 465–472. doi:10.1016/j.pec.2008.07.024

Bright, T. J., Wong, A., Dhurjati, R., Bristow, E., Bastian, L., Coeytaux, R. R.,...Lobach, D. (2012). Effect of clinical decision-support systems: A systematic review. *Annals of Internal Medicine, 157*(1), 29–43. doi:10.7326/0003-4819-157-1-201207030-00450

Brocklehurst, P., Price, J., Glenny, A. M., Tickle, M., Birch, S., Mertz, E., & Grytten, J. (2013). The effect of different methods of remuneration on the behaviour of primary care dentists. *Cochrane Database of Systematic Reviews, 2013*(11), 1–68. doi:10.1002/14651858.CD009853.pub2

Brody, A. A., Barnes, K., Ruble, C., & Sakowski, J. (2012). Evidence-based practice councils: Potential path to staff nurse empowerment and leadership growth. *Journal of Nursing Administration, 42*(1), 28–33. doi:10.1097/NNA.0b013e31823c17f5

Brosey, L. A., & March, K. S. (2015). Effectiveness of structured hourly nurse rounding on patient satisfaction and clinical outcomes. *Journal of Nursing Care Quality, 30*(2), 153–159. doi:10.1097/NCQ.0000000000000086

Brouwers, M. C., Kho, M. E., Browman, G. P., Burgers, J. S., Cluzeau, F., Feder, G.,...Zitzelsberger, L. (2010). AGREE II: Advancing guideline development, reporting and evaluation in health care. *Canadian Medical Association Journal, 182*(18), E839–E842. doi:10.1503/cmaj.090449

Brown, C., Wickline, M. A., Ecoff, L., & Glaser, D. (2009). Nursing practice, knowledge, attitudes, and perceived barriers to evidence-based practice at an academic medical center. *Journal of Advanced Nursing, 65*(2), 371–381. doi:10.1111/j.1365-2648.2008.04878.x

Brummel, N. E., Vasilevskis, E. E., Han, J. H., Boehm, L., Pun, B. T., & Ely, E. W. (2013). Implementing delirium screening in the ICU: Secrets to success. *Critical Care Medicine, 41*(9), 2196–2208. doi:10.1097/CCM.0b013e31829a6f1e

Bruno, T. O., Hicks, C. B., Naggie, S., Wohl, D. A., Albrecht, H., Thielman, N. M.,...Weyer, D. (2014). VISION: A regional performance improvement initiative for HIV health care providers. *Journal of Continuing Education in the Health Professions, 34*(3), 171–178. doi:10.1002/chp.21248

Brunsveld-Reinders, A. H., Arbous, M. S., Kuiper, S. G., & de Jonge, E. (2015). A comprehensive method to develop a checklist to increase safety of intra-hospital transport of critically ill patients. *Critical Care, 19*(214), 1–10. doi:10.1186/s13054-015-0938-1

Burke, J. G., Lich, K. H., Neal, J. W., Meissner, H. I., Yonas, M., & Mabry, P. L. (2015). Enhancing dissemination and implementation research using systems science methods. *International Journal of Behavioral Medicine, 22*(3), 283–291. doi:10.1007/s12529-014-9417-3

Burkitt, K. H., Sinkowitz-Cochran, R. L., Obrosky, D. S., Cuerdon, T., Miller, L. J., Jain, R.,...Fine, M. J. (2010). Survey of employee knowledge and attitudes before and after a multicenter Veterans' Administration quality improvement initiative to reduce nosocomial methicillin-resistant *Staphylococcus aureus* infections. *American Journal of Infection Control, 38*(4), 274–282. doi:10.1016/j.ajic.2009.08.019

Burman, M. E., Robinson, B., & Hart, A. M. (2013). Linking evidence-based nursing practice and patient-centered care through patient preferences. *Nursing Administrative Quarterly, 37*(3), 231–241. doi:10.1097/NAQ.0b013e318295ed6b

Busby, L. T., Sheth, S., Garey, J., Ginsburg, A., Flynn, T., Willen, M. A., . . . Beveridge, R. (2011). Creating a process to standardize regimen order sets within an electronic health record. *Journal of Oncology Practice, 7*(4), e8–e14. doi:10.1200/JOP.2011.000275

Butz, A. M., Kohr, L., & Jones, D. (2004). Developing a successful poster presentation. *Journal of Pediatric Health Care, 18*(1), 45–48. doi:10.1016/j.pedhc.2003.08.006

Bycel, J. (2014). Emphasize "stats & passion" in elevator pitches. *Nonprofit Communications Report, 12*(9), 4.

Byrnes, M. C., Schuerer, D. J. E., Schallom, M. E., Sona, C. S., Mazuski, J. E., Taylor, B. E., . . . Coopersmith, C. M. (2009). Implementation of a mandatory checklist of protocols and objectives improves compliance with a wide range of evidence-based intensive care unit practices. *Critical Care Medicine, 37*(10), 2775–2781. doi:10.1097/CCM.0b013e3181a96379

Caccia, N., Nakajima, A., & Kent, N. (2015). Competency-based medical education: The wave of the future. *Journal of Obstetrics & Gynaecology Canada, 37*(4), 349–353. doi:10.1016/S1701-2163(15)30286-3

Cahill, N. E., Murch, L., Cook, D., Heyland, D. K., & Canadian Critical Care Trials Group. (2014). Implementing a multifaceted tailored intervention to improve nutrition adequacy in critically ill patients: Results of a multicenter feasibility study. *Critical Care, 18*(R96), 1–13. doi:10.1186/cc13867

Caminiti, C., Scoditti, U., Diodati, F., & Passalacqua, R. (2005). How to promote, improve and test adherence to scientific evidence in clinical practice. *BMC Health Services Research, 5*(62), 1–11. doi:10.1186/1472-6963-5-62

Carayon, P., Wetterneck, T. B., Rivera-Rodriguez, A. J., Hundt, A. S., Hoonakker, P., Holden, R., & Gurses, A. P. (2014). Human factors systems approach to healthcare quality and patient safety. *Applied Ergonomics, 45*(1), 14–25. doi:10.1016/j.apergo.2013.04.023

Carayon, P., Xie, A., & Kianfar, S. (2014). Human factors and ergonomics as a patient safety practice. *BMJ Quality & Safety, 23*(3), 196–205. doi:10.1136/bmjqs-2013-001812

Carey, R. G. (2002). Constructing powerful control charts. *Journal of Ambulatory Care Management, 25*(4), 64–70.

Carey, R. G., & Lloyd, R. C. (2001). *Measuring quality improvement in healthcare: A guide to statistical process control applications.* Milwaukee, WI: ASQ Quality Press.

Carlfjord, S., Lindberg, M., Bendtsen, P., Nilsen, P., & Andersson, A. (2010). Key factors influencing adoption of an innovation in primary health care: A qualitative study based on implementation theory. *BMC Family Practice, 11*(60), 1–11. doi:10.1186/1471-2296-11-60

Carpenter, C. R., & Sherbino, J. (2010). How does an "opinion leader" influence my practice? *CJEM, 12*(5), 431–434. doi:10.1017/S1481803500012586

Cavalcanti, A. B., Bozza, F. A., Machado, F. R., Salluh, J. I. F., Campagnucci, V. P., Vendramim, P., . . . Berwanger, O. (2016). Effect of a quality improvement intervention with daily round checklists, goal setting, and clinician prompting on mortality of critically ill patients: A randomized clinical trial. *Journal of the American Medical Association, 315*(14), 1480–1490. doi:10.1001/jama.2016.3463

Centers for Disease Control and Prevention (CDC). (n.d.) Evaluation plan template. Retrieved from https://www.cdc.gov/asthma/program_eval/appendixf_evaluation_plan_outline.doc

Centers for Disease Control and Prevention (CDC). (2002). Guideline for hand hygiene in health-care settings: Recommendations of the healthcare infection control practices advisory committee and the HICPAC/SHEA/APIC/IDSA hand hygiene taskforce. *Morbidity and Mortality Weekly Report, 51*(RR-16), 1–56.

Centers for Disease Control and Prevention (CDC). (2010). *Simply put: A guide for creating easy-to-understand materials.* Retrieved from http://www.cdc.gov/healthliteracy/pdf/simply_put.pdf

Centers for Disease Control and Prevention (CDC). (2015a). National health initiatives, strategies, and action plans. Retrieved from https://www.cdc.gov/stltpublichealth/strategy/index.html

Centers for Disease Control and Prevention (CDC). (2015b). Reminder systems and strategies for increasing childhood vaccination rates. Retrieved from https://www.cdc.gov/vaccines/hcp/admin/reminder-sys.html

Centers for Disease Control and Prevention (CDC). (2016a). Appendix F. Individual Evaluation Plan Outline. Retrieved from https://www.cdc.gov/asthma/program_eval/guide.htm

Centers for Disease Control and Prevention (CDC). (2016b). STEADI materials for your older adult patients. Retrieved from https://www.cdc.gov/steadi/patient.html

Centers for Disease Control and Prevention (CDC). (2017a). Data & statistics. Retrieved from https://www.cdc.gov/DataStatistics/

Centers for Disease Control and Prevention (CDC). (2017b). National Center for Emerging and Zoonotic Infectious Diseases (NCEZID). Retrieved from https://www.cdc.gov/ncezid/

Centers for Disease Control and Prevention (CDC). (2017c). The National Institute for Occupational Safety and Health (NIOSH). Retrieved from https://www.cdc.gov/niosh/topics/emerginfectdiseases/default.html

Centers for Medicare & Medicaid Services (CMS). (2017). Hospital value-based purchasing. Retrieved from https://www.cms.gov/Medicare/Quality-Initiatives-Patient-Assessment-Instruments/hospital-value-based-purchasing/index.html?redirect=/Hospital-Value-Based-Purchasing

Chalkidou, K., Lord, J., Fischer, A., & Littlejohns, P. (2008). Evidence-based decision making: When should we wait for more information? *Health Affairs, 27*(6), 1642–1653. doi:10.1377/hlthaff.27.6.1642

Champagne, F., Lemieux-Charles, L., Duranceau, M.-F., MacKean, G., & Reay, T. (2014). Organizational impact of evidence-informed decision making training initiatives: A case study comparison of two approaches. *Implementation Science, 9*(53), 1–14. doi:10.1186/1748-5908-9-53

Chan, A. J., Chan, J., Cafazzo, J. A., Rossos, P. G., Tripp, T., Shojania, K., . . . Easty, A. C. (2012). Order sets in health care: A systematic review of their effects. *International Journal of Technology Assessment in Health Care, 28*(3), 235–240. doi:10.1017/S0266462312000281

Chan, M. F., Ho, A., & Day, M. C. (2008). Investigating the knowledge, attitudes and practice patterns of operating room staff towards standard and transmission-based precautions: Results of a cluster analysis. *Journal of Clinical Nursing, 17*(8), 1051–1062. doi:10.1111/j.1365-2702.2007.01998.x

Chang, C. S. (2014). Moderating effects of nurses' organizational justice between organizational support and organizational citizenship behaviors for evidence-based practice. *Worldviews on Evidence-Based Nursing, 11*(5), 332–340. doi:10.1111/wvn.12054

Chapman, R., Rahman, A., Courtney, M., & Chalmers, C. (2017). Impact of teamwork on missed care in four Australian hospitals. *Journal of Clinical Nursing, 26*(1–2), 170–181. doi:10.1111/jocn.13433

Cheifetz, O., Park Dorsay, J., Hladysh, G., Macdermid, J., Serediuk, F., & Woodhouse, L. J. (2014). CanWell: Meeting the psychosocial and exercise needs of cancer survivors by translating evidence into practice. *Psycho-Oncology, 23*(2), 204–215. doi:10.1002/pon.3389

Chou, A. F., Vaughn, T. E., McCoy, K. D., & Doebbeling, B. N. (2011). Implementation of evidence-based practices: Applying a goal commitment framework. *Health Care Management Review, 36*(1), 4–17. doi:10.1097/HMR.0b013e3181dc8233

Chou, R., Gordon, D. B., de Leon-Casasola, O. A., Rosenberg, J. M., Bickler, S., Brennan, T., . . . Wu, C. L. (2016). Management of postoperative pain: A clinical practice guideline from the American Pain Society, the American Society of Regional Anesthesia and Pain Medicine, and the American Society of Anesthesiologists' Committee on Regional Anesthesia, Executive Committee, and Administrative Council. *Journal of Pain, 17*(2), 131–157. doi:10.1016/j.jpain.2015.12.008

Clay-Williams, R., Nosrati, H., Cunningham, F. C., Hillman, K., & Braithwaite, J. (2014). Do large-scale hospital- and system-wide interventions improve patient outcomes: A systematic review. *BMC Health Services Research, 14*(369), 1–13. doi:10.1186/1472-6963-14-369

Clinkard, D., Moult, E., Holden, M., Davison, C., Ungi, T., Fichtinger, G., & McGraw, R. (2015). Assessment of lumbar puncture skill in experts and nonexperts using checklists and quantitative tracking of needle trajectories: Implications for competency-based medical education. *Teaching and Learning in Medicine, 27*(1), 51–56. doi:10.1080/10401334.2014.979184

Clutter, P. C., Reed, C., Cornett, P. A., & Parsons, M. L. (2009). Action planning strategies to achieve quality outcomes. *Critical Care Nursing Quarterly, 32*(4), 272–284. doi:10.1097/CNQ.0b013e3181bad30f

Cohen, E. E. W., LaMonte, S. J., Erb, N. L., Beckman, K. L., Sadeghi, N., Hutcheson, K. A., . . . Pratt-Chapman, M. L. (2016). American Cancer Society head and neck cancer survivorship care guideline. *CA: A Cancer Journal for Clinicians, 66*(3), 203–239. doi:10.3322/caac.21343

Cole, A. M., Esplin, A., & Baldwin, L. (2015). Adaptation of an evidence-based colorectal cancer screening program using the consolidated framework for implementation research. *Preventing Chronic Disease, 12*, E213. doi:10.5888/pcd12.150300

Colón-Emeric, C., Toles, M., Cary, M. P., Jr., Batchelor-Murphy, M., Yap, T., Song, Y., . . . Anderson, R. A. (2016). Sustaining complex interventions in long-term care: A qualitative study of direct care staff and managers. *Implementation Science, 11*(94), 1–10. doi:10.1186/s13012-016-0454-y

Condly, S., Clark, R., & Stolovitch, H. (2003). The effects of incentives on workplace performance: A meta-analytic review of research studies 1. *Performance Improvement Quarterly, 16*(3), 46–63. doi:10.1111/j.1937-8327.2003.tb00287.x

Conklin, J., Lusk, E., Harris, M., & Stolee, P. (2013). Knowledge brokers in a knowledge network: The case of Seniors Health Research Transfer Network knowledge brokers. *Implementation Science, 8*(7), 1–10.

Connor, B. T. (2014). Differentiating research, evidence-based practice, and quality improvement. *American Nurse Today, 9*(6). Retrieved from https://www.americannursetoday.com/differentiating-research-evidence-based-practice-and-quality-improvement/

Conroy, K. M., Elliott, D., & Burrell, A. R. (2013). Developing content for a process-of-care checklist for use in intensive care units: A dual-method approach to establishing construct validity. *BMC Health Services Research, 13*(380), 1–10. doi:10.1186/1472-6963-13-380

Conway, L. J., Riley, L., Saiman, L., Cohen, B., Alper, P., & Larson, E. L. (2014). Implementation and impact of an automated group monitoring and feedback system to promote hand hygiene among health care personnel. *Joint Commission Journal on Quality and Patient Safety, 40*(9), 408–417. doi:10.1016/S1553-7250(14)40053-9

Costantino, G., Montano, N., & Casazza, G. (2015). When should we change our clinical practice based on the results of a clinical study? Searching for evidence: PICOS and PubMed. *Internal and Emergency Medicine, 10*(4), 525–527. doi:10.1007/s11739-015-1225-5

Crowe, C., Bobrow, B. J., Vadeboncoeur, T. F., Dameff, C., Stolz, U., Silver, A., . . . Spaite, D. W. (2015). Measuring and improving cardiopulmonary resuscitation quality inside the emergency department. *Resuscitation, 93,* 8–13. doi:10.1016/j.resuscitation.2015.04.031

Cullen, L. (2013). Pain assessment for older adults. In M. Farrington (Series Ed.), *EBP to Go: Accelerating evidence-based practice series.* Iowa City, IA: Office of Nursing Research, Evidence-Based Practice and Quality, Department of Nursing Services and Patient Care, University of Iowa Hospitals and Clinics.

Cullen, L., & Adams, S. L. (2012). Planning for implementation of evidence-based practice. *Journal of Nursing Administration, 42*(4), 222–230. doi:10.1097/NNA.0b013e31824ccd0a

Cullen, L., Baumler, S., Farrington, M., Dawson, C., Folkmann, P., & Brenner, L. (in press). Oral care for symptom management in head and neck cancer. *American Journal of Nursing.*

Cullen, L., Dawson, C. J., & Williams, K. (2010). Evidence-based practice: Strategies for nursing leaders. In D. Huber (Ed.), *Leadership and nursing care management* (4th ed., pp. 367–386, 851–855). Maryland Heights, MO: Elsevier Saunders.

Cullen, L., Greiner, J., Greiner, J., Bombei, C., & Comried, L. (2005). Excellence in evidence-based practice: Organizational and unit exemplars. *Critical Care Nursing Clinics of North America, 17*(2), 127–142. doi:10.1016/j.ccell.2005.01.002

Cullen, L., Hanrahan, K., Neis, N., Farrington, M., Laffoon, T., & Dawson, C. (in press). Evidence-based practice: Strategies for nursing leaders. In D. Huber (Ed.), *Leadership and nursing care management* (6th ed.). Philadelphia, PA: Elsevier.

Cullen, L., Hanrahan, K., Tucker, S., Rempel, G., & Jordan, K. (2012). *Evidence-based practice building blocks: Comprehensive strategies, tools, and tips.* Iowa City, IA: Nursing Research and Evidence-Based Practice Office, Department of Nursing Services and Patient Care, University of Iowa Hospitals and Clinics.

Cullen, L., Prickett, K., Lower, J., Ostrander, K., Pollpeter, W., Stillings, S., . . . Smith, K. (2013, April). *Evidence-based patient preference for pain assessment among hospitalized older adults.* Poster session presented at the 20th Annual University of Iowa Hospitals and Clinics Evidence-Based Practice Conference, Coralville, IA.

Cullen, L., Smelser, J., Wagner, M., & Adams, S. (2012). Evidence into practice: Using research findings to create practice recommendations. *Journal of PeriAnesthesia Nursing, 27*(5), 343–351. doi:10.1016/j.jopan.2012.07.006

Cullen, L., & Titler, M. G. (2004). Promoting evidence-based practice: An internship for staff nurses. *Worldviews on Evidence-Based Nursing, 1*(4), 215–223. doi:10.1111/j.1524-475X.2004.04027.x

Cullen, L., Titler, M., & Drahozal, R. (1999). Family and pet visitation in the critical care unit. *Critical Care Nurse, 19*(3), 84–87.

Cullen, L., Titler, M., & Drahozal, R. (2003). Family and pet visitation in the critical care unit. *Critical Care Nurse, 23*(5), 62–66.

Cullen, L., Wagner, M., Matthews, G., & Farrington, M. (2017). Evidence into practice: Integration within an organizational infrastructure. *Journal of PeriAnesthesia Nursing, 32*(3), 247–256. doi:10.1016/j.jopan.2017.02.003

Curran, E., Harper, P., Loveday, H., Gilmour, H., Jones, S., Benneyan, J.J., . . . Pratt, R. (2008). Results of a multicentre randomised controlled trial of statistical process control charts and structured diagnostic tools to reduce ward-acquired meticillin-resistant *Staphylococcus aureus*: The CHART project. *Journal of Hospital Infection, 70*(2), 127–135. doi:10.1016/j.jhin.2008.06.013

The DAISY Foundation. (2017). What is the DAISY Award? Retrieved from https://www.daisyfoundation.org/daisy-award

Dalto, J. (2013, February 18). Tips for writing instructional and training material [Web log post]. Retrieved from http://blog.convergencetraining.com/tips-for-writing-instructional-and-training-material

Dang, D., Melnyk, B., Fineout-Overholt, E., Ciliska, D., DiCenso, A., Cullen, L., . . . Stevens, K. (2015). Models to guide implementation of evidence-based practice. In B. Melnyk & E. Fineout-Overholt (Eds.), *Evidence-based practice in nursing & healthcare: A guide to best practice* (3rd ed., pp. 274–315). Philadelphia, PA: Lippincott, Williams & Wilkins.

Davidson, J. E., & Brown, C. (2014). Evaluation of nurse engagement in evidence-based practice. *AACN Advanced Critical Care, 25*(1), 43–55. doi:10.1097/NCI.0000000000000006

Davies, B., Tremblay, D., & Edwards, N. (2010). Sustaining evidence-based practice systems and measuring the impacts. In D. Bick & I. Graham (Eds.), *Evaluating the impact of implementing evidence-based practice* (pp. 168-188). United Kingdom: Wiley-Blackwell.

Davis-Ajami, M. L., Costa, L., & Kulik, S. (2014). Gap analysis: Synergies and opportunities for effective nursing leadership. *Nursing Economic$, 32*(1), 17–25.

Deberg, J., & Egeland, M. (2014). Hospital noise: How librarians can help. *Journal of Hospital Librarianship, 14*(2), 120–139. doi:10.1080/15323269.2014.888512

Deblois, S., & Lepanto, L. (2016). Lean and Six Sigma in acute care: A systematic review of reviews. *International Journal of Health Care Quality Assurance, 29*(2), 192–208. doi:10.1108/IJHCQA-05-2014-0058

Deitrick, L. M., Baker, K., Paxton, H., Flores, M., & Swavely, D. (2012). Hourly rounding: Challenges with implementation of an evidence-based process. *Journal of Nursing Care Quality, 27*(1), 13–19. doi:10.1097/NCQ.0b013e318227d7dd

De Leon, E., Fuentes, L. W., & Cohen, J. E. (2014). Characterizing periodic messaging interventions across health behaviors and media: Systematic review. *Journal of Medical Internet Research, 16*(3), e93. doi:10.2196/jmir.2837

Delmore, B., Lebovits, S., Baldock, P., Suggs, B., & Ayello, E. A. (2011). Pressure ulcer prevention program: A journey. *Journal of Wound, Ostomy, and Continence Nursing, 38*(5), 505–513. doi:10.1097/WON.0b013e31822ad2ab

Dempsey, A. F., Pyrzanowski, J., Brewer, S., Barnard, J., Sevick, C., & O'Leary, S. T. (2015). Acceptability of using standing orders to deliver human papillomavirus vaccines in the outpatient obstetrician/gynecologist setting. *Vaccine, 33*(15), 1773–1779. doi:10.1016/j.vaccine.2015.02.044

Denenberg, R., & Curtiss, C. P. (2016). Appropriate use of opioids in managing chronic pain. *American Journal of Nursing, 116*(7), 26–38. doi:10.1097/01.NAJ.0000484931.50778.6f

Denning, P., & Dew, N. (2012). The profession of IT: The myth of the elevator pitch. *Communications of the ACM, 55*(6), 38–40. doi:10.1145/2184319.2184333

Deochand, N., & Deochand, M. E. (2016). Brief report on hand-hygiene monitoring systems: A pilot study of a computer-assisted image analysis technique. *Journal of Environmental Health, 78*(10), 14–20.

De Sanctis, V., Bossi, P., Sanguineti, G., Trippa, F., Ferrari, D., Bacigalupo, A., . . . Lalla, R. V. (2016). Mucositis in head and neck cancer patients treated with radiotherapy and systemic therapies: Literature review and consensus statements. *Critical Reviews in Oncology/Hematology, 100*, 147–166. doi:10.1016/j.critrevonc.2016.01.010

Deuster, S., Roten, I., & Muehlebach, S. (2010). Implementation of treatment guidelines to support judicious use of antibiotic therapy. *Journal of Clinical Pharmacy and Therapeutics, 35*(1), 71–78. doi:10.1111/j.1365-2710.2009.01045.x

Devalia, B. (2010). Adherence to protocol during the acute management of diabetic ketoacidosis: Would specialist involvement lead to better outcomes? *International Journal of Clinical Practice, 64*(11), 1580–1582. doi:10.1111/j.1742-1241.2010.02348.x

de Visser, R. O. (2015). Personalized feedback based on a drink-pouring exercise may improve knowledge of, and adherence to, government guidelines for alcohol consumption. *Alcoholism Clinical & Experimental Research, 39*(2), 317–323. doi:10.1111/acer.12623

de Vos, M. L. G., van der Veer, S. N., Graafmans, W. C., de Keizer, N. F., Jager, K. J., Westert, G. P., & van der Voort, P. H. J. (2013). Process evaluation of a tailored multifaceted feedback program to improve the quality of intensive care by using quality indicators. *BMJ Quality & Safety, 22*(3), 233–241. doi:10.1136/bmjqs-2012-001375

Dixon, M.-N., & Keasling, M. (2014). Development of a therapeutic hypothermia protocol: Implementation for postcardiac arrest STEMI patients. *Critical Care Nursing Quarterly, 37*(4), 377–383. doi:10.1097/CNQ.0000000000000037

Dixon-Woods, M., Amalberti, R., Goodman, S., Bergman, B., & Glasziou, R. (2011). Problems and promises of innovation: Why healthcare needs to rethink its love/hate relationship with the new. *BMJ Quality & Safety, 20*(Suppl. 1), i47–i51. doi:10.1136/bmjqs.2010.046227

Dobbins, M., Robeson, P., Ciliska, D., Hanna, S., Cameron, R., O'Mara, L., . . . Mercer, S. (2009). A description of a knowledge broker role implemented as part of a randomized controlled trial evaluating three knowledge translation strategies. *Implementation Science, 4*(23), 1–9. doi:10.1186/1748-5908-4-23

Doebbeling, B. N., & Flanagan, M. E. (2011). Emerging perspectives on transforming the healthcare system: Redesign strategies and a call for needed research. *Medical Care, 49*(12 Suppl. 1), S59–S64. doi:10.1097/MLR.0b013e31821b57eb

Dogherty, E. J., Harrison, M. B., & Graham, I. D. (2010). Facilitation as a role and process in achieving evidence-based practice in nursing: A focused review of concept and meaning. *Worldviews on Evidence-Based Nursing, 7*(2), 76–89. doi:10.1111/j.1741-6787.2010.00186.x

Dogherty, E. J., Harrison M. B., Graham I. D., Vandyk, A. D., & Keeping-Burke, L. (2013). Turning knowledge into action at the point-of-care: The collective experience of nurses facilitating the implementation of evidence-based practice. *Worldviews on Evidence-Based Nursing, 10*(3), 129–139. doi:10.1111/wvn.12009

Dole, N. (2009, March). *Accurate blood pressure measurement of the obese arm: A staff nurse case example of evidence-based practice.* Paper presented at the 34th annual conference of the American Academy of Ambulatory Care Nursing, Philadelphia, PA.

Dole, N., Griffin, E., Flansburg, C., Happel, B., Burstain, T., Denning, N., . . . Goerdt, C. (2011, February). *Accurate blood pressure monitoring in the obese patient.* Paper presented at the Advanced Practice Institute: Promoting Adoption of Evidence-Based Practice, Iowa City, IA.

Dolezal, D., Cullen, L., Harp, J., & Mueller, T. (2011). Implementing preoperative screening of undiagnosed obstructive sleep apnea. *Journal of PeriAnesthesia Nursing, 26*(5), 338–342. doi:10.1016/j.jopan.2011.07.003

Dow, A. W., DiazGranados, D., Mazmanian, P. E., & Retchin, S. M. (2013). Applying organizational science to health care: A framework for collaborative practice. *Academic Medicine, 88*(7), 952–957. doi:10.1097/ACM.0b013e31829523d1

Doyle, C., Howe, C., Woodcock, T., Myron, R., Phekoo, K., McNicholas, C., . . . Bell, D. (2013). Making change last: Applying the NHS institute for innovation and improvement sustainability model to healthcare improvement. *Implementation Science, 8*(127), 1–10. doi:10.1186/1748-5908-8-127

Doyon, S., Perreault, M., Marquis, C., Gauthier, J., Lebel, D., Bailey, B., . . . Bussières, J. F. (2009). Quantitative evaluation of a clinical intervention aimed at changing prescriber behaviour in response to new guidelines. *Journal of Evaluation in Clinical Practice, 15*(6), 1111–1117. doi:10.1111/j.1365-2753.2009.01259.x

Drenkard, K. (2012). Strategy as solution: Developing a nursing strategic plan. *Journal of Nursing Administration, 42*(5), 242–243. doi:10.1097/NNA.0b013e318252efef

Drexel, C., Merlo, K., Basile, J. N., Watkins, B., Whitfield, B., Katz, J. M., . . . Sullivan, T. (2011). Highly interactive multisession programs impact physician behavior on hypertension management: Outcomes of a new CME model. *Journal of Clinical Hypertension, 13*(2), 97–105. doi:10.1111/j.1751-7176.2010.00399.x

Driessen, M. T., Groenewoud, K., Proper, K., Anema, J. R., Bongers, P. M., & van der Beek, A. J. (2010). What are possible barriers and facilitators to implementation of a participatory ergonomics programme? *Implementation Science, 5*(64), 1–9. doi:10.1186/1748-5908-5-64

Drouin, D., Campbell, N. R., & Kaczorowski, J. (2006). Implementation of recommendations on hypertension: The Canadian Hypertension Education Program. *Canadian Journal of Cardiology, 22*(7), 595–598.

Dückers, M. L., Wagner, C., Vos, L., & Groenewegen, P. P. (2011). Understanding organisational development, sustainability, and diffusion of innovations within hospitals participating in a multilevel quality collaborative. *Implementation Science, 6*(18), 1–10. doi:10.1186/1748-5908-6-18

Duff, J., Walker, K., & Omari, A. (2011). Translating venous thromboembolism (VTE) prevention evidence into practice: A multdisciplinary evidence implementation project. *Worldviews on Evidence-Based Nursing, 8*(1), 30–39. doi:10.1111/j.1741-6787.2010.00209.x

Duffy, J. R., Culp, S., Sand-Jecklin, K., Stroupe, L., & Lucke-Wold, N. (2016). Nurses' research capacity, use of evidence, and research productivity in acute care. *Journal of Nursing Administration, 45*(3), 158–164. doi:10.1097/NNA.0000000000000176

Duffy, J. R., Thompson, D., Hobbs, T., Niemeyer-Hackett, N. L., & Elpers, S. (2011). Evidence-based nursing leadership: Evaluation of a joint academic-service journal club. *Journal of Nursing Administration, 41*(10), 422–427. doi:10.1097/NNA.0b013e31822edda6

Durand, M.-A., Witt, J., Joseph-Williams, N., Newcombe, R. G. Politi, M. C., Sivell, S., & Elwyn, G. (2015). Minimum standards for the certification of patient decision support interventions: Feasibility and application. *Patient Education and Counseling, 98*(4), 462–468. doi:10.1016/j.pec.2014.12.009

Dyrkorn, R., Gjelstad, S., Espnes, K. A., & Lindbæk, M. (2016). Peer academic detailing on use of antibiotics in acute respiratory tract infections. A controlled study in an urban Norwegian out-of-hours service. *Scandinavian Journal of Primary Health Care, 34*(2), 180–185. doi:10.3109/02813432.2016.1163035

Edwards, J. C., Feldman, P. H., Sangl, J., Polakoff, D., Stern, G., & Casey, D. (2007). Sustainability of partnership projects: A conceptual framework and checklist. *Joint Commission Journal on Quality and Patient Safety, 33*(Suppl. 12), 37–47. doi:10.1016/S1553-7250(07)33122-X

Eid, T., & Bucknall, T. (2008). Documenting and implementing evidence-based post-operative pain management in older patients with hip fractures. *Journal of Orthopaedic Nursing, 12*(2), 90–98. doi:10.1016/j.joon.2008.07.003

Eldredge, J. D., Carr, R., Broudy, D., & Voorhees, R. E. (2008). The effect of training on question formulation among public health practitioners: Results from a randomized controlled trial. *Journal of the Medical Library Association, 96*(4), 299–309. doi:10.3163/1536-5050.96.4.005

Ellen, M. E., Léon, G., Bouchard, G., Lavis, J. N., Ouimet, M., & Grimshaw, J. M. (2013). What supports do health system organizations have in place to facilitate evidence-informed decision-making? A qualitative study. *Implementation Science, 8*(84), 1–19. doi:10.1186/1748-5908-8-84

Ellerbee, S. M. (2009). An artistic view of posters . . . reprinted with permission from The Oklahoma Nurses Association. *Newborn and Infant Nursing Reviews, 9*(2), 109–110.

Ellis, J. (2006). All inclusive benchmarking. *Journal of Nursing Management, 14*(5), 377–383. doi:10.1111/j.1365-2934.2006.00596.x

Elsey, H., Khanal, S., Manandhar, S., Sah, D., Baral, S. C., Siddiqi, K., & Newell, J. N. (2016). Understanding implementation and feasibility of tobacco cessation in routine primary care in Nepal: A mixed methods study. *Implementation Science, 11*(104), 1–12. doi:10.1186/s13012-016-0466-7

Elwyn, G., Scholl, I., Tietbohl, C., Mann, M., Edwards, A. G. K., Clay, K., . . . Frosch, D. (n.d.). The implementation of patient decision support interventions into routine clinical practice: A systematic review. Retrieved from http://www.ipdas.ohri.ca/IPDAS-Implementation.pdf

Erasmus, V., Kuperus, M. N., Richardus, J. H., Vos, M. C., Oenema, A., & van Beeck, E. F. (2010). Improving hand hygiene behavior of nurses using action planning: A pilot study in the intensive care unit and surgical ward. *Journal of Hospital Infections, 76*(2), 161–164. doi:10.1016/j.jhin.2010.04.024

Esposito, D., Heeringa, J., Bradley, K., Croake, S., & Kimmey, L. (2015). PCORI dissemination and implementation framework. Retrieved from http://www.pcori.org/sites/default/files/PCORI-Dissemination-Implementation-Framework.pdf

Estabrooks, C., Chong, H., Brigidear, K., & Profetto-McGrath, J. (2005). Profiling Canadian nurses' preferred knowledge sources for clinical practice. *Canadian Journal of Nursing Research, 37*(2), 118–140.

Estabrooks, C. A., Squires, J. E., Hayduk, L., Morgan, D., Cummings, G. G., Ginsburg, L., . . . Norton, P. G. (2015). The influence of organizational context on best practice use by care aides in residential long-term care settings. *Journal of the American Medical Directors Association, 16*(6), 537.e1–e10. doi:10.1016/j.jamda.2015.03.009

Ettorchi-Tardy, A., Levif, M., & Michel, P. (2012). Benchmarking: A method for continuous quality improvement in health. *Healthcare Policy, 7*(4), e101–119. doi:10.12927/hcpol.2012.22872

Everett, L. Q., & Sitterding, M. C. (2011). Transformational leadership required to design and sustain evidence-based practice: A system exemplar. *Western Journal of Nursing Research, 33*(3), 398–426. doi:10.1177/0193945910383056

Ezziane, Z., Maruthappu, M., Gawn, L., Thompson, E. A., Athanasiou, T., & Warren, O.J. (2012). Building effective clinical teams in healthcare. *Journal of Health Organization and Management, 26*(4–5), 428–436. doi:10.1108/14777261211251508

Fabry, D. (2015). Hourly rounding: Perspectives and perceptions of the frontline nursing staff. *Journal of Nursing Management, 23*(2), 200–210. doi:10.1111/jonm.12114

Facchiano, L., & Hoffman Snyder, C. (2012). Evidence-based practice for the busy nurse practitioner: Part three: Critical appraisal process. *Journal of the American Academy of Nurse Practitioners, 24*(12), 704–715. doi:10.1111/j.1745-7599.2012.00752.x

Fakhry, M., Hanna, G. B., Anderson, O., Holmes, A., & Nathwani, D. (2012). Effectiveness of an audible reminder on hand hygiene adherence. *American Journal of Infection Control, 40*(4), 320–323. doi:10.1016/j.ajic.2011.05.023

Farley, K., Hanbury, A., & Thompson, C. (2014). Gathering opinion leader data for a tailored implementation intervention in secondary healthcare: A randomised trial. *BMC Medical Research Methodology, 14*(38), 1–7. doi:10.1186/1471-2288-14-38

Farrell, M. (2016). Use of iPhones by nurses in an acute care setting to improve communication and decision-making processes: Qualitative analysis of nurses' perspectives on iPhone use. *JMIR mHealth uHealth, 4*(2), e43. doi:10.2196/mhealth.5071

Farrington, M., Bruene, D., & Wagner, M. (2015). Pain management prior to nasogastric tube placement: Atomized lidocaine. *ORL – Head and Neck Nursing, 33*(1), 8–16.

Farrington, M., Cullen, L., & Dawson, C. (2010). Assessment of oral mucositis in adult and pediatric oncology patients: An evidence-based approach. *ORL – Head and Neck Nursing, 28*(3), 8–15.

Farrington, M., Cullen, L., & Dawson, C. (2013). Evidence-based oral care for oral mucositis. *ORL – Head and Neck Nursing, 31*(3), 6–15.

Farrington, M., Cullen, L., & Dawson, C. (2014). Cryotherapy is a simple nursing intervention for oral mucositis. *ORL – Head and Neck Nursing, 32*(20), 13–15.

Farrington, M., Hanson, A., Laffoon, T., & Cullen, L. (2015). Low-dose ketamine infusions for postoperative pain in opioid-tolerant orthopaedic spine patients. *Journal of PeriAnesthesia Nursing, 30*(4), 338–345. doi:10.1016/j.jopan.2015.03.005

Farrington, M., Lang, S., Cullen, L., & Stewart, S. (2009). Nasogastric tube placement in pediatric and neonatal patients. *Pediatric Nursing, 3*(1), 17–24.

Federal Plain Language Guidelines. (2011, March). Retrieved from http://www.plainlanguage.gov/howto/guidelines/FederalPLGuidelines/FederalPLGuidelines.pdf

Fernandez, N., Dory, V., Ste-Marie, L. G., Chaput, M., Charlin, B., & Boucher, A. (2012). Varying conceptions of competence: An analysis of how health sciences educators define competence. *Medical Education, 46*(4), 357–365. doi:10.1111/j.1365-2923.2011.04183.x

Fineout-Overholt, E., Gallagher-Ford, L., Mazurek Melnyk, B., & Stillwell, S. B. (2011). Evidence-based practice, step by step: Evaluating and disseminating the impact of an evidence-based intervention: Show and tell. *American Journal of Nursing, 111*(7), 56–59. doi:10.1097/01.NAJ.0000399317.21279.47

Fischer, M. A. (2016). Academic detailing in diabetes: Using outreach education to improve the quality of care. *Current Diabetes Reports, 16*(10), 98. doi:10.1007/s11892-016-0785-8

Fishbein, A. B., Tellez, I., Lin, H., Sullivan, C., & Groll, M. E. (2011). Glow gel hand washing in the waiting room: A novel approach to improving hand hygiene education. *Infection Control and Hospital Epidemiology, 32*(7), 661–666. doi:10.1086/660359

Fisher, A. (2014, January 23). Does anybody really need a one-minute "elevator pitch"? [Web log post]. *Fortune.* Retrieved from http://fortune.com/2014/01/23/does-anybody-really-need-a-one-minute-elevator-pitch

Fisher, D., Cochran, K. M., Provost, L. P., Patterson, J., Bristol, T., Metzguer, K., ... McCaffrey, M. J. (2013). Reducing central line-associated bloodstream infections in North Carolina NICUs. *Pediatrics, 132*(6), 1–8. doi:10.1542/peds.2013-2000

Fishman, S. M., Young, H. M., Lucas Arwood, E., Chou, R., Herr, K., Murinson, B. B., ... Strassels, S. A. (2013). Core competencies for pain management: Results of an interprofessional consensus summit. *Pain Medicine, 14*(7), 971–981. doi:10.1111/pme.12107

Fleiszer, A. R., Semenic, S. E., Ritchie, J. A., Richer, M. C., & Denis, J. L. (2016a). A unit-level perspective on the long-term sustainability of a nursing best practice guidelines program: An embedded multiple case study. *International Journal of Nursing Studies, 53,* 204–218. doi:10.1016/j.ijnurstu.2015.09.004

Fleiszer, A. R., Semenic, S. E., Ritchie, J. A., Richer, M. C., & Denis, J. L. (2016b). Nursing unit leaders' influence on the long-term sustainability of evidence-based practice improvements. *Journal of Nursing Management, 24*(3), 309–318. doi:10.1111/jonm.12320

Fleuren, M. A. H., Paulussen, T. G. W. M., van Dommelen, P., & Van Buuren, S. (2014). Towards a measurement instrument for determinants of innovations. *International Journal for Quality in Health Care, 26*(5), 501–510. doi:10.1093/intqhc/mzu060

Fleuren, M. A. H., van Dommelen, P., & Dunnink, T. (2015). A systematic approach to implementing and evaluating clinical guidelines: The results of fifteen years of Preventive Child Health Care guidelines in the Netherlands. *Social Science & Medicine, 136–137,* 35–43. doi:10.1016/j.socscimed.2015.05.001

Flodgren, G., Eccles, M. P., Shepperd, S., Scott, A., Parmelli, E., & Beyer, F. R. (2011). An overview of reviews evaluating the effectiveness of financial incentives in changing healthcare professional behaviours and patient outcomes. *Cochrane Database of Systematic Reviews, 2011*(7), 1–96. doi:10.1002/14651858. CD009255

Flodgren, G., Gonçalves-Bradley, D. C., & Pomey, M.-P. (2016). External inspection of compliance with standards for improved healthcare outcomes. *Cochrane Database of Systematic Reviews, 2016*(12), 1–50. doi:10.1002/14651858.CD008992.pub3

Flodgren, G., Parmelli, E., Doumit, G., Gattellari, M., O'Brien, M. A., Grimshaw, J., & Eccles, M. P. (2011). Local opinion leaders: Effects on professional practice and health care outcomes. *Cochrane Database of Systematic Reviews, 8*, 1–71. doi:10.1002/14651858.CD000125.pub4

Flodgren, G., Rojas-Reyes, M. X., Cole, N., & Foxcroft, D. R. (2012). Effectiveness of organisational infrastructures to promote evidence-based nursing practice. *Cochrane Database of Systematic Review, 2*, 1–48. doi:10.1002/14651858.CD002212.pub2

Flowchart (n.d.) Retrieved 2017 from https://en.wikipedia.org/wiki/Flowchart

Flynn, M. G., & McGuinness, C. (2011). Hospital clinicians' information behavior and attitudes towards the 'clinical informationist': An Irish survey. *Health Information and Libraries Journal, 28*(1), 23–32. doi:10.1111/j.1471-1842.2010.00917.x

Foote, J. M., Conley, V., Williams, J. K., McCarthy, A. M., & Countryman, M. (2015). Academic and institutional review board collaboration to ensure ethical conduct of Doctor of Nursing Practice projects. *Journal of Nursing Education, 54*(7), 372–377. doi:10.3928/01484834-20150617-03

Förberg, U., Unbeck, M., Wallin, L., Johansson, E., Petzold, M., Ygge, B., & Ehrenberg, A. (2016). Effects of computer reminders on complications of peripheral venous catheters and nurses' adherence to a guideline in paediatric care—A cluster randomised study. *Implementation Science, 11*(10), 1–13. doi:10.1186/s13012-016-0375-9

Ford, J. H., II, Krahn, D., Wise, M., & Oliver, K. A. (2011). Measuring sustainability within the Veterans Administration Mental Health System Redesign initiative. *Quality Management in Health Care. 20*(4), 263–279. doi:10.1097/QMH.0b013e3182314b20

Forsberg, E., Ziegert, K., Hult, H., & Fors, U. (2014). Clinical reasoning in nursing, a think-aloud study using virtual patients—A base for an innovative assessment. *Nurse Education Today, 34*(4), 538–542. doi:10.1016/j.nedt.2013.07.010

Forsner, T., Wistedt, A. A., Brommels, M., Jansky, I., Ponce de Leon, A., & Forsell, Y. (2010). Supported local implementation of clinical guidelines in psychiatry: A two-year follow-up. *Implementation Science, 5*(4), 1–11. doi:10.1186/1748-5908-5-4

Forsyth, D. M., Wright, T. L., Scherb, C. A., & Gaspar, P. M. (2010). Disseminating evidence-based practice projects: Poster design and evaluation. *Clinical Scholars Review, 3*(1), 14–21. doi:10.1891/1939-2095.3.1.14

Fourney, A. M., & Williams, M. L. (2003). Formative evaluation of an intervention to increase compliance to HIV therapies: The ALP project. *Health Promotion Practice, 4*(2), 165–170. doi:10.1177/1524839902250771

Foy, R., MacLennan, G., Grimshaw, J., Penney, G., Campbell, M., & Grol, R. (2002). Attributes of clinical recommendations that influence change in practice following audit and feedback. *Journal of Clinical Epidemiology, 55*(7), 717–722. doi:10.1016/S0895-4356(02)00403-1

Frasure, J. (2014). The effectiveness of four translation strategies on nurses' adoption of an evidence-based bladder protocol. *Journal of Neuroscience Nursing, 46*(4), 218–226. doi:10.1097/JNN.0000000000000069

Frølich, A. (2012). *Identifying organisational principles and management practices important to the quality of health care services for chronic conditions* (Doctoral thesis, University of Copenhagen, Copenhagen, Denmark). Retrieved from http://www.danmedj.dk/portal/pls/portal/!PORTAL.wwpob_page.show?_docname=8760869.PDF

Frost, S. A., Alogso, M.-C., Metcalfe, L., Lynch, J. M., Hunt, L., Sanghavi, R., . . . Hillman, K. M. (2016). Chlorhexidine bathing and health care-associated infections among adult intensive care patients: A systematic review and meta-analysis. *Critical Care, 20*(1), 379. doi:10.1186/s13054-016-1553-5

Gagliardi, A. R., Marshall, C., Huckson, S., James, R., & Moore, V. (2015). Developing a checklist for guideline implementation planning: Review and synthesis of guideline development and implementation advice. *Implementation Science, 10*(19), 1–9. doi:10.1186/s13012-015-0205-5

Gainforth, H. L., Latimer-Cheung, A. E., Athanasopoulos, P., Moore, S., & Martin Ginis, K. A. (2014). The role of interpersonal communication in the process of knowledge mobilization within a community-based organization: A network analysis. *Implementation Science, 9*(59), 1–8. doi:10.1186/1748-5908-9-59

Gandhi, T., Graydon-Baker, E., Huber, C., Whittemore, A., & Gustafson, M. (2005). Closing the loop: Follow-up and feedback in a patient safety program. *Joint Commission Journal on Quality & Patient Safety, 31*(11), 614-621. doi:10.1016/S1553-7250(05)31079-8

Ganz, F. D., Ofra, R., Khalaila, R., Levy, H., Arad, D., Kolpak, O., . . . Benbenishty, J. (2013). Translation of oral care practice guidelines into clinical practice by intensive care unit nurses. *Journal of Nursing Scholarship, 45*(4), 355–362. doi:10.1111/jnu.12039

Gardner, G., Gardner, A., & O'Connell, J. (2014). Using the Donabedian framework to examine the quality and safety of nursing service innovation. *Journal of Clinical Nursing, 23*(1–2), 145–155. doi:10.1111/jocn.12146

Gardner, K., Jr., Kanaskie, M. L., Knehans, A. C., Salisbury, S., Doheny, K. K., & Schirm, V. (2016). Implementing and sustaining evidence based practice through a nursing journal club. *Applied Nursing Research, 31*, 139–145.

Gattinger, H., Stolt, M., Hantikainen, V., Köpke, S., Senn, B., & Leino-Kilpi, H. (2015). A systematic review of observational instruments used to assess nurses' skills in patient mobilisation. *Journal of Clinical Nursing, 24*(5–6), 640–661. doi:10.1111/jocn.12689

Gawande, A. (2010). *The checklist manifesto: How to get things done.* London, UK: Picador.

Gawlinski, A., & Rutledge, D. (2008). Selecting a model for evidence-based practice changes: A practical approach. *AACN Advanced Critical Care, 19*(3), 291–300. doi:10.1097/01.AACN.0000330380.41766.63

Genco, E. K., Forster, J. E., Flaten, H., Goss, F., Heard, K. J., Hoppe, J., & Monte, A. A. (2016). Clinically inconsequential alerts: The characteristics of opioid drug alerts and their utility in preventing adverse drug events in the emergency department. *Annals of Emergency Medicine, 67*(2), 240–248.e3. doi:10.1016/j.annemergmed.2015.09.020

George, E. L., & Tuite, P. (2008). A process for instituting best practice in the intensive care unit. *Indian Journal of Critical Care Medicine, 12*(2), 82–87. doi:10.4103/0972-5229.42562

Gerhardt, W. E., Schoettker, P. J., Donovan, E. F., Kotagal, U. R., & Muething, S. E. (2007). Putting evidence-based clinical practice guidelines into practice: An academic pediatric center's experience. *The Joint Commission Journal on Quality and Patient Safety, 33*(4), 226–235. doi:10.1016/S1553-7250(07)33027-4

Gerrish, K., McDonnell, A., Nolan, M., Guillaume, L., Kirshbaum, M., & Tod, A. (2011). The role of advanced practice nurses in knowledge brokering as a means of promoting evidence-based practice among clinical nurses. *Journal of Advanced Nursing, 67*(9), 2004–2014. doi:10.1111/j.1365-2648.2011.05642.x

Gifford, W., Davies, B., Tourangeau, A., & Lefebre, N. (2011). Developing team leadership to facilitate guide utilization: Planning and evaluating a 3-month intervention strategy. *Journal of Nursing Management, 19*(1), 121–132. doi:10.1111/j.1365-2834.2010.01140.x

Gift, R. G., & Mosel, D. (1994). *Benchmarking in health care.* Chicago, IL: American Hospital Publishing, Inc.

Giguère, A., Légaré, F., Grimshaw, J., Turcotte, S., Fiander, M., Grudniewicz, A., . . . Gagnon, M.-P. (2012). Printed educational materials: Effects on professional practice and healthcare outcomes. *Cochrane Database of Systematic Reviews, 10,* 1–199. doi:10.1002/14651858.CD004398.pub3

Gilbertson, H. R., Rogers, E. J., & Ukoumunne, O. C. (2011). Determination of a practical pH cutoff level for reliable confirmation of nasogastric tube placement. *Journal of Parenteral & Enteral Nutrition, 35*(4), 540–544. doi:10.1177/0148607110383285

Gillaizeau, F., Chan, E., Trinquart, L., Colombet, I., Walton, R. T., Rège-Walther, M., . . . Durieux, P. (2013). Computerized advice on drug dosage to improve prescribing practice. *Cochrane Database of Systematic Reviews, 11,* 1–208. doi:10.1002/14651858.CD002894.pub3

Gillespie, B. M., & Marshall, A. (2015). Implementation of safety checklists in surgery: A realist synthesis of evidence. *Implementation Science, 10*(137), 1–14. doi:10.1186/s13012-015-0319-9

Global Health Workforce Alliance. (2008). Guidelines: Incentives for health professionals. Retrieved from http://www.who.int/workforcealliance/documents/Incentives_Guidelines%20EN.pdf

Gnanasampanthan, V., Porten, L., & Bissett, I. (2014). Improving surgical intravenous fluid management: A controlled educational study. *ANZ Journal of Surgery, 84*(12), 932–936. doi:10.1111/ans.12751

Golden, S. H., Hager, D., Gould, L. J., Mathioudakis, N., & Pronovost, P. J. (2017). A gap analysis needs assessment tool to drive a care delivery and research agenda for integration of care and sharing of best practices across a health system. *Joint Commission Journal on Quality & Patient Safety, 43*(1), 18-28. doi:10.1016/j.jcjq.2016.10.004

Graan, S. M., Botti, M., Wood, B., & Redley, B. (2016). Nursing handover from ICU to cardiac ward: Standardised tools to reduce safety risks. *Australian Critical Care, 29*(3), 165–171. doi:10.1016/j.aucc.2015.09.002

Grad, R. M., Pluye, P., Mercer, J., Marlow, B., Beauchamp, M. E., Shulha, M., . . . Wood-Dauphinee, S. (2008). Impact of research-based synopses delivered as daily e-mail: A prospective observational study. *Journal of the American Medical Informatics Association, 15*(2), 240–245. doi:10.1197/jamia.M2563

GRADE Working Group. (2016). Home. Retrieved from http://gradeworkinggroup.org

Grant, A. M., & Hofmann, D. A. (2011). It's not all about me: Motivating hand hygiene among health care professionals by focusing on patients. *Psychological Science, 22*(12), 1494–1499. doi:10.1177/0956797611419172

Green, A. E., & Aarons, G. A. (2011). A comparison of policy and direct practice stakeholder perceptions of factors affecting evidence-based practice implementation using concept mapping. *Implementation Science, 6*(104), 1–12. doi:10.1186/1748-5908-6-104

Greenhalgh, T., Robert, G., Macfarlane, F., Bate, P., & Kyriakidou, O. (2004). Diffusion of innovations in service organizations: Systematic review and recommendations. *Milbank Quarterly, 82*(4), 581–629. doi:10.1111/j.0887-378X.2004.00325.x

Grimshaw, J. M., Thomas, R. E., MacLennan, G., Fraser, C., Ramsay, C. R., Vale, L., . . . Donaldson, C. (2004). Effectiveness and efficiency of guideline dissemination and implementation strategies. *Health Technology Assessment, 8*(6), 1–72.

Grol, R., & Grimshaw, J. (2003). From best evidence to best practice: Effective implementation of change in patients' care. *The Lancet, 362*(9391), 1225–1230. doi:10.1016/S0140-6736(03)14546-1

Grol, R., & Wensing, M. (2004). What drives change? Barriers to and incentives for achieving evidence-based practice. *Medical Journal of Australia, 180*(Suppl. 6), S57–S60.

Groot-Jensen, S., Kiessling, A., Zethraeus, N., Bjornstedt-Bennermo, M., & Henriksson, P. (2016). Cost-effectiveness of case-based training for primary care physicians in evidence-based medicine of patients with coronary heart disease. *European Journal of Preventive Cardiology, 23*(4), 420–427. doi:1177/2047487315583798

Grove, S. K., Gray, J. R., & Burns, N. (2014). *Understanding nursing research: Building an evidence-based practice* (6th ed.). St. Louis, MO: Elsevier Saunders.

Gruen, R. L., Elliott, J. H., Nolan, M. L., Lawton, P. D., Parkhill, A., McLaren, C. J., & Lavis J. N. (2008). Sustainability science: An integrated approach for health-programme planning. *The Lancet, 372*(9649), 1579–1589. doi:10.1016/S0140-6736(08)61659-1

Gugiu, P. C., & Gugiu, M. R. (2010). A critical appraisal of standard guidelines for grading levels of evidence. *Evaluation & the Health Professions, 33*(3), 233–255. doi:10.1177/0163278710373980

Gunningberg, L., Fogelberg-Dahm, M., & Ehrenberg, A. (2009). Improved quality and comprehensiveness in nursing documentation of pressure ulcers after implementing an electronic health record in hospital care. *Journal of Clinical Nursing, 18*(11), 1557–1564. doi:10.1111/j.1365-2702.2008.02647.x

Gussgard, A. M., Jokstad, A., Hope, A. J., Wood, R., & Tenenbaum, H. (2015). Radiation-induced mucositis in in patients with head and neck cancer: Should the signs or the symptoms be measured? *Journal of the Canadian Dental Association, 81.*

Guyatt, G. H., Oxman, A. D., Akl, E. A., Kunz, R., Vist, G., Brozek, J., . . . Schünemann, H. J. (2011). GRADE guidelines. 1. Introduction—GRADE evidence profiles and summary of findings tables. *Journal of Clinical Epidemiology, 64*(4), 383–394. doi:10.1016/j.jclinepi.2010.04.026

Guyatt, G. H., Oxman, A. D., Kunz, R., Falck-Ytter, Y., Vist, G. E., Liberati, A., & Schünemann, H. J. (2008). GRADE: Going from evidence to recommendations. *BMJ, 336*(7652), 1049–1051. doi:10.1136/bmj.39493.646875.AE

Hageman, M. G., Ring, D. C., Gregory, P. J., Rubash, H. E., & Harmon, L. (2015). Do 360-degree feedback survey results relate to patient satisfaction measures? *Clinical Orthopaedics and Related Research, 473*(5), 1590–1597. doi:10.1007/s11999-014-3981-3

Häggman-Laitila, A., Mattila, L.-R., & Melender, H.-L. (2016). A systematic review of journal clubs for nurses. *Worldviews on Evidence-Based Nursing, 13*(2), 163–171. doi:10.1111/wvn.12131

Halawa, N. (2014). Evidence-based medicine: The conundrum of grading systems. *The Consultant Pharmacist, 29*(8), 536–546. doi:10.4140/TCP.n.2014.536

Haley, M., Lettis, A., Rose, P. M., Jenkins, L. S., Glasziou, P., & Rose, P. W. (2012). Implementing evidence in practice: Do action lists work? *Education for Primary Care, 23*(2), 107–114. doi:10.1080/14739879.2012.11494085

Hall, A. B., Montero, J., Cobian, J., & Regan, T. (2015). The effects of an electronic order set on vancomycin dosing in the ED. *American Journal of Emergency Medicine, 33*(1), 92–94. doi:10.1016/j.ajem.2014.09.049

Hamilton, J., & Edgar, L. (1992). A survey examining nurses' knowledge of pain control. *Journal of Pain and Symptom Management, 7*(1), 18–26. doi:10.1016/0885-3924(92)90103-O

Hannon, B. J. (n.d.). *Quality Quips: It's a jungle out there* [Unpublished manuscript]. Quality Improvement and Safety Committee, Department of Nursing Services and Patient Care, University of Iowa Hospitals and Clinics, Iowa City, United States.

Hanrahan, K. (n.d.) Evaluation of the environment of care in a children's hospital. Unpublished grant application. University of Iowa Hospitals and Clinics.

Hanrahan, K. (2012). Hyaluronidase for IV extravasation evidence-based guideline. In A. M. McCarthy (Series Ed.), *Series on evidence-based practice for children and families.* Iowa City, IA: The University of Iowa College of Nursing, Office for Nursing Research.

Hanrahan, K. (2013). Hyaluronidase for treatment of intravenous extravasations: Implementation of an evidence-based guideline in a pediatric population. *Journal for Specialists in Pediatric Nursing, 18*(3), 253–262. doi:10.1111/jspn.12035

Hanrahan, K., Marlow, K. L., Aldrich, C., & Hiatt, A. M. (2012). *Dissemination of nursing knowledge: Tips and resources.* Iowa City, IA: University of Iowa College of Nursing.

Hanrahan, K., Wagner, M., Matthews, G., Stewart, S., Dawson, C., Greiner, J., . . . Williamson, A. (2015). Sacred cow gone to pasture: A systematic evaluation and integration of evidence-based practice. *Worldviews on Evidence-Based Nursing, 12*(1), 3–11. doi:10.1111/wvn.12072

Harris, C., & Turner, T. (2011). Centre for Clinical Effectiveness: Evidence-based answers to clinical questions for busy clinicians. Retrieved from http://www.monashhealth.org/images/CCE_Website/CCE_Resources/Finding_the_Evidence_BusyClinicians2014.pdf

Harris, J. K., Erwin, P. C., Smith, C., & Brownson, R. C. (2015). The diffusion of evidence-based decision making among local health department practitioners in the United States. *Journal of Public Health Management and Practice, 21*(2), 134–140. doi:10.1097/PHH.0000000000000129

Harrison, M. B., Graham, I. D., van den Hoek, J., Dogherty, E. J., Carley, M. E., & Angus, V. (2013). Guideline adaptation and implementation planning: A prospective observational study. *Implementation Science, 8*(49), 1–14. doi:10.1186/1748-5908-8-49

Harron, A., & Titterington, J. (2016). Use of outcome measurement by paediatric AHPs in Northern Ireland. *International Journal of Language & Communication Disorders, 51*(4), 487–492. doi:10.1111/1460-6984.12224

Harvard Business Review. (2004). *Harvard business essentials: Managing projects large and small: The fundamental skills to deliver on budget and on time.* Boston, MA: Harvard Business School Press.

Harvey, G., & Kitson, A. (2016). PARIHS revisited: From heuristic to integrated framework for the successful implementation of knowledge into practice. *Implementation Science, 11*(33), 1–13. doi:10.1186/s13012-016-0398-2

Hauck, S., Winsett, R. P., & Kuric, J. (2013). Leadership facilitation strategies to establish evidence-based practice in an acute care hospital. *Journal of Advanced Nursing, 69*(3), 664–674. doi:10.1111/j.1365-2648.2012.06053.x

Haxton, D., Doering, J., Gingras, L., & Kelly, L. (2012). Implementing skin-to-skin contact at birth using the Iowa Model: Applying evidence to practice. *Nursing for Women's Health, 16*(3), 220–230. doi:10.1111/j.1751-486X.2012.01733.x

Haynes, A. B., Weiser, T. G., Berry, W. R., Lipsitz, S. R., Breizat, A. H., Dellinger, E. P., . . . Gawande, A. A. (2009). A surgical safety checklist to reduce morbidity and mortality in a global population. *New England Journal of Medicine, 360*(5), 491–499. doi:10.1056/NEJMsa0810119

Haynes, R. B., Devereaux, P. J., & Guyatt, G. H. (2002). Clinical expertise in the era of evidence-based medicine and patient choice. *Evidence-Based Medicine, 7*(2), 36–38. doi:10.1136/ebm.7.2.36

Hefner, J. L., Tripathi, R. S., Abel, E. E., Farneman, M., Galloway, J., & Moffatt-Bruce, S. D. (2016). Quality improvement intervention to decrease prolonged mechanical ventilation after coronary artery bypass surgery. *American Journal of Critical Care, 25*(5), 423–430. doi:10.4037/ajcc2016165

Heneghan, C. (2011). Considerable uncertainty remains in the evidence for primary prevention of cardiovascular disease [Editorial]. *Cochrane Database of Systematic Reviews,* (1). doi:10.1002/14651858.ED000017

Henneman, E. A., Kleppel, R., & Hinchey, K. T. (2013). Development of a checklist for documenting team and collaborative behaviors during multidisciplinary bedside rounds. *Journal of Nursing Administration, 43*(5), 280–285. doi:10.1097/NNA.0b013e31828eebfb

Herr, K., Bojoro, K., Steffensmeier, J., & Rakel, B. (2006). Acute pain management in older adults evidence-based practice guideline. In M. Titler (Ed.), *Series on evidence-based practice.* Iowa City, IA: University of Iowa College of Nursing, Research Translation and Dissemination Core.

Herr, K., St. Marie, B., Gordon, D. B., Paice, J. A., Watt-Watson, J., Stevens, B. J., . . . Young, H. M. (2015). An interprofessional consensus of core competencies for prelicensure education in pain management: Curriculum application for nursing. *The Journal of Nursing Education, 54*(6), 317–327. doi:10.3928/01484834-20150515-02

Herr, K., Titler, M., Fine, P. G., Sanders, S., Cavanaugh, J. E., Swegle, J., . . . Forcucci, C. (2012). The effect of a Translating Research Into Practice (TRIP)-cancer intervention on cancer pain management in older adults in hospice. *Pain Medicine, 13*(8), 1004–1017. doi:10.1111/j.1526-4637.2012.01405.x

Herzer, K., Niessen, L., Constenla, D., Ward, W., & Pronovost, P. (2014). Cost-effectiveness of a quality improvement programme to reduce central line-associated bloodstream infections in intensive care units in the USA. *BMJ Open, 4*(9), e006065. doi:10.1136/bmjopen-2014-006065

Higuchi, K. S., Davies, B. L., Edwards, N., Ploeg, J., & Virani, T. (2011). Implementation of clinical guidelines for adults with asthma and diabetes: A three-year follow-up evaluation of nursing care. *Journal of Clinical Nursing, 20*(9–10), 1329–1338. doi:10.1111/j.1365-2702.2010.03590.x

Hiller, A., Farrington, M., Forman, J., McNulty, H., & Cullen, L. (in press). Evidence-based nurse-driven algorithm for intrapartum bladder care. *Journal of PeriAnesthesia Nursing*.

Hilligoss, B., & Moffatt-Bruce, S. D. (2014). The limits of checklists: Handoff and narrative thinking. *BMJ Quality & Safety, 23*(7), 528–533. doi:10.1136/bmjqs-2013-002705

Hockenberry, M. (2014). Quality improvement and evidence-based practice change projects and the institutional review board: Is approval necessary? *Worldviews on Evidence-Based Nursing, 11*(4), 217–218. doi:10.1111/wvn.12049

Hoke, L., & Guarracino, D. (2016). Beyond socks, signs, and alarms: A reflective accountability model for fall prevention. *American Journal of Nursing, 116*(1), 42–47. doi:10.1097/01.NAJ.0000476167.43671.00

Holland, K., & Watson, R. (2012). *Writing for publication in nursing and healthcare: Getting it right.* Chichester, West Sussex: Wiley-Blackwell.

Holleman, G., Poot, E., Mintjes-de Groot, J., & van Achterberg, T. (2009). The relevance of team characteristics and team directed strategies in the implementation of nursing innovations: A literature review. *International Journal of Nursing Studies, 46*(9), 1256–1264. doi:10.1016/j.ijnurstu.2009.01.005

Holmes, B. J., Schellenberg, M., Schell, K., & Scarrow, G. (2014). How funding agencies can support research use in healthcare: An online province-wide survey to determine knowledge translation training needs. *Implementation Science, 9*(71), 1–10. doi:10.1186/1748-5908-9-71

Holt, D., Bouder, F., Elemuwa, C., Gaedicke, G., Khamesipour, A., Kisler, B., . . . Rath, B. (2016). The importance of the patient voice in vaccination and vaccine safety—Are we listening? *Clinical Microbiology and Infection, 22*(Suppl. 5), S146–S153. doi:10.1016/j.cmi.2016.09.027

Hoogendam, A., de Vries Robbe, P. F., & Overbeke, A. J. (2012). Comparing patient characteristics, type of intervention, control, and outcome (PICO) queries with unguided searching: A randomized controlled crossover trial. *Journal of the Medical Library Association, 100*(2), 121–126. doi:10.3163/1536-5050.100.2.010

Hopkinson, S. G., & Jennings, B. M. (2013). Interruptions during nurses' work: A state-of-the-science review. *Research in Nursing & Health, 36*(1), 38–53. doi:10.1002/nur.21515

Horn, S. D., Sharkey, S. S., Hudak, S., Gassaway, J., James, R., & Spector, W. (2010). Pressure ulcer prevention in long-term-care facilities: A pilot study implementing standardized nurse aide documentation and feedback reports. *Advances in Skin & Wound Care, 23*(3), 120–131. doi:10.1097/01.ASW.0000363516.47512.67

Horsley, T., O'Neill, J., & Campbell, C. (2009). The quality of questions and use of resources in self-directed learning: Personal learning projects in the maintenance of certification. *Journal of Continuing Education in the Health Professions, 29*(2), 91–97. doi:10.1002/chp.20017

Hsu, C. P., Chiang, C. Y., Chang, C. W., Huang, H. C., & Chen, C. C. (2015). Enhancing the commitment of nurses to the organisation by means of trust and monetary reward. *Journal of Nursing Management, 23*(5), 567–76. doi:10.1111/jonm.12180

Huang, X., Lin, J., & Demner-Fushman, D. (2006). Evaluation of PICO as a knowledge representation for clinical questions. *Proceedings of the AMIA Annual Symposium, USA, 2006* 350–363.

Huddleston, P., & Gray, J. (2016a). Describing nurse leaders' and direct care nurses' perceptions of a healthy work environment in acute care settings, Part 2. *Journal of Nursing Administration, 46*(9), 462–467. doi:10.1097/NNA.0000000000000376

Huddleston, P., & Gray, J. (2016b). Measuring nurse leaders' and direct care nurses' perceptions of a healthy work environment in an acute care setting, Part 1: A pilot study. *Journal of Nursing Administration, 46*(7–8), 373–378. doi:10.1097/NNA.0000000000000361

Huddleston, P., Mancini, M. E., & Gray, J. (2017). Measuring nurse leaders' and direct care nurses' perceptions of a healthy work environment in acute care settings, Part 3: Healthy Work Environment Scales for nurse leaders and direct care nurses. *Journal of Nursing Administration, 47*(3), 140–146. doi:10.1097/NNA.0000000000000456

Huether, K., Abbott, L., Cullen, L., Cullen, L., & Gaarde, A. (2016). Energy Through Motion: An evidence-based exercise program to reduce cancer-related fatigue and improve quality of life. *Clinical Journal of Oncology Nursing, 20*(3), E60–E70. doi:10.1188/16.CJON.E60-E70

Hughes, A. (2010). 8 rules for perfecting your pitch. *Black Enterprise, 41*(1), 100.

Hughes, R. G. (2008a). Nurses at the sharp end of patient care. In R. Hughes (Ed.), *Patient safety and quality: An evidence-based handbook for nurses*. Rockville, MD: Agency for Healthcare Research and Quality. Retrieved from http://www.ahrq.gov/qual/nurseshdbk

Hughes, R. G. (2008b). Tools and strategies for quality improvement and patient safety. In R. Hughes (Ed.), *Patient safety and quality: An evidence-based handbook for nurses* (Chapter 4). Rockville, MD: Agency for Healthcare Research and Quality. Retrieved from http://www.ahrq.gov/qual/nurseshdbk

Huis, A., Holleman, G., van Achterberg, T., Grol, R., Schoonhoven, L., & Hulscher, M. (2013). Explaining the effects of two different strategies for promoting hand hygiene in hospital nurses: A process evaluation alongside a cluster randomized controlled trial. *Implementation Science, 8*(41), 1–13. doi:10.1186/1748-5908-8-41

Huis, A., Schoonhoven, L., Grol, R., Donders, R., Hulscher, M., & van Achterberg, T. (2013). Impact of a team and leaders-directed strategy to improve nurses' adherence to hand hygiene guidelines: A cluster randomised trial. *International Journal of Nursing Studies, 50*(4), 464–474. doi:10.1016/j.ijnurstu.2012.08.004

Hulscher, M. E., Schouten, L. M., Grol, R. P., & Buchan, H. (2013). Determinants of success of quality improvement collaboratives: What does the literature show? *BMJ Quality & Safety, 22*(1), 19–31. doi:10.1136/bmjqs-2011-000651

Hysong, S. J. (2009). Meta-analysis: Audit and feedback features impact effectiveness on care quality. *Medical Care, 47*(3), 356–363. doi:10.1097/MLR.0b013e3181893f6b

Hysong, S. J., Kell, H. J., Petersen, L. A., Campbell, B. A., & Trautner, B. W. (2016). Theory-based and evidence-based design of audit and feedback programmes: Examples from two clinical intervention studies. *BMJ Quality & Safety, 26*(4), 323–334. doi:10.1136/bmjqs-2015-004796

Hysong, S. J., Knox, M. K., & Haidet, P. (2014). Examining clinical performance feedback in patient-aligned care teams. *Journal of General Internal Medicine, 29*(Suppl. 2), 667–674. doi:10.1007/s11606-013-2707-7

Hysong, S. J., Simpson, K., Pietz, K., SoRelle, R., Smitham, K. B., & Petersen, L. A. (2012). Financial incentives and physician commitment to guideline-recommended hypertension management. *American Journal of Managed Care, 18*(10), e378–391.

Hysong, S. J., Teal, C. R., Khan, M. J., & Haidet, P. (2012). Improving quality of care through improved audit and feedback. *Implementation Science, 7*(45), 1–10. doi:10.1186/1748-5908-7-45

Immunization Action Coalition. (2015). Using standing orders for administering vaccines: What you should know. Retrieved from http://www.immunize.org/standing-orders

Infusion Nurses Society. (2011). Infusion nursing standards of practice. *Journal of Infusion Nursing, 34*(Suppl. 1), 1–115.

Ingersoll, G. L., Witzel, P. A., Berry, C., & Qualls, B. (2010). Meeting Magnet research and evidence-based practice expectations through hospital based research centers. *Nursing Economics, 28*(4), 226–235.

Innis, J., & Berta, W. (2016). Routines for change: How managers can use absorptive capacity to adopt and implement evidence-based practice. *Journal of Nursing Management, 24*(6), 718–724. doi:10.1111/jonm.12368

Institute for Healthcare Improvement [IHI Open School]. (2014a, May 5). Whiteboard: Control charts [Video file]. Retrieved from https://www.youtube.com/watch?v=9kmbIj5zRtA

Institute for Healthcare Improvement [IHI Open School]. (2014b, May 5). Whiteboard: Static vs dynamic data [Video file]. Retrieved from http://www.ihi.org/education/ihiopenschool/resources/Pages/AudioandVideo/Whiteboard10.aspx

Institute for Healthcare Improvement (IHI). (2015). The science of improvement on a whiteboard! [Web log post]. Retrieved from http://www.ihi.org/education/IHIOpenSchool/resources/Pages/BobLloydWhiteboard.aspx

Institute for Healthcare Improvement (IHI). (2017). How to improve. Science of improvement: Establishing measures. Retrieved from http://www.ihi.org/resources/Pages/HowtoImprove/ScienceofImprovementEstablishingMeasures.aspx

Institute for Safe Medication Practices. (2010). ISMP's guidelines for standard order sets. Retrieved from http://www.ismp.org/tools/guidelines/standardordersets.pdf

Institute for Safe Medication Practices. (2013, September 19). ISMP Medication Safety Alert: Small effort, big payoff: Automated maximum dose alerts with hard stops. Retrieved from http://www.ismp.org/Newsletters/acutecare/showarticle.aspx?id=59

Institute of Medicine (IOM). (2004). *Patient safety: Achieving a new standard of care.* Washington, DC: The National Academies Press.

Institute of Medicine (IOM). (2010a). *Clinical data as the basic staple of health learning: Creating and protecting a public good: Workshop summary.* Washington, DC: The National Academies Press.

Institute of Medicine (IOM). (2010b). *The future of nursing: Leading change, advancing health.* Washington, DC: The National Academies Press.

Institute of Medicine (IOM). (2011a). *Clinical practice guidelines we can trust.* Washington, DC: The National Academies Press.

Institute of Medicine (IOM). (2011b). *Finding what works in healthcare: Standards for systematic reviews.* Washington, DC: The National Academies Press.

Institute of Medicine (IOM). (2011c). *Relieving pain in America: A blueprint for transforming prevention, care, education, and research.* Washington, DC: The National Academies Press.

Institute of Medicine (IOM). (2015a). *Best care at lower cost.* Washington, DC: The National Academies Press.

Institute of Medicine (IOM). (2015b). *Integrating research in practice: Health system leaders working toward high-value care: Workshop summary.* Washington, DC: The National Academies Press.

International Committee of Medical Journal Editors. (2017). Defining the roles of authors and contributors. Retrieved from http://www.icmje.org/recommendations/browse/roles-and-responsibilities/defining-the-role-of-authors-and-contributors.html

International Patient Decision Aid Standards (IPDAS) Collaboration. (2005). IPDAS 2005: Criteria for judging the quality of patient decision aids. Retrieved from http://ipdas.ohri.ca/IPDAS_checklist.pdf

International Patient Decision Aid Standards Steering Committee. (2013). The IPDAS story. Retrieved from http://ipdas.ohri.ca/IPDAS_story.pdf

Iowa Model Collaborative. (2017). Iowa Model of Evidence-Based Practice: Revisions and validation. *Worldviews on Evidence-Based Nursing, 14*(3), 175–182. doi:10.1111/wvn.12223

Iowa State University. (n.d.). Revised Bloom's Taxonomy. Retrieved from http://www.celt.iastate.edu/teaching/effective-teaching-practices/revised-blooms-taxonomy

Ipsos MORI Social Research Institute. (2009). Understanding your stakeholders: A best practice guide for the public sector. Retrieved from http://www.fundacionseres.org/Lists/Informes/Attachments/667/understanding-stakeholders.pdf

Ireland, S., Kirkpatrick, H., Boblin, S., & Robertson, K. (2013). The real world journey of implementing fall prevention best practices in three acute care hospitals: A case study. *Worldviews on Evidence-Based Nursing, 10*(2), 95–103. doi:10.1111/j.1741-6787.2012.00258.x

Issel, L. M. (2014). *Health program planning: A practical, systematic approach for community health* (3rd ed.). Burlington, MA: Jones & Bartlett Learning.

Ivers, N., Jamtvedt, G., Flottorp, S., Young, J. M., Odgaard-Jensen, J., French, S. D., . . . Oxman, A. D. (2012). Audit and feedback: Effects on professional practice and healthcare outcomes. *Cochrane Database of Systematic Reviews, 2012*(6), 1–229. doi:10.1002/14651858.CD000259.pub3

Ivers, N. M., Grimshaw, J. M., Jamtvedt, G., Flottorp, S., O'Brien, M. A., French, S. D., . . . Odgaard-Jensen, J. (2014). Growing literature, stagnant science? Systematic review, meta-regression and cumulative analysis of audit and feedback interventions in health care. *Journal of General Internal Medicine, 29*(11), 1534–1541. doi:10.1007/s11606-014-2913-y

Jackson, S., Bombei, C., Stenger, A., Bowman, A., & Cullen., L. (n.d.). *Probiotic use to prevent antibiotic-associated diarrhea and* Clostridium difficile *diarrhea in the medical intensive care unit (MICU).* Unpublished manuscript, University of Iowa Hospitals and Clinics, Iowa City, Iowa.

Jacobs, J. A., Duggan, K., Erwin, P., Smith, C., Borawski, E., Compton, J., . . . Brownson, R. C. (2014). Capacity building for evidence-based decision making in local health departments: Scaling up an effective training approach. *Implementation Science, 9*(124), 1–11. doi:10.1186/s13012-014-0124-x

Jamal, A., Temsah, M.-H., Khan, S. A., Al-Eyadhy, A., Koppel, C., & Chiang, M. F. (2016). Mobile phone use among medical residents: A cross-sectional multicenter survey in Saudi Arabia. *JMIR mHealth uHealth, 4*(2), e61. doi:10.2196/mhealth.4904

Jankowski, I. M., & Nadzam, D. M. (2011). Identifying gaps, barriers, and solutions in implementing pressure ulcer prevention programs. *Joint Commission Journal on Quality & Patient Safety, 37*(6) 253–264. doi:10.1016/S1553-7250(11)37033-X

Jansson, M. M., Syrjälä, H. P., Ohtonen, P. P., Meriläinen, M. H., Kyngäs, H. A., & Ala-Kokko, T. I. (2016). Randomized, controlled trial of the effectiveness of simulation education: A 24-month follow-up study in a clinical setting. *American Journal of Infection Control, 44*(4), 387–393. doi:10.1016/j.ajic.2015.10.035

Jeffs, L., Beswick, S., Lo, J., Campbell, H., Ferris, E., & Sidani, S. (2013). Defining what evidence is, linking it to patient outcomes, and making it relevant to practice: Insight from clinical nurses. *Applied Nursing Research, 26*(3), 105–109. doi:10.1016/j.apnr.2013.03.002

Jeffs, L., MacMillan, K., McKey, C., & Ferris, E. (2009). Nursing leaders' accountability to narrow the safety chasm: Insights and implications from the collective evidence based on health care safety. *Nursing Leadership, 22*(1), 86–98. doi:10.12927/cjnl.2009.20615

Johnson, J. E., Smith, A. L., & Mastro, K. A. (2012). From Toyota to the bedside: Nurses can lead the lean way in health care reform. *Nursing Administration Quarterly, 36*(3), 234–242. doi:10.1097/NAQ.0b013e318258c3d5

Johnson, K. A., Ford, J. H., II, & McCluskey, M. (2012). Promoting new practices to increase access to and retention in addiction treatment: An analysis of five communication channels. *Addictive Behaviors, 37*(11), 1193–1197. doi:10.1016/j.addbeh.2012.05.019

Johnson, K., Grossman, C., Anau, J., Greene, S., Kimbel, K., Larson, E., & Newton, K. (2015). *Integrating research into health care systems: executives' views* [Discussion Paper]. Washington, DC: Institute of Medicine. Retrieved from https://nam.edu/perspectives-2015-integrating-research-into-health-care-systems-executives-views

Johnson, K., Tuzzio, L., Renz, A., Baldwin, L.-M., & Parchman, M. (2016). Decision-to-implement worksheet for evidence-based interventions: From the WWAMI Region Practice and Research Network. *Journal of the American Board of Family Medicine, 29*(5), 553–562. doi:10.3122/jabfm.2016.05.150327

Johnson, M. J., & May, C. R. (2015). Promoting professional behaviour change in healthcare: What interventions work, and why? A theory-led overview of systematic reviews. *BMJ Open, 5*(9), e008592. doi:10.1136/bmjopen-2015-008592

Jones, K. R. (2010). Rating the level, quality, and strength of the research evidence. *Journal of Nursing Care Quality, 25*(4), 304–312. doi:10.1097/NCQ.0b013e3181db8a44

Jones, T. R., & Coke, L. (2016). Impact of standardized new medication education program on postdischarge patients' knowledge and satisfaction. *Journal of Nursing Administration, 46*(10), 535–540. doi:10.1097/NNA.0000000000000398

Kaasalainen, S., Ploeg, J., Donald, F., Coker, E., Brazil, K., Martin-Misener, R., . . . Hadjistavropoulos, T. (2015). Positioning clinical nurse specialists and nurse practitioners as change champions to implement a pain protocol in long-term care. *Pain Management Nursing, 16*(2), 78–88. doi:10.1016/j.pmn.2014.04.002

Kaasalainen, S., Williams, J., Hadjistavropoulos, T., Thorpe, L., Whiting, S., Neville, S., & Tremeer, J. (2010). Creating bridges between researchers and long-term care homes to promote quality of life for residents. *Qualitative Health Research, 20*(12), 1689–1704. doi:10.1177/1049732310377456

Kahle, D. (2016, April 27). The incredible power of an elevator speech. *Kahle Wisdom.* Retrieved from http://www.davekahle.com/wordpressblogs/2016/04/27/incredible-power-elevator-speech

Kaissi, A. A., & Begun, J. W. (2008). Strategic planning processes and hospital financial performance. *Journal of Healthcare Management, 53*(3), 197–209.

Kalman, Y. M., & Ravid, G. (2015). Filing, piling, and everything in between: The dynamics of e-mail inbox management. *Journal of the Association for Information Science & Technology, 66*(12), 2540–2552. doi:10.1002/asi.23337

Kane, R. L., Johnson, P. E., Town, R. J., & Butler, M. (2004). *Economic incentives for preventive care.* (Evidence Report/Technology Assessment No. 101). Retrieved from AHRQ website: http://archive.ahrq.gov/downloads/pub/evidence/pdf/ecinc/ecinc.pdf

Kartin, P. T., Tasci, S., Soyuer, S., & Elmali, F. (2014). Effect of an oral mucositis protocol on quality of life of patients with head and neck cancer treated with radiation therapy. *Clinical Journal of Oncology Nursing, 18*(6), E118–E125. doi:10.1188/14.CJON.E118-E125

Kastner, M., Bhattacharyya, O., Hayden, L., Makarski, J., Estey, E., Durocher, L., . . . Brouwers, M. (2015). Guideline uptake is influenced by six implementability domains for creating and communicating guidelines: A realist review. *Journal of Clinical Epidemiology, 68*(5), 498–509. doi:10.1016/j.jclinepi.2014.12.013

Katz, D. A., Holman, J. E., Johnson, S. R., Hillis, S. L., Adams, S. L., Fu, S. S., . . . Weg, M. W. (2014). Implementing best evidence in smoking cessation treatment for hospitalized veterans: Results from the VA-BEST trial. *Joint Commission Journal on Quality & Patient Safety, 40*(11), 493–502. doi:10.1016/S1553-7250(14)40064-3

Katz, D. A., Stewart, K., Paez, M., Holman, J., Adams, S. L., Web, M. W V., . . . Ono, S. (2016). "Let me get you a nicotine patch": Nurses' perceptions of implementing smoking cessation guidelines for hospitalized veterans. *Military Medicine, 181*(4), 373–382. doi:10.7205/MILMED-D-15-00101

Keefe, D. M., Schubert, M. M., Elting, L. S., Sonis, S. T., Epstein, J. B., Raber-Durlacher, J. E., . . . Peterson, D. E. (2007). Updated clinical practice guidelines for the prevention and treatment of mucositis. *Cancer, 109*(5), 820–831. doi:10.1002/cncr.22484

Kelly, K. P., Guzzetta, C. E., Mueller-Burke, D., Nelson, K., DuVal, J., Hinds, P. S., & Robinson, N. (2011). Advancing evidence-based nursing practice in a children's hospital using competitive awards. *Western Journal of Nursing Research, 33*(3), 306–332. doi:10.1177/0193945910379586

Kemper, C., Blackburn, C., Doyle, J. A., & Hyman, D. (2013). Engaging patients and families in system-level improvement: A safety imperative. *Nursing Administrative Quarterly, 37*(3), 203–215. doi:10.1097/NAQ.0b013e318295f61e

Kenny, K. J., Baker, L., Lanzon, M., Stevens, L. R., & Yancy, M. (2008). An innovative approach to peer review for the advanced practice nurse—A focus on critical incidents. *Journal of the American Academy of Nurse Practitioners, 20*(7), 376–381. doi:10.1111/j.1745-7599.2008.00335.x

KhanAcademy. (2016). Creating a histogram. Retrieved from https://www.khanacademy.org/math/ccsixth-grade-math/cc-6th-data-statistics/histograms/v/histograms-intro

Khan, I. A., Mehta, N. J., Gowda, R. M., Sacchi, T. J., & Vasavada, B. C. (2004). Reinforcement as a means for quality improvement in management of coronary syndromes: Adherence to evidence-based medicine. *International Journal of Cardiology, 95*(2–3), 281–283. doi:10.1016/j.ijcard.2003.04.043

Khong, P. C., Holroyd, E., & Wang, W. (2015). A critical review of the theoretical frameworks and the conceptual factors in the adoption of clinical decision support systems. *Computer, Informatics, Nursing, 33*(12), 555–570. doi:10.1097/CIN.0000000000000196

Kim, H. Y., Lee, W. K., Na, S., Roh, Y. H., Shin, C. S., & Kim, J. (2016). The effects of chlorhexidine gluconate bathing on health care-associated infection in intensive care units: A meta-analysis. *Journal of Critical Care, 32*, 126-–137. doi:10.1016/j.jcrc.2015.11.011

Kimber, C., & Grimmer-Somers, K. (2011). Preventing osteoporosis-related fractures from happening (again). *International Journal of Orthopaedic & Trauma Nursing, 15*(3), 121–135. doi:10.1016/j.ijotn.2010.12.001

King, S., Carbonaro, M., Greidanus, E., Ansell, D., Foisy-Doll, C., & Magus, S. (2014). Dynamic and routine interprofessional simulations: Expanding the use of simulation to enhance interprofessional competencies. *Journal of Allied Health, 43*(3), 169–175.

Kirchhoff, K. T. (1999). Strategies in research utilization, one form of evidence-based practice. In M. A. Mateo & K. T. Kirchhoff (Eds.), *Using and conducting nursing research in the clinical settings* (pp. 56–63). Philadelphia, PA: W. B. Saunders.

Kirchhoff, K. (2009). Design of questionnaires and structured interviews. In M. Mateo & K. Kirchhoff (Eds.), *Research for advanced practice nurses: From evidence to practice* (pp. 167–185). New York, NY: Springer Publishing Company.

Kis, E., Szegesdi, I., Dobos, E., Nagy, E., Boda, K., Kemény, L., & Horvath, A. R. (2010). Quality assessment of clinical practice guidelines for adaptation in burn injury. *Burns, 36*(5), 606–615. doi:10.1016/j.burns.2009.08.017

Knowlton, K., Kulkarni, S. P., Azhar, G. S., Mavalankar, D., Jaiswal, A., Connolly, M., . . . Ahmedabad Heat and Climate Study Group. (2014). Development and implementation of South Asia's first heat-health action plan in Ahmedabad (Gujarat, India). *International Journal of Environmental Research and Public Health, 11*(4), 3473–3492. doi:10.3390/ijerph110403473

Knudsen, H. K., & Roman, P. M. (2015). Innovation attributes and adoption decisions: Perspectives from leaders of a national sample of addiction treatment organizations. *Journal of Substance Abuse Treatment, 49*, 1–7. doi:10.1016/j.jsat.2014.08.003

Koffel, J. B. (2015). Use of recommended search strategies in systematic reviews and the impact of librarian involvement: A cross-sectional survey of recent authors. *PLoS ONE, 10*(5), e0125931. doi:10.1371/journal.pone.0125931

Korhonen, A., Ojanperä, H., Puhto, T., Järvinen, R., Kejonen, P., & Holopainen, A. (2015). Adherence to hand hygiene—Significance of measuring fidelity. *Journal of Clinical Nursing, 24*(21–22), 3197–3205. doi:10.1111/jocn.12969

Kortteisto, T., Kaila, M., Komulainen, J., Mäntyranta, T., & Rissanen, P. (2010). Healthcare professionals' intentions to use clinical guidelines: A survey using the theory of planned behaviour. *Implementation Science, 5*(51), 1–10. doi:10.1186/1748-5908-5-51

Kosse, N. M., Brands, K., Bauer, J. M., Hortobagyi, T., & Lamoth, C. J. C. (2013). Sensor technologies aiming at fall prevention in institutionalized old adults: A synthesis of current knowledge. *International Journal of Medical Informatics, 82*(9), 743–752. doi:10.1016/j.ijmedinf.2013.06.001

Kouzes, J. M., & Posner, B. Z. (2012). *The leadership challenge: How to make extraordinary things happen in organizations* (5th ed.). San Francisco, CA: Jossey-Bass.

Krahn, M., & Naglie, G. (2008). The next step in guideline development: Incorporating patient preferences. *JAMA, 300*(4), 436–438. doi:10.1001/jama.300.4.436

Krill, C., Staffileno, B. A., & Raven, C. (2012). Empowering staff nurses to use research to change practice for safe patient handling. *Nursing Outlook, 60*(3), 157–162.e1. doi:10.1016/j.outlook.2011.06.005

Kristensen, H. K., & Hounsgaard, L. (2013). Implementation of coherent, evidence-based pathways in Danish rehabilitation practice. *Disability and Rehabilitation, 35*(23), 2021–2028. doi:10.3109/09638288.2013.768301

Kristensen, H., & Hounsgaard, L. (2014). Evaluating the impact of audits and feedback as methods for implementation of evidence in stroke rehabilitation. *British Journal of Occupational Therapy, 77*(5), 251–259. doi:10.4276/030802214X13990455043520

Krom, Z. R., Batten, J., & Bautista, C. (2010). A unique collaborative nursing evidence-based practice initiative using the Iowa Model: A clinical nurse specialist, a health science librarian, and a staff nurse's success story. *Clinical Nurse Specialist, 24*(2), 54–59. doi:10.1097/NUR.0b013e3181cf5537

Krueger, R. A., & Casey, M. A. (2000). *Focus groups: A practical guide for applied research.* Thousand Oaks, CA: Sage Publications, Inc.

Kruglikova, I., Grantcharov, T. P., Drewes, A. M., & Funch-Jensen, P. (2010). The impact of constructive feedback on training in gastrointestinal endoscopy using high-fidelity virtual-reality simulation: A randomised controlled trial. *Gut, 59*(2), 181–185. doi:10.1136/gut.2009.191825

Kushner, J. A., Lawrence, H. P., Shoval, I., Kiss, T. L., Devins, G. M., Lee, L., & Tenenbaum, H. C. (2008). Development and validation of a Patient-Reported Oral Mucositis Symptom (PROMS) scale. *Journal of the Canadian Dental Association, 74*(1), 59.

Kwok, Y. L. A., Callard, M., & McLaws, M.-L. (2015). An automated hand hygiene training system improves hand hygiene technique but not compliance. *American Journal of Infection Control, 43*(8), 821–825. doi:10.1016/j.ajic.2015.04.201

Lachance, C. (2014). Nursing journal clubs: A literature review on the effective teaching strategy for continuing education and evidence-based practice. *Journal of Continuing Education in Nursing, 45*(12), 559–565. doi:10.3928/00220124-20141120-01

Lahmann, N. A., Halfens, R. J., & Dassen, T. (2010). Impact of prevention structures and processes on pressure ulcer prevalence in nursing homes and acute-care hospitals. *Journal of Evaluation in Clinical Practice, 16*(1), 50–56. doi:10.1111/j.1365-2753.2008.01113.x

Laibhen-Parkes, N. (2014). Evidence-based practice competence: A concept analysis. *International Journal of Nursing Knowledge, 25*(3), 173–182. doi:10.1111/2047-3095.12035

Lalla, R. V., Saunders, D. P., & Peterson, D. E. (2014). Chemotherapy or radiation-induced oral mucositis. *Dental Clinics of North America, 58*(2), 341–349. doi:10.1016/j.cden.2013.12.005

Landis-Lewis, Z., Brehaut, J. C., Hochheiser, H., Douglas, G. P., & Jacobson, R. S. (2015). Computer-supported feedback message tailoring: Theory-informed adaptation of clinical audit and feedback for learning and behavior change. *Implementation Science, 10*(12), 1–12. doi:10.1186/s13012-014-0203-z

Lang, R. L. N. (2012). *Evaluating the effectiveness of nurse-focused computerized clinical decision support on urinary catheter practice guidelines* (Nursing Thesis and Capstone Projects, paper 128). Retrieved from http://digitalcommons.gardner-webb.edu/nursing_etd/128

Langley, A., & Denis, J.-L. (2011). Beyond evidence: The micropolitics of improvement. *BMJ Quality and Safety, 20*(Suppl. 1), i43–i46. doi:10.1136/bmjqs.2010.046482

Larson, D. B., Donnelly, L. F., Podberesky, D. J., Merrow, A. C., Sharpe, R. E., Jr., & Kruskal, J. B. (2016). Peer feedback, learning, and improvement: Answering the call of the Institute of Medicine report on diagnostic error. *Radiology, 283*(1), 231–241. doi:10.1148/radiol.2016161254

Larson, E. L., Patel, S. J., Evans, D., & Saiman, L. (2013). Feedback as a strategy to change behaviour: The devil is in the details. *Journal of Evaluation in Clinical Practice, 19*(2), 230–234. doi:10.1111/j.1365-2753.2011.01801.x

LaRue, E. M., Draus, P., & Klem, M. L. (2009). A description of a web-based education tool for understanding the PICO framework in evidence-based practice with a citation ranking system. *Computers, Informatics, Nursing, 27*(1), 44–49. doi:10.1097/NCN.0b013e31818dd3d7

Lau, R., Stevenson, F., Ong, B. N., Dziedzic, K., Treweek, S., Eldridge, S., . . . Murray, E. (2016). Achieving change in primary care—Causes of the evidence to practice gap: Systematic reviews of reviews. *Implementation Science, 11*(40), 1–39. doi:10.1186/s13012-016-0396-4

Laurikainen, E., Rintala, E., Kaarto, A. M., & Routamaa, M. (2016). Adherence to surgical hand rubbing directives in a hospital district of Southwest Finland. *Infectious Diseases, 48*(2), 116–121. doi:10.3109/23744235.2015.1089591

Lavoie-Tremblay, M., O'Connor, P., Lavigne, G. L., Briand, A., Biron, A., Baillargeon, S., . . . Cyr, G. (2015). Effective strategies to spread redesigning care processes among healthcare teams. *Journal of Nursing Scholarship, 47*(4), 328–337. doi:10.1111/jnu.12141

Lawn, J. (2008, December 1). Want to have impact? Strive for brevity. *Food Management.* Retrieved from http://www.food-management.com/market-trends-amp-opinions/want-have-impact-strive-brevity

Lawton, R., Heyhoe, J., Louch, G., Ingleson, E., Glidewell, L., Willis, T. A., . . . Foy, R. (2016). Using the theoretical domains framework (TDF) to understand adherence to multiple evidence-based indicators in primary care: A qualitative study. *Implementation Science, 11*(113), 1–16. doi:10.1186/s13012-016-0479-2

Lee, H. L., Huang, S. H., & Huang, C. M. (2016). Evaluating the effect of three teaching strategies on student nurses' moral sensitivity. *Nursing Ethics.* doi:10.1177/0969733015623095

Lee, M. C., Johnson, K. L., Newhouse, R. P., & Warren, J. I. (2013). Evidence-based practice process quality assessment: EPQA guidelines. *Worldviews on Evidence-Based Nursing, 10*(3), 140–149. doi:10.1111/j.1741-6787.2012.00264.x

Lee, R. L., & Lee, P. H. (2014). To evaluate the effects of a simplified hand washing improvement program in schoolchildren with mild intellectual disability: A pilot study. *Research in Developmental Disabilities, 35*(11), 3014–3025. doi:10.1016/j.ridd.2014.07.016

Lehotsky, A., Szilagyi, L., Ferenci, T., Kovacs, L., Pethes, R., Weber, G., & Haidegger, T. (2015). Quantitative impact of direct, personal feedback on hand hygiene technique. *Journal of Hospital Infection, 91*(1), 81–84. doi:10.1016/j.jhin.2015.05.010

Leicher, V., & Mulder, R. H. (2016). Development of vignettes for learning and professional development. *Gerontology & Geriatrics Education, 12,* 1–17. doi:10.1080/02701960.2016.1247065

Lekan, D., Hendrix, C. C., McConnell, E. S., & White, H. (2010). The Connected Learning Model for disseminating evidence-based care practices in clinical settings. *Nurse Education in Practice, 10*(4), 243–248. doi:10.1016/j.nepr.2009.11.013

Leone, A. F., Standoli, F., & Hirth, V. (2009). Implementing a pain management program in a long-term care facility using a quality improvement approach. *Journal of the American Medical Directors Association, 10*(1), 67–73. doi:10.1016/j.jamda.2008.08.003

Leslie, M. S., Erickson-Owens, D., & Cseh, M. (2015). The evolution of individual maternity care providers to delayed cord clamping: Is it the evidence? *Journal of Midwifery & Women's Health, 60*(5), 561–569. doi:10.1111/jmwh.12333

Lessard, L., Bareil, C., Lalonde, L., Duhamel, F., Hudon, E., Goudreau, J., & Lévesque, L. (2016). External facilitators and interprofessional facilitation teams: A qualitative study of their roles in supporting practice change. *Implementation Science, 11*(97), 1–12. doi:10.1186/s13012-016-0458-7

Leung, K., Trevena, L., & Waters, D. (2014). Systematic review of instruments for measuring nurses' knowledge, skills and attitudes for evidence-based practice. *Journal of Advanced Nursing, 70*(10), 2181–2195. doi:10.1111/jan.12454

Leung, K., Trevena, L., & Waters, D. (2016). Development of a competency framework for evidence-based practice in nursing. *Nurse Education Today, 39,* 189–196. doi:10.1016/j.nedt.2016.01.026

Levchenko, A. I., Boscart, V. M., & Fernie, G. R. (2014). Automated monitoring: A potential solution for achieving sustainable improvement in hand hygiene practices. *Computers, Informatics, Nursing, 32*(8), 397–403. doi:10.1097/CIN.0000000000000067

Levin, R. F., & Chang. A. (2014). Tactics for teaching evidence-based practice: Determining the level of evidence of a study. *Worldviews on Evidence-Based Nursing, 11*(1), 75–78. doi:10.1111/wvn.12023

Liberating Structures. (n.d.). Introduction. Retrieved from http://www.liberatingstructures.com

Liddy, C., Hogg, W., Singh, J., Taljaard, M., Russell, G., Armstrong, C. D., . . . Grimshaw, J. M. (2015). A real-world stepped wedge cluster randomized trial of practice facilitation to improve cardiovascular care. *Implementation Science, 10*(150), 1–11. doi:10.1186/s13012-015-0341-y

Liddy, C., Johnston, S., Nash, K., Irving, H., & Davidson, R. (2016). Implementation and evolution of a regional chronic disease self-management program. *Canadian Journal of Public Health, 107*(2), e194–e201. doi:10.17269/cjph.107.5126

Likert, R. (1932). A technique for the measurement of attitudes. *Archives of Psychology, 22*(140), 1–55.

Lindamer, L. A., Lebowitz, B., Hough, R. L., Garcia, P., Aguirre, A., Halpain, M. C., . . . Jeste, D. V. (2009). Establishing an implementation network: Lessons learned from community-based participatory research. *Implementation Science, 4*(17), 1–7. doi:10.1186/1748-5908-4-17

Lipman, P. D., Lange, C. J., Cohen, R. A., & Peterson, K. A. (2014). A mixed-methods study of research dissemination across practice-based research networks. *Journal of Ambulatory Care Management, 37*(2), 179–188. doi:10.1097/JAC.0000000000000018

Lipmanowicz, H., & McCandless, K. (2014). *The surprising power of liberating structures: Simple rules to unleash a culture of innovation*. Seattle, WA: Liberating Structures Press.

Li-Ying, J., Paunova, M., & Egerod, I. (2016). Knowledge sharing behaviour and intensive care nurse innovation: The moderating role of control of care quality. *Journal of Nursing Management, 24*(7), 943–953. doi:10.1111/jonm.12404

Lockett, A., El Enany, N., Currie, G., Oborn, E., Barrett, M., Racko, G., . . . Waring J. (2014). A formative evaluation of collaboration for leadership in applied health research and care (CLAHRC): Institutional entrepreneurship for service innovation. *Health Services and Delivery Research, 2*(31). doi:10.3310/hsdr02310

Long, J. C., Cunningham, F. C., & Braithwaite, J. (2013). Bridges, brokers, and boundary spanners in collaborative networks: A systematic review. *BMC Health Services Research, 13*(158), 1–13. doi:10.1186/1472-6963-13-158

Long, L. E., Burkett, K., & McGee, S. (2009). Promotion of safe outcomes: Incorporating evidence into policies and procedures. *Nursing Clinics of North America, 44*(1), 57–70. doi:10.1016/j.cnur.2008.10.013

Lovaglio, P. G. (2012). Benchmarking strategies for measuring the quality of healthcare: Problems and prospects. *Scientific World Journal*, (2012). doi:10.1100/2012/606154

Lowson, K., Jenks, M., Filby, A., Carr, L., Campbell, B., & Powell, J. (2015). Examining the implementation of NICE guidance: Cross-sectional survey of the use of NICE interventional procedures guidance by NHS Trusts. *Implementation Science, 10*(93), 1–9. doi:10.1186/s13012-015-0283-4

Lugtenberg, M., Burgers, J. S., Han, D., & Westert, G. P. (2014). General practitioners' preferences for interventions to improve guideline adherence. *Journal of Evaluation in Clinical Practice, 20*(6), 820–826. doi:10.1111/jep.12209

Luke, M. M., & Alavosius, M. (2011). Adherence with universal precautions after immediate, personalized performance feedback. *Journal of Applied Behavior Analysis, 44*(4), 967–971. doi:10.1901/jaba.2011.44-967

Maas, M. J., van der Wees, P. J., Braam, C., Koetsenruijter, J., Heerkens, Y. F., van der Vleuten, C. P. M., & Nijhuis-van der Sanden, M. W. G. (2015). An innovative peer assessment approach to enhance guideline adherence in physical therapy: Single-masked, cluster-randomized controlled trial. *Physical Therapy, 95*(4), 600–612. doi:10.2522/ptj.20130469

Maas, M. J., van Dulmen, S. A., Sagasser, M. H., Heerkens, Y. F., van der Vleuten, C. P., Nijhuis-van der Sanden, M. W., & van der Wees, P. J. (2015). Critical features of peer assessment of clinical performance to enhance adherence to a low back pain guideline for physical therapists: A mixed methods design. *BMC Medical Education, 15*(203), 1–12. doi:10.1186/s12909-015-0484-1

Mader, E. M., Fox, C. H., Epling, J. W., Noronha, G. J., Swanger, C. M., Wisniewski, A. M., . . . Morley, C. P. (2016). A practice facilitation and academic detailing intervention can improve cancer screening rates in primary care safety net clinics. *Journal of the American Board of Family Medicine, 29*(5), 533–542. doi:10.3122/jabfm.2016.05.160109

Madsen, D., Sebolt, T., Cullen, L., Folkedahl, B., Mueller, T., Richardson, C., & Titler, M. (2005). Listening to bowel sounds: An evidence-based practice project. *American Journal of Nursing, 105*(12), 40–50. doi:10.1097/00000446-200512000-00029

Magers, T. L. (2014). An EBP mentor and unit-based EBP team: A strategy for successful implementation of a practice change to reduce catheter-associated urinary tract infections. *Worldviews on Evidence-Based Nursing, 11*(5), 341–343. doi:10.1111/wvn.12056

Mahanes, D., Quatrara, B. D., & Shaw, K. D. (2013). APN-led nursing rounds: An emphasis on evidence-based nursing care. *Intensive and Critical Care Nursing, 29*(5), 256–260. doi:10.1016/j.iccn.2013.03.004

Maher, L., Gustafson, D., & Evans, A. (2010). NHS sustainability model. Retrieved from http://www.qihub. scot.nhs.uk/media/162236/sustainability_model.pdf

Majid, S., Foo, S., Luyt, B., Zhang, X., Theng, Y. L., Chang, Y. K, & Mokhtar, I. A. (2011). Adopting evidence-based practice in clinical decision making: Nurses' perceptions, knowledge and barriers. *Journal of the Medical Library Association, 99*(3), 229–236. doi:10.3163/1536-5050.99.3.010

Makic, M. B. F., Lovett, K., & Azam, M. F. (2012). Placement of an esophageal temperature probe by nurses. *AACN Advanced Critical Care, 23*(1), 24–31. doi:10.1097/NCI.0b013e31823324f3

Makic, M. B., Rauen, C., Watson, R., & Poteet, A. W. (2014). Examining the evidence to guide practice: Challenging practice habits. *Critical Care Nurse, 34*(2), 28–45. doi:10.4037/ccn2014262

Manika, D., Ball, J. G., & Stout, P. A. (2014). Factors associated with the persuasiveness of direct-to-consumer advertising on HPV vaccination among young women. *Journal of Health Communication, 19*(11), 1232–1247. doi:10.1080/10810730.2013.872727

Manley, B. J., Gericke, R. K., Brockman, J. A., Robles, J., Raup, V. T., & Bhayani, S. B. (2014). The pitfalls of electronic health orders: Development of an enhanced institutional protocol after a preventable patient death. *Patient Safety in Surgery, 8*(1), 39. doi:10.1186/s13037-014-0039-0

Mann-Salinas, E., Hayes, E., Robbins, J., Sabido, J., Feider, L., Allen, D., & Yoder, L. (2014). A systematic review of the literature to support an evidence-based precepting program. *Burns, 40*(3), 374–387. doi:10.1016/j.burns.2013.11.008

Marshall, A. P., West, S. H., & Aitken, L. M. (2013). Clinical credibility and trustworthiness are key characteristics used to identify colleagues from whom to seek information. *Journal of Clinical Nursing, 22*(9–10), 1424–1433. doi:10.1111/jocn.12070

Marshall, N., Spooner, M., Galvin, P. L., Ti, J. P., McElvaney, N. G., & Lee, M. J. (2011). Informatics in radiology: Evaluation of an e-learning platform for teaching medical students competency in ordering radiologic examinations. *Radiographics, 31*(5), 1463–1474. doi:10.1148/rg.315105081

Matthew-Maich, N., Ploeg, J., Dobbins, M., & Jack, S. (2013). Supporting the uptake of nursing guidelines: What you really need to know to move nursing guidelines into practice. *Worldviews on Evidence-Based Nursing, 10*(2), 104–115. doi:10.1111/j.1741-6787.2012.00259.x

Mauger, B., Marbella, A., Pines, E., Chopra, R., Black, E. R., & Aronson, N. (2014). Implementing quality improvement strategies to reduce healthcare-associated infections: A systematic review. *American Journal of Infection Control, 42*(Suppl. 10), S274–S283. doi:10.1016/j.ajic.2014.05.031

Maurer, J., & Harris, K. M. (2014). Issuance of patient reminders for influenza vaccination by US-based primary care physicians during the first year of universal influenza vaccination recommendations. *American Journal of Public Health, 104*(6), e60–e62. doi:10.2105/AJPH.2014.301888

May, L. J., Longhurst, C. A., Pageler, N. M., Wood, M. S., Sharek, P. J., & Zebrack, C. M. (2014). Optimizing care of adults with congenital heart disease in a pediatric cardiovascular ICU using electronic clinical decision support*. *Pediatric Critical Care Medicine, 15*(5), 428–434. doi:10.1097/PCC.0000000000000124

Mayer, J., Mooney, B., Gundlapalli, A., Harbarth, S., Stoddard, G. J., Rubin, M. A. . . . Samore, M. H. (2011). Dissemination and sustainability of a hospital-wide hand hygiene program emphasizing positive reinforcement. *Infection Control & Hospital Epidemiology, 32*(1), 59–66. doi:10.1086/657666

McCaffery, M., & Ferrell, B. R. (1997). Nurses' knowledge of pain assessment and management: How much progress have we made? *Journal of Pain and Symptom Management, 14*(3), 175–188. doi:S088539249700170X

McCormack, B., Rycroft-Malone, J., DeCorby, K., Hutchinson, A. M., Bucknall, T., Kent, B., . . . Wilson, V. (2013). A realist review of interventions and strategies to promote evidence-informed healthcare: A focus on change agency. *Implementation Science, 8*(107), 1–12. doi:10.1186/1748-5908-8-107

McDowell, D. S., & McComb, S. A. (2014). Safety checklist briefings: A systematic review of the literature. *AORN Journal, 99*(1), 125–137. doi:10.1016/j.aorn.2013.11.015

McGillis Hall, L., Lalonde, M., Dales, L., Peterson, J., & Cripps, L. (2011). Strategies for retaining midcareer nurses. *Journal of Nursing Administration, 41*(12), 531–537. doi:10.1097/NNA.0b013e3182378d6c

McGreevey, J. D., (2013). Order sets in electronic health records: Principles of good practice. *Chest, 143*(1), 228–235. doi:10.1378/chest.12-0949

McGregor, D., Rankin, N., Butow, P., York, S., White, K., Phillips, J., . . . Shaw, T. (2017). Closing evidence-practice gaps in lung cancer: Results from multi-methods priority setting in the clinical context. *Asia-Pacific Journal of Clinical Oncology, 13*(1), 28–36. doi:10.1111/ajco.12499

McKee, C., Berkowitz, I., Cosgrove, S. E., Bradley, K., Beers, C., Perl, T. M., . . . Miller, M. R. (2008). Reduction of catheter-associated bloodstream infections in pediatric patients: Experimentation and reality. *Pediatric Critical Care Medicine, 9*(1), 40–46. doi:10.1097/01.PCC.0000299821.46193.A3

McKeever, S., Kinney, S., Lima, S., & Newall, F. (2016). Creating a journal club competition improves paediatric nurses' participation and engagement. *Nurse Education Today, 37*, 173–177. doi:10.1016/j.nedt.2015.11.017

McKibbon, K. A., & Marks, S. (2001). Posing clinical questions: Framing the question for scientific inquiry. *AACN Clinical Issues, 12*(4), 477–481. doi:10.1097/00044067-200111000-00004

McLennon, S. (2005). Persistent pain management evidence-based practice guideline. In M. Titler (Ed.), *Series on evidence-based practice.* Iowa City, IA: University of Iowa College of Nursing, Research Translation and Dissemination Core.

Medicare. (n.d.-a). Find & compare doctors, hospitals, & other providers. Retrieved from https://www.medicare.gov/forms-help-and-resources/find-doctors-hospitals-and-facilities/quality-care-finder.html

Medicare. (n.d.-b). Hospital compare. Retrieved from https://www.medicare.gov/hospitalcompare/search.html?

Medicare. (n.d.-c). Hospital value-based purchasing. Retrieved from https://www.medicare.gov/hospitalcompare/data/hospital-vbp.html

Melnyk, B. M., & Fineout-Overholt, E. (2010). *Evidence-based practice in nursing and healthcare. A guide to best practice* (2nd ed.). Philadelphia, PA: Lippincott Williams & Wilkins.

Melnyk, B. M., Fineout-Overholt, E., Gallagher-Ford, L., & Stillwell, S. B. (2011). Evidence-based practice, step by step: Sustaining evidence-based practice through organizational policies and an innovative model. *American Journal of Nursing, 111*(9), 57–60. doi:10.1097/01.NAJ.0000405063.97774.0e

Melnyk, B. M., Gallagher-Ford, L., Thomas, B. K., Troseth, M., Wyngarden, K., & Szalacha, L. (2016). A study of chief nurse executives indicates low prioritization of evidence-based practice and shortcomings in hospital performance metrics across the United States. *Worldviews on Evidence-Based Nursing, 13*(1), 6–14. doi:10.1111/wvn.12133

Menendez, M. E., van Hoorn, B. T., Mackert, M., Donovan, E. E., Chen, N. C., & Ring, D. (2017). Patients with limited health literacy ask fewer questions during office visits with hand surgeons. *Clinical Orthopaedics and Related Research, 475*(5), 1291–1297. doi:10.1007/s11999-016-5140-5

Michetti, C., Fakhry, S., Ferguson, P., Cook, A., Moore, F., Gross, R., & AAST Ventilator-Associated Pneumonia Investigators. (2012). Ventilator-associated pneumonia rates at major trauma centers compared with a national benchmark: A multi-institutional study of the AAST. *Journal of Trauma & Acute Care Surgery, 72*(5), 1165–1173. doi:10.1097/TA.0b013e31824d10fa

Microsoft . (n.d.). Create a histogram. Retrieved from https://support.offi ce.com/en-us/article/Create-ahistogram-B6814E9E-5860-4113-BA51-E3A1B9EE1BBE

Middaugh, D. J. (2015). The voice—of email. *MEDSURG Nursing, 24*(4), 277–278.

Miech, E. (2016). Inside help: A systematic review of champions in healthcare-related implementation. Retrieved from http://www.hsrd.research.va.gov/for_researchers/cyber_seminars/archives/video_archive.cfm?SessionID=1160

Milat, A. J., Bauman, A., & Redman, S. (2015). Narrative review of models and success factors for scaling up public health interventions. *Implementation Science, 10*(113), 1–11. doi:10.1186/s13012-015-0301-6

Mind Tools. (2016). Action plans: Small-scale planning. Retrieved from https://www.mindtools.com/pages/article/newHTE_04.htm

Mitchell, M. D., Lavenberg, J. G., Trotta, R. L., & Umscheid, C. A. (2014). Hourly rounding to improve nursing responsiveness. *Journal of Nursing Administration, 44*(9), 462–472. doi:10.1097/NNA.0000000000000101

Moch, S. D., Quinn-Lee, L., Gallegos, C., & Sortedahl, C. K. (2015). Navigating evidence-based practice projects: The faculty role. *Nursing Education Perspectives, 36*(2), 128–130. doi:10.5480/12-1014.1

Mohammed, M. A., Worthington, P., & Woodall, W. H. (2008). Plotting basic control charts: Tutorial notes for healthcare practitioners. *Quality & Safety in Health Care, 17*(2), 137–145. doi:10.1136/qshc.2004.012047

Mold, J. W., Aspy, C. B., Smith, P. D., Zink, T., Knox, L., Lipman, P. D., . . . Cohen, R. (2014). Leveraging practice-based research networks to accelerate implementation and diffusion of chronic kidney disease guidelines in primary care practices: A prospective cohort study. *Implementation Science, 9*(169), 1–11. doi:10.1186/s13012-014-0169-x

Mold, J. W., Fox, C., Wisniewski, A., Lipman, P. D., Krauss, M. R., Harris, D. R., . . . Gonin, R. (2014). Implementing asthma guidelines using practice facilitation and local learning collaboratives: A randomized controlled trial. *Annals of Family Medicine, 12*(3), 233–240. doi:10.1370/afm.1624

Montini, T., & Graham, I. D. (2015). "Entrenched practices and other biases": Unpacking the historical, economic, professional, and social resistance to de-implementation. *Implementation Science, 10*(24), 1–8. doi:10.1186/s13012-015-0211-7

Montori, V. M., Brito, J. P., & Murad, M. H. (2013). The optimal practice of evidence-based medicine: Incorporating patient preferences in practice guidelines. *JAMA, 310*(23), 2503–2504. doi:10.1001/jama.2013.281422

Moore, H. (2014). Improving kangaroo care policy and implementation in the neonatal intensive care. *Journal of Neonatal Nursing, 21*(4), 157–160. doi:10.1016/j.jnn.2014.11.001

Morgan, J. L., Baggari, S. R., Chung, W., Ritch, J., McIntire, D. D., & Sheffield, J. S. (2015). Association of a best-practice alert and prenatal administration with tetanus toxoid, reduced diphtheria toxoid, and acellular pertussis vaccination rates. *Obstetrics and Gynecology, 126*(2), 333–337. doi:10.1097/AOG.0000000000000975

Morris, Z. S., & Clarkson, P. J. (2009). Does social marketing provide a framework for changing healthcare practice? *Health Policy, 91*(2), 135–141. doi:10.1016/j.healthpol.2008.11.009

Morrison, R. S., & Peoples, L. (1999). Using focus group methodology in nursing. *Journal of Continuing Education in Nursing, 30*(2), 62–65.

Morrow, R. W., Tattelman, E., Purcell, J. M., King, J., & Fordis, M. (2016). Academic peer detailing—The preparation and experience of detailers involved in a project to disseminate a comparative effectiveness module. *Journal of Continuing Education in the Health Professions, 36*(2), 123–126. doi:10.1097/CEH.0000000000000067

Moss, J. M., Bryan, W. E., III, Wilkerson, L. M., Jackson, G. L., Owenby, R. K., Van Houtven, C., . . . Hastings, S. N. (2016). Impact of clinical pharmacy specialists on the design and implementation of a quality improvement initiative to decrease inappropriate medications in a Veterans Affairs emergency department. *Journal of Managed Care & Specialty Pharmacy, 22*(1), 74–80. doi:10.18553/jmcp.2016.22.1.74

Murad, M. H., Montori, V. M., Ioannidis, J. P. A., Jaeschke, R., Devereaux, P. J., Kameshwar, P., . . . Guyatt, G. (2014). How to read a systematic review and meta-analysis and apply the results to patient care: Users' guide to the medical literature. *JAMA, 312*(2), 171–179. doi:10.1001/jama.2014.5559

Murphy, N. (2015). Advancing the interdisciplinary collaborative health team model: Applying democratic professionalism, implementation science, and therapeutic alliance to enact social justice practice. *Advances in Nursing Science, 38*(3), 215–226. doi:10.1097/ANS.0000000000000079

Mwaniki, P., Ayieko, P., Todd, J., & English, M. (2014). Assessment of paediatric inpatient care during a multifaceted quality improvement intervention in Kenyan district hospitals—Use of prospectively collected case record data. *BMC Health Services Research, 14*(312), 1–10. doi:10.1186/1472-6963-14-312

MySecretMathTutor. (2011, September 1). Re: Statistics–How to make a histogram [Video file]. Retrieved from https://www.youtube.com/watch?v=KCH_ZDygrm4

Nancarrow, S. A., Booth, A., Ariss, S., Smith, T., Enderby, P., & Roots, A. (2013). Ten principles of good interdisciplinary team work. *Human Resources for Health, 11*. doi:10.1186/1478-4491-11-19

Nasby, D. (2009). Nursing research grand rounds. *Differentiating research and quality improvement.* Rochester, MN: Mayo Clinic.

National Cancer Institute. (n.d.). NCI-designated cancer centers. Retrieved from https://www.cancer.gov/research/nci-role/cancer-centers

National Guideline Clearinghouse (NGC). (2011). Home. Retrieved from http://www.guideline.gov

National Health Service. (n.d.-a.). Quality and service improvement tools: Statistical process control (SPC). Retrieved November 28, 2016 from http://webarchive.nationalarchives.gov.uk/20121108103848/http://www.institute.nhs.uk/quality_and_service_improvement_tools/quality_and_service_improvement_tools/statistical_process_control.html

National Health Service. (n.d.-b.). Quality and service improvement tools: variation–an overview. Retrieved from http://webarchive.nationalarchives.gov.uk/20121108105624/http://www.institute.nhs.uk/quality_and_service_improvement_tools/quality_and_service_improvement_tools/variation_-_an_overview.html

National Health Service. (n.d.-c.). Run chart rules for interpretation. Retrieved from http://www.qihub.scot.nhs.uk/media/529936/run%20chart%20rules.pdf

National Health Service. (2010). Explanation of statistical process control charts: Changes to the presentation of information in the *Staphylococcus aureus* bacteremia quarterly reports. Retrieved from http://www.wales.nhs.uk/sites3/page.cfm?orgid=379&pid=13438

National Public Radio Books. (2010, January 5). Atul Gawande's "checklist" for surgery success. Retrieved from http://www.npr.org/templates/story/story.php?storyId=122226184

Nayback-Beebe, A. M., Forsythe, T., Funari, T., Mayfield, M., Thomas, W., Smith, K. K., ... Scott, P. (2013). Using evidence-based leadership initiatives to create a healthy nursing work environment. *Dimensions of Critical Care Nursing, 32*(4), 166–173. doi:10.1097/DCC.0b013e3182998121

Neis, N. (2015). *No lion around: PICU mobility protocol.* Unpublished manuscript, 2013–2014 Evidence-Based Practice Staff Nurse Internship, Department of Nursing Services and Patient Care, University of Iowa Hospitals and Clinics, Iowa City, Iowa.

Nelson, B. (2016). You get what you reward: A research-based approach to employee recognition. In M. Grawitch, & D. Ballard (Eds.), *The psychologically healthy workplace: Building a win-win environment for organizations and employees.* Washington, DC: American Psychological Association.

Nemeth, L. (2014). Performance appraisal. In D. Huber (Ed.), *Leadership and nursing care management* (5th ed., pp. 399–409). St. Louis, MO: Elsevier Saunders.

Neufeld, N. J., Fernández, M. G., Christo, P. J., & Williams, K. A. (2013). Positive recognition program increases compliance with medication reconciliation by resident physicians in an outpatient clinic. *American Journal of Medical Quality, 28*(1), 40–45. doi:10.1177/1062860612443550

Nevin, D. J., Mrklas, K. J., Holodinsky, J. K., Straus, S. E., Hemmelgarn, B. R., Jeffs, L. P., & Stelfox, H. T. (2015). Towards understanding the de-adoption of low-value clinical practices: A scoping review. *BMC Medicine, 13*(1), 1–21. doi:10.1186/s12916-015-0488-z

NHSScotland Quality Improvement Hub. (2016). Run chart overview. Retrieved from https://qi.elft.nhs.uk/resource/run-charts/

Niederhauser, A., Lukas, C. V., Parker, V., Ayello, E. A., Zulkowski, K., & Berlowitz, D. (2012). Comprehensive programs for preventing pressure ulcers: A review of the literature. *Advances in Skin & Wound Care, 25*(4), 167–188. doi:10.1097/01.ASW.0000413598.97566.d7

Noordman, J., van der Weijden, T., & van Dulmen, S. (2014). Effects of video-feedback on the communication, clinical competence and motivational interviewing skills of practice nurses: A pre-test post-test control group study. *Journal of Advanced Nursing, 70*(10), 2272–2283. doi:10.1111/jan.12376

Nordqvist, C., Timpka, T., & Lindqvist, K. (2009). What promotes sustainability in Safe Community programmes? *BMC Health Services Research, 9*(4), 1–9. doi:10.1186/1472-6963-9-4

Northcutt, S. (n.d.). *What is a security thought leader.* Retrieved from http://www.sans.edu/research/security-laboratory/article/sec-thought-leader

Novak, I., & McIntyre, S. (2010). The effect of education with workplace supports on practitioners' evidence-based practice knowledge and implementation behaviors. *Australian Occupational Therapy Journal, 57*(6), 386–393. doi:10.1111/j.1440-1630.2010.00861.x

O'Brien, M. A., Rogers, S., Jamtvedt, G., Oxman, A. D., Odgaard-Jensen, J., Kristoffersen, D. T., . . . Harvey, E. L. (2007). Educational outreach visits: Effects on professional practice and health care outcomes. *Cochrane Database of Systematic Reviews, 4,* 1–82. doi:10.1002/14651858.cd000409.pub2

Odedra, K., & Hitchcock, J. (2012). Implementation of nursing grand rounds at a large acute hospital trust. *British Journal of Nursing, 21*(3), 182–185. doi:10.12968/bjon.2012.21.3.182

Ofek Shlomai, N., Rao, S., & Patole, S. (2015). Efficacy of interventions to improve hand hygiene compliance in neonatal units: A systematic review and meta-analysis. *European Journal of Clinical Microbiology & Infectious Diseases, 34*(5), 887–897. doi:10.1007/s10096-015-2313-1

Office for Human Research Protections (OHRP). (n.d.). Quality improvement activities FAQs. Retrieved from https://www.hhs.gov/ohrp/regulations-and-policy/guidance/faq/quality-improvement-activities/index.html

Office for Human Research Protections (OHRP). (2009, January 15). Title 45: Public welfare DHHS, part 46: Protection of human subjects. Retrieved from http://www.hhs.gov/ohrp/humansubjects/guidance/45cfr46.html#46.102

Ogier, M. E. (1998). *Reading research: How to make research more approachable* (2nd ed.). Oxford, UK: Bailliere Tindall/Elsevier Science.

O'Leary, D. F., & Mhaolrúnaigh, S. N. (2012). Information-seeking behavior of nurses: Where is information sought and what processes are followed? *Journal of Advanced Nursing, 68*(2), 379–390. doi:10.1111/j.1365-2648.2011.05750.x

Olsen, B. F., Rustøen, T., Sandvik, L., Miaskowski, C., Jacobsen, M., & Valeberg, B. T. (2015). Implementation of a pain management algorithm in intensive care units and evaluation of nurses' level of adherence with the algorithm. *Heart & Lung, 44*(6), 528–533. doi:10.1016/j.hrtlng.2015.08.001

Oman, K. S., Duran, C., & Fink, R. (2008). Evidence-based policy and procedures: An algorithm for success. *Journal of Nursing Administration, 38*(1), 47–51. doi:10.1097/01.NNA.0000295634.18463.4d

Open Society Foundations. (2013). Case studies: Examples of successful advocacy efforts in different settings around the world. Retrieved from http://naloxoneinfo.org/case-studies/standing-orders

O'Rourke, T. P., Girardi, G. J., Balaskas, T. N., Havlisch, R. A., Landstrom, G., Kirby, B., . . . Simpson, K. R. (2011). Implementation of a system-wide policy for labor induction. *MCN, The American Journal of Maternal Child Nursing, 36*(5), 305–311. doi:10.1097/NMC.0b013e3182069e12

Overdyk, F. J., Dowling, O., Newman, S., Glatt, D., Chester, M., Armellino, D., . . . DiCapua, J. F. (2016). Remote video auditing with real-time feedback in an academic surgical suite improves safety and efficiency metrics: A cluster randomised study. *BMJ Quality & Safety, 25*(12). doi:10.1136/bmjqs-2015-004226

Oxman, A. D., Sackett, D. L., & Guyatt, G. H. (1993). Users' guides to the medical literature: I. How to get started. The Evidence-Based Medicine Working Group. *JAMA, 270*(17), 2093–2095. doi:10.1001/jama.1993.03510170083036

Page, I., Hardy, G., Fairfield, J., Orr, D., & Nichani, R. (2011). Implementing surviving sepsis guidelines in a district general hospital. *Journal of the Royal College of Physicians of Edinburgh, 41*(4), 309–315. doi:10.4997/JRCPE.2011.405

Painter, M. (2013). Improving incentives. Prologue: You can't buy heroes: Aligning physician incentives doesn't do it. Robert Wood Johnson Foundation. Retrieved from http://www.hci3.org/wp-content/uploads/files/files/IssueBrief-HCI3-RWJF-2013-08-07.pdf

Pankratz, M., Hallfors, D., & Cho, H. (2002). Measuring perceptions of innovation adoption: The diffusion of a federal drug prevention policy. *Health Education Research, 17*(3), 315–326. doi:10.1093/her/17.3.315

Panzano, P. C., Sweeney, H. A., Seffrin, B., Massatti, R., & Knudsen, K. J. (2012). The assimilation of evidence-based healthcare innovations: A management-based perspective. *Journal of Behavioral Health Services & Research, 39*(4), 397–416. doi:10.1007/s11414-012-9294-y

Panzarella, K. J. (2003). *Assessing clinical competency in the health sciences* (Doctoral dissertation). Retrieved from State University of New York at Buffalo. (Volume 64–04, section A, p. 1211).

Parry, G. J., Carson-Stevens, A., Luff, D. F., McPherson, M. E., & Goldmann, D. A. (2013). Recommendations for evaluation of health care improvement initiatives. *Academic Pediatrics, 13*(Suppl. 6), S23–S30. doi:10.1016/j.acap.2013.04.007

Pasero, C., Quinlan-Colwell, A., Rae, D., Broglio, K., & Drew, D. (2016). American Society for Pain Management nursing position statement: Prescribing and administering opioid doses based solely on pain intensity. *Pain Management Nursing, 17*(3), 170–180. doi:10.1016/j.pmn.2016.03.001

Pashaeypoor, S., Ashktorab, T., Rassouli, M., & Alavi-Majd, H. (2016). Predicting the adoption of evidence-based practice using "Rogers diffusion of innovation model." *Contemporary Nurse, 52*(1), 85–94. doi:10.1080/10376178.2016.1188019

Payne, V. L., & Hysong, S. J. (2016). Model depicting aspects of audit and feedback that impact physicians' acceptance of clinical performance feedback. *BMC Health Services Research, 16*(260), 1–12. doi:10.1186/s12913-016-1486-3

Pearson, A. (2014). Evidence synthesis and its role in evidence-based health care. *The Nursing Clinics of North America, 49*(4), 453–460. doi:10.1016/j.cnur.2014.08.001

Peek, C. J. (2003). An evidence-based "elevator speech" for a practical world. *Families, Systems and Health, 21*(2), 135–139. doi:10.1037/1091-7527.21.2.135

Pelletier, L. G., & Sharp, E. (2008). Persuasive communication and proenvironmental behaviours: How message tailoring and message framing can improve the integration of behaviours through self-determined motivation. *Canadian Psychology, 49*(3), 210–217. doi:10.1037/a0012755

Peltan, I. D., Shiga, T., Gordon, J. A., & Currier, P. F. (2015). Simulation improves procedural protocol adherence during central venous catheter placement: A randomized controlled trial. *Simulation in Healthcare, 10*(5), 270–276. doi:10.1097/SIH.0000000000000096

Perla, R. J., Provost, L. P., Murray, S. K. (2011). The run chart: A simple analytical tool for learning from variation in healthcare processes. *BMJ Quality & Safety, 20*, 46–51. doi:10.1136/bmjqs.2009.037895

Perri-Moore, S., Kapsandoy, S., Doyon, K., Hill, B., Archer, M., Shane-McWhorter, L., . . . Zeng-Treitler, Q. (2016). Automated alerts and reminders targeting patients: A review of the literature. *Patient Education and Counseling, 99*(6), 953–959. doi:10.1016/j.pec.2015.12.010

Perry, S. B., Zeleznik, H., & Breisinger, T. (2014). Supporting clinical practice behavior change among neurologic physical therapists: A case study in knowledge translation. *Journal of Neurologic Physical Therapy, 38*(2), 134–143. doi:10.1097/NPT.0000000000000034

Peter, S., & Gill, F. (2009). Development of a clinical practice guideline for testing nasogastric tube placement. *Journal for Specialists in Pediatric Nursing, 14*(1), 3–11. doi:10.1111/j.1744-6155.2008.00161.x

Petersen, L. A., Simpson, K., Pietz, K., Urech, T. H., Hysong, S. J., Profit, J., . . . Woodard, L. D. (2013). Effects of individual physician-level and practice-level financial incentives on hypertension care: A randomized trial. *JAMA, 310*(10), 1042–1050. doi:10.1001/jama.2013.276303

Petitti, D. B., Teutsch, S. M., Barton, M. B., Sawaya, G. F., Ockene, J. K., & DeWitt, T. (2009). Update on the methods of the U.S. Preventive Services Task Force: Insufficient evidence. *Annals of Internal Medicine, 150*(3), 199–205. doi:10.7326/0003-4819-150-3-200902030-00010

Pezzolesi, C., Manser, T., Schifano, F., Kostrzewski, A., Pickles, J., Harriet, N., . . . Dhillon, S. (2013). Human factors in clinical handover: Development and testing of a "handover performance tool" for doctors' shift handovers. *International Journal for Quality in Health Care, 25*(1), 58–65. doi:10.1093/intqhc/mzs076

Piscotty, R. J., Kalisch, B., Gracey-Thomas, A., & Yarandi, H. (2015). Electronic nursing care reminders: Implications for nursing leaders. *Journal of Nursing Administration, 45*(5), 239–242. doi:10.1097/NNA.0000000000000192

Ploeg, J., Skelly, J., Rowan, M., Edwards, N., Davies, B., Grinspun, D., . . . Downey, A. (2010). The role of nursing best practice champions in diffusing practice guidelines: A mixed methods study. *Worldviews on Evidence-Based Nursing, 7*(4), 238–251. doi:10.1111/j.1741-6787.2010.00202.x

Poock, A. (2016, October). *Evidence-based nutrition screening for adult oncology patients in an ambulatory setting.* Presented at the Advanced Practice Institute: Promotion Adoption of Evidence-Based Practice, University of Iowa Hospitals and Clinics, Department of Nursing Services and Patient Care, Iowa City, IA.

Popovski, Z., Mercuri, M., Main, C., Sne, N., Walsh, K., Sung, M., . . . Mertz, D. (2015). Multifaceted intervention to optimize antibiotic use for intra-abdominal infections. *Journal of Antimicrobial Chemotherapy, 70*(4), 1226–1229. doi:10.1093/jac/dku498

Porter-O'Grady, T., Alexander, D. R., Blaylock, J., Minkara, N., & Surel, D. (2006). Constructing a team model: Creating a foundation for evidence-based teams. *Nursing Administration Quarterly, 30*(3), 211–220. doi:10.1097/00006216-200607000-00005

Portz, D., & Johnston, M. P. (2014). Implementation of an evidence-based education practice change for patients with cancer. *Clinical Journal of Oncology Nursing, 18*(5), 36–40. doi:10.1188/14.CJON.S2.36-40

Poulsen, M. N., Vandenhoudt, H., Wyckoff, S. C., Obong'o, C. O., Ochura, J., Njika, G., . . . Miller, K. S. (2010). Cultural adaptation of a U.S. evidence-based parenting intervention for rural Western Kenya: From parents matter! To families matter! *AIDS Education and Prevention, 22*(4), 273–285. doi:10.1521/aeap.2010.22.4.273

Powell, B. J., McMillen, J. C., Proctor, E. K., Carpenter, C. R., Griffey, R. T., Bunger, A. C., . . . York, J. L. (2012). A compilation of strategies for implementing clinical innovations in health and mental health. *Medical Care Research and Review, 69*(2), 123–157. doi:10.1177/1077558711430690

Prasad, V., & Ioannidis, J. P. (2014). Evidence-based de-implementation for contradicted, unproven, and aspiring healthcare practices. *Implementation Science, 9*(1), 1–5. doi:10.1186/1748-5908-9-1

Preferred Reporting Items for Systematic Reviews and Meta-Analyses (PRISMA). (2015). PRISMA statement. Retrieved from http://www.prisma-statement.org/

Prince, R. A., & Rogers, B. (2012, March 16). What is a thought leader? *Forbes.* Retrieved from https://www.forbes.com/sites/russprince/2012/03/16/what-is-a-thought-leader/#4c1119557da0

Proctor, E. K., Powell, B. J., & McMillen, J. C. (2013). Implementation strategies: Recommendations for specifying and reporting. *Implementation Science, 8*(139), 1–11. doi:10.1186/1748-5908-8-139

Pronovost, P. J., Demski, R., Callender, T., Winner, L., Miller, M. R., Austin, J. M., . . . National Leadership Core Measures Work Groups. (2013). Demonstrating high reliability on accountability measures at The Johns Hopkins Hospital. *The Joint Commission Journal on Quality and Patient Safety, 39*(12), 531–544. doi:10.1016/S1553-7250(13)39069-2

Pryse, Y. M. (2012). *Using evidence based practice: The relationship between work environment, nursing leadership, and nurses at the bedside* (Doctoral dissertation, Indiana University). Retrieved from https://scholarworks.iupui.edu/handle/1805/3220

Pryse, Y., McDaniel, A., & Schafer, J. (2014). Psychometric analysis of two new scales: The evidence-based practice nursing leadership and work environment scales. *Worldviews on Evidence-Based Nursing, 11*(4), 240–247. doi:10.1111/wvn.12045

Przybyl, H., Androwich, I., & Evans, J. (2015). Using high-fidelity simulation to assess knowledge, skills, and attitudes in nurses performing CRRT. *Nephrology Nursing Journal, 42*(2), 135–147.

Puetz, B. (2014). Strategic management. In D. Huber (Ed.), *Leadership and nursing care management* (5th ed.). St. Louis, MO: Elsevier Saunders.

Pusic, M. V., Boutis, K., Pecaric, M. R., Savenkov, O., Beckstead, J. W., & Jaber, M. Y. (2016). A primer on the statistical modelling of learning curves in health professions education. *Advances in Health Sciences Education.* doi:10.1007/s10459-016-9709-2

Puterman, M. L., Zhang, Y., Aydede, S. K., Palmer, B., MacLeod, S., Bavafa, H., & MacKenzie, J. (2013). "If you're not keeping score, you're just practicing": A Lean healthcare program evaluation framework. *Healthcare Quarterly, 16*(2), 23–30.

Putzer, G. J., & Park, Y. (2012). Are physicians likely to adopt emerging mobile technologies? Attitudes and innovation factors affecting smartphone use in the southeastern United States. *Perspectives in Health Information Management, 9*(Spring), 1b.

Qaseem, A., Snow, V., Owens, D. K., Shekelle, P., & Clinical Guidelines Committee of the American College of Physicians. (2010). The development of clinical practice guidelines and guidance statements of the American College of Physicians: Summary of methods. *Annals of Internal Medicine, 153*(3), 194–199. doi:10.7326/0003-4819-153-3-201008030-00010

QSEN Institute. (2012). Graduate QSEN competencies. Retrieved from http://qsen.org/competencies/graduate-ksas

Rabin, B. A., Brownson, R. C., Haire-Joshu, D., Kreuter, M. W., & Weaver, N. L. (2008). A glossary for dissemination and implementation research in health. *Journal of Public Health Management and Practice, 14*(2), 117–123. doi:10.1097/01.PHH.0000311888.06252.bb

Raja, A. S., Ip, I. K., Dunne, R. M., Schuur, J. D., Mills, A. M., & Khorasani, R. (2015). Effects of performance feedback reports on adherence to evidence-based guidelines in use of CT for evaluation of pulmonary embolism in the emergency department: A randomized trial. *American Journal of Roentgenology, 205*(5), 936–940. doi:10.2214/AJR.15.14677

Rangachari, P., Madaio, M., Rethemeyer, K., Wagner, P., Hall, L., Roy, S., & Rissing, P. (2014). Role of communication content and frequency in enabling evidence-based practices. *Quality Management in Health Care, 23*(1), 43–58. doi:10.1097/QMH.0000000000000017

Rankin, N. M., McGregor, D., Butow, P. N., White, K., Phillips, J. L., Young, J. M., . . . Shaw, T. (2016). Adapting the nominal group technique for priority setting of evidence-practice gaps in implementation science. *BMC Medical Research Methodology, 16*(110), 1–9. doi:10.1186/s12874-016-0210-7

Rash, C. J., DePhillipps, D., McKay, J. R., Drapkin, M., & Petry, N. M. (2013). Training workshops positively impact beliefs about contingency management in a nationwide dissemination effort. *Journal of Substance Abuse Treatment, 45*(3), 306–312. doi:10.1016/j.jsat.2013.03.003

Rashidian, A., Eccles, M. P., & Russell, I. (2008). Falling on stony ground? A qualitative study of implementation of clinical guidelines' prescribing recommendations in primary care. *Health Policy, 85*(1), 148–161.

Rassin, M., Kurzweil, Y., & Maoz, Y. (2015). Identification of the learning styles and "on-the-job" learning methods implemented by nurses for promoting their professional knowledge and skills. *International Journal of Nursing Education Scholarship, 12*(1), 75–81.doi:10.1515/ijnes-2015-0006

Registered Nurses' Association of Ontario. (2007). *Assessment and management of pain: Supplement.* Toronto, Ontario, Canada: Registered Nurses' Association of Ontario.

Registered Nurses' Association of Ontario. (2012). *Toolkit: Implementation of best practice guidelines* (2nd ed.). Toronto, ON: Registered Nurses' Association of Ontario.

Registered Nurses' Association of Ontario. (2013). *Developing and sustaining nursing leadership best practice guideline* (2nd ed.). Toronto, ON: Registered Nurses' Association of Ontario.

Reich, J. A., Goodstein, M. E., Callahan, S. E., Callahan, K. M., Crossley, L. W., Doron, S. I., . . . Nasraway, Jr., S. A. (2015). Physician report cards and rankings yield long-lasting hand hygiene compliance exceeding 90%. *Critical Care, 19.* doi:10.1186/x13054-015-1008-4

Research Toolkit. (2013). Primary Care Evidence Review Toolkit. Retrieved from http://researchtoolkit.org/index.php/disseminating-and-closing-research/disseminating-and-measuring-impact/item/7117-primary-care-evidence-review-toolkit

Reynolds, S. S., McLennon, S. M., Ebright, P. R., Murray, L. L., & Bakas, T. (2016). Program evaluation of neuroscience competency programs to implement evidence-based practices. *Journal of Evaluation in Clinical Practice, 23*(1), 149–155. doi:10.1111/jep.12654

Reynolds, S. S., Murray, L. L., McLennon, S. M., & Bakas, T. (2016). Implementation of a stroke competency program to improve nurses' knowledge of and adherence to stroke guidelines. *Journal of Neuroscience Nursing, 48*(6), 328–335.

Rice, M. (2010). Evidence-based practice problems: Form and focus. *Journal of the American Psychiatric Nurses Association, 16*(5), 307–314. doi:10.1177/1078390310374990

Richardson, J., & Tjoelker, R. (2012). Beyond the central line-associated bloodstream infection bundle: The value of the clinical nurse specialist in continuing evidence-based practice changes. *Clinical Nurse Specialist, 26*(4), 205–211. doi:10.1097/NUR.0b013e31825aebab

Richardson, W. S., Wilson, M. C., Nishikawa, J., & Hayward, R. S. (1995). The well-built clinical question: A key to evidence-based decisions. *ACP Journal Club, 123*(3), A12–A13. doi:10.7326/ACPJC-1995-123-3-A12

Rios, L., Ye, C., & Thabane, L. (2010). Association between framing of the research question using the PICOT format and reporting quality of randomized controlled trials. *BMC Medical Research Methodology, 10*(11), 1–8. doi:10.1186/1471-2288-10-11

Robert Wood Johnson Foundation. (2010). How to display comparative information that people can understand and use. Retrieved from http://www.rwjf.org/en/library/research/2010/07/how-to-display-comparative-information-that-people-can-understan.html

Robert Wood Johnson Foundation. (2013). Quality/equality glossary. Retrieved from http://www.rwjf.org/en/library/research/2013/04/quality-equality-glossary.html

Robinson, L., Paull, D. E., Mazzia, L. M., Falzetta, L., Hay, J., Neily, J., . . . Bagian, J. P. (2010). The role of the operating room nurse manager in the successful implementation of preoperative briefings and postoperative debriefings in the VHA Medical Team Training Program. *Journal of PeriAnesthesia Nursing, 25*(5), 302–306. doi:10.1016/j.jopan.2010.07.003

Robinson, S. T., & Kirsch, J. R. (2015). Lean strategies in the operating room. *Anesthesia Clinics, 33*(4), 713–730. doi:10.1016/j.anclin.2015.07.010

Rodriguez, L., Jung, H. S., Goulet, J. A., Cicalo, A., Machado-Aranda, D. A., & Napolitano, L. M. (2014). Evidence-based protocol for prophylactic antibiotics in open fractures: Improved antibiotic stewardship with no increase in infection rates. *Journal of Trauma and Acute Care Surgery, 77*(3), 400–407. doi:10.1097/TA.0000000000000398

Rogers, E. (2003). *Diffusion of innovations* (5th ed.). New York, NY: The Free Press.

Rondinelli, J., Ecker, M., Crawford, C., Seelinger, C., & Omery, A. (2012). Hourly rounding implementation: A multisite description of structures, processes, and outcomes. *Journal of Nursing Administration, 42*(6), 326–332. doi:10.1097/NNA.0b013e31824ccd43

Rosen, B. L., Goodson, P., Thompson, B., & Wilson, K. L. (2015). School nurses' knowledge, attitudes, perceptions of role as opinion leader, and professional practice regarding human papillomavirus vaccine for youth. *Journal of School Health, 85*(2), 73–81. doi:10.1111/josh.12229

Rosen, M. A., & Pronovost, P. J. (2014). Advancing the use of checklists for evaluating performance in health care. *Academic Medicine, 89*(7), 963–965. doi:10.1097/ACM.0000000000000285

Rosenthal, D. I., Mendoza, T. R., Chambers, M. S., Burkett, V. S., Garden, A. S., Hessell, A. C., . . . Cleeland, C. S. (2008). The M. D. Anderson symptom inventory—Head and neck module, a patient-reported outcome instrument, accurately predicts the severity of radiation-induced mucositis. *International Journal of Radiation Oncology, Biology, Physics, 72*(5), 1355–1361. doi:10.1016/j.ijrobp.2008.02.072

Rosenzweig, M., Giblin, J., Mickle, M., Morse, A., Sheehy, P., Sommer, V., & Bridging the Gap Working Group. (2012). Bridging the gap: A descriptive study of knowledge and skill needs in the first year of oncology nurse practitioner practice. *Oncology Nursing Forum, 39*(2), 195–201. doi:10.1188/12. ONF.195-201

Roush, K. (2017a). Becoming a published writer. *American Journal of Nursing, 117*(3), 63-66. doi:10.1097/01.NAJ.0000513291.04075.82

Roush, K. (2017b). Writing your manuscript: Structure and style. *American Journal of Nursing, 117*(4), 56–61. doi:10.1097/01.NAJ.0000515234.28924.7d

Royal College of Nursing. (2007). Developing and sustaining effective teams. Retrieved from https:// my.rcn.org.uk/__data/assets/pdf_file/0003/78735/003115.pdf

Ruhe, M. C., Weyer, S. M., Zronek, S., Wilkinson, A., Wilkinson, P. S., & Stange, K. C. (2005). Facilitating practice change: Lessons from the STEP-UP clinical trial. *Preventive Medicine, 40*(6), 729–734. doi:10.1016/j.ypmed.2004.09.015

Rushmer, R. K., Hunter, D. J., & Steven, A. (2014). Using interactive workshops to prompt knowledge exchange: A realist evaluation of a knowledge to action initiative. *Public Health, 128*(6), 552–560. doi:10.1016/j.puhe.2014.03.012

Russell, N. C. C., Wallace, L. M., & Ketley, D. (2011). Evaluation and measurement for improvement in service-level quality improvement initiatives. *Health Services Management Research, 24*(4), 182–189. doi:10.1258/hsmr.2011.011010

Sackett, D. L., Rosenberg, W. M., Gray, J. A., Haynes, R. B., & Richardson, W. S. (1996). Evidence based medicine: What it is and what it isn't. *British Medical Journal, 312*(7023), 71–72. doi:10.1136/ bmj.312.7023.71

Sackett, D. L., Straus, S. E., Richardson, W. S., Rosenberg, W., & Haynes, R. B. (2000). *Evidence-based medicine: How to practice and teach EBM* (2nd ed.). London, UK: Churchill Livingstone.

Sadler, B. L., Joseph, A., Keller, A., & Rostenberg, B. (2009). IHI Innovation Series white paper.: Using evidence-based environmental design to enhance safety and quality. Retrieved from http://www.ihi. org/resources/Pages/IHIWhitePapers/UsingEvidenceBasedEnvironmentalDesignWhitePaper.aspx

Salaripour, M., & Perl, T. (2013). The effectiveness and the retention level of the competency-based training for infection prevention and control practices. *The Canadian Journal of Infection Control, 28*(1), 13–17.

Salbach, N. M., Veinot, P., Jaglal, S. B., Bayley, M., & Rolfe, D. (2011). From continuing education to personal digital assistants: What do physical therapists need to support evidence-based practice in stroke management? *Journal of Evaluation in Clinical Practice, 17*(4), 786–793. doi:10.1111/ j.1365.2753.2010.01456.x

Sandström, B., Borglin, G., Nilsson, R., & Willman, A. (2011). Promoting the implementation of evidence-based practice: A literature review focusing on the role of nursing leadership. *Worldviews on Evidence-Based Nursing, 8*(4), 212–223. doi:10.1111/j.1741-6787.2011.00216.x

Saunders, H., & Vehviläinen-Julkunen, K. (2016). The state of readiness for evidence-based practice among nurses: An integrative review. *International Journal of Nursing Studies, 56,* 128–140. doi:10.1016/j.ijnurstu.2015.10.018

Saver, C. (2014). *Anatomy of writing for publication for nurses* (2nd ed.). Indianapolis, IN: Sigma Theta Tau International.

Schaffer, M. A., Sandau, K. E., & Diedrick, L. (2013). Evidence-based practice models for organizational change: Overview and practical applications. *Journal of Advanced Nursing, 69*(5), 1197–1209. doi:10.1111/j.1365-2648.2012.06122.x

Schardt, C., Adams, M. B., Owens, T., Keitz, S., & Fontelo, P. (2007). Utilization of the PICO framework to improve searching PubMed for clinical questions. *BMC Medical Informatics and Decision Making, 7*(16), 1–6. doi:10.1186/1472-6947-7-16

Schifalacqua, M. M., Shepard, A., & Kelley, W. (2012). Evidence-based practice: Cost-benefit of large system implementation. *Quality Management in Health Care, 21*(2), 74–80. doi:10.1097/QMH.0b013e31824d196f

Schifalacqua, M., Costello, C., & Denman, W. (2009). Roadmap for planned change, part 1: Change leadership and project management. *Nurse Leader, 7*(2), 26–29. doi:10.1016/j.mnl.2009.01.003

Schmaltz, S. (2011). A selection of statistical process control tools used in monitoring health care performance. Rockville, MD: Agency for Healthcare Research and Quality. Retrieved from http://qualitymeasures.ahrq.gov/expert/expert-commentary.aspx?id=16454

Schmidt, T. (2009). *Strategic project management made simple.* Hoboken, NJ: Wiley & Sons, Inc.

Schmittdiel, J. A., Adams, S. R., Goler, N., Sanna, R. S., Boccio, M., Bellamy, D. J., . . . Ferrara, A. (2017). The impact of telephonic wellness coaching on weight loss: A "Natural Experiments for Translation in Diabetes (NEXT-D)" study. *Obesity, 25*(2), 352–356. doi:10.1002/oby.21723

Schoville, R. R., Shever, L. L., Calarco, M. M., & Tschannen, D. (2014). A cost-benefit analysis: Electronic clinical procedural resource supporting evidence-based practice. *Nursing Economic$, 32*(5), 241–247.

Schreiner, M., Kudrna, B., & Kenney, C. (2015). How undergraduate students can contribute to EBP. *Nursing Management, 46*(9), 21–23. doi:10.1097/01.NUMA.0000470777.48225.b5

Schroeter, K. (2008). *Competence literature review.* Retrieved from http://www.cc-institute.org/docs/default-document-library/2011/10/19/competence_lit_review.pdf?Status=Master

Schweickert, P. A., Gaughen, J. R., Kreitel, E. M., Shephard, T. J., Solenski, N. J., & Jensen, M. E. (2016). An overview of antithrombotics in ischemic stroke. *Nurse Practitioner, 41*(6), 48–55. doi:10.1097/01.NPR.0000483077.47966.6e

Scott, A., Sivey, P., Ait Ouakrim, D., Willenberg, L., Naccarella, L., Furler, J., & Young, D. (2011). The effect of financial incentives on the quality of health care provided by primary care physicians. *Cochrane Database of Systematic Reviews, 2011*(9), 1–61. doi:10.1002/14651858.CD008451.pub2

Sebastián-Viana, T., Losa-Iglesias, M., González-Ruiz, J. M., Lema-Lorenzo, I., Núñez-Crespo, F. J., Salvadores Fuentes, P., . . . ARCE Team. (2016). Reduction in the incidence of pressure ulcers upon implementation of a reminder system for health-care providers. *Applied Nursing Research, 29,* 107–112. doi:10.1016/j.apnr.2015.05.018

Sehr, J., Eisele-Hlubocky, L., Junker, R., Johns, E., Birk, D., & Gaehle, K. (2013). Family pet visitation. *American Journal of Nursing, 113*(12), 54–59. doi:10.1097/01.NAJ.0000438869.75401.21

Selker, H., Grossman, C., Adams, A., Goldmann, D., Dezii, C., Meyer, G., . . . Platt, R. (2011). *The common rule and continuous improvement in health care: A learning health system perspective.* Washington, DC: Institute of Medicine.

Shah, B. R., Bhattacharyya, O., Yu, C. H. Y., Mamdani, M. M., Parsons, J. A., Straus, S. E., & Zwarenstein, M. (2014). Effect of an educational toolkit on quality of care: A pragmatic cluster randomized trial. *PLoS Medicine, 11*(2). doi:10.1371/journal.pmed.1001588

Shah, P. N., Narayanaswamy, R., & Khobragade. (2016). Anesthesia workstation ventilator malfunction due to accidental misplacement of a nasogastric tube. *Journal of Anaesthesiology Clinical Pharmacology, 32*(1), 116–117. doi:10.4103/0970-9185.173375

Shalom, E., Shahar, Y., Parmet, Y., & Lunenfeld, E. (2015). A multiple-scenario assessment of the effect of a continuous-care, guideline-based decision support system on clinicians' compliance to clinical guidelines. *International Journal of Medical Informatics, 84*(4), 248–262. doi:10.1016/j.ijmedinf.2015.01.004

Shapiro, S. E., & Donaldson, N. A. (2008). Evidence-based practice for advanced practice emergency nurses, part III: Planning, implementing, and evaluating an evidence-based small test of change. *Advanced Emergency Nursing Journal, 30*(3), 222–232. doi:10.1097/01.TME.0000334374.36905.69

Sheakley, M. L., Gilbert, G. E., Leighton, K., Hall, M., Callender, D., & Pederson, D. (2016). A brief simulation intervention increasing basic science and clinical knowledge. *Medical Education Online, 21.* doi:10.3402/meo.v21.30744

Shimizu, Y., & Shimanouchi, S. (2006). Effective components of staff and organizational development for client outcomes by implementation of action plans in home care. *International Medical Journal, 13*(3), 175–183.

Shirey, M. R., Hauck, S. L., Embree, J. L., Kinner, T. J., Schaar, G. L., Phillips, L. A., . . . McCool, I. A. (2011). Showcasing differences between quality improvement, evidence-based practice, and research. *Journal of Continuing Education in Nursing, 42*(2), 57–70. doi:10.3928/00220124-20100701-01

Shoemaker, L. K., & Fischer, B. (2011). Creating a nursing strategic planning framework based on evidence. *Nursing Clinics of North America, 46*(1), 11–25. doi:10.1016/j.cnur.2010.10.007

Shojania, K. G., Jennings, A., Mayhew, A., Ramsay, C. R., Eccles, M. P., & Grimshaw, J. (2009). The effects of on-screen, point of care computer reminders on processes and outcomes of care. *Cochrane Database of Systematic Reviews, 2009*(3), 1–70. doi:10.1002/14651858.CD001096.pub2

Shojania, K. G., Jennings, A., Mayhew, A., Ramsay, C., Eccles, M., & Grimshaw, J. (2010). Effect of point-of-care computer reminders on physician behaviour: A systematic review. *Canadian Medical Association Journal, 182*(5), E216–E225. doi:10.1503/cmaj.090578

Sidani, S., Manojlovich, M., Doran, D., Fox, M., Covell, C. L., Kelly, H., . . . McAllister, M. (2016). Nurses' perceptions of interventions for the management of patient-oriented outcomes: A key factor for evidence-based practice. *Worldviews on Evidence-Based Nursing, 13*(1), 66–74. doi:10.1111/wvn.12129

Siedlecki, S. L. (2017). How to create a poster that attracts an audience. *American Journal of Nurses, 117*(3), 48–54. doi:10.1097/01.NAJ.0000513287.29624.7e

Siering, U., Eikermann, M., Hausner, E., Hoffman-Eßer, W., & Neugebauer, E. A. (2013). Appraisal tools for clinical practice guidelines: A systematic review. *PLoS ONE, 8*(12), e82915. doi:10.1371/journal. pone.0082915

Sigma Theta Tau International 2005-2007 Research and Scholarship Advisory Committee. (2008). Sigma Theta Tau International position statement on evidence-based practice. February 2007 summary. *Worldviews on Evidence-Based Nursing, 5*(2), 57–59. doi:10.1111/j.1741-6787.2008.00118.x

Simpson, D. (2016). "Going up?" A sport psychology consultant's guide to the elevator speech. *Journal of Sport Psychology in Action, 7*(2), 109–120. doi:10.1080/21520704.2016.1182091

Siriwardena, A. N., & Gillam, S. (2014). Evaluating improvement. *Quality in Primary Care, 22*(2), 63–70.

Six Sigma study guide (2014, January 20). Run chart: Creation, analysis, & rules. Retrieved from http://sixsigmastudyguide.com/run-chart

Sleutel, M. R., Barbosa-Leiker, C., & Wilson, M. (2015). Psychometric testing of the Health Care Evidence-Based Practice Assessment Tool. *Journal of Nursing Measurement, 23*(3), 485–498. doi:10.1891/1061-3749.23.3.485

Smith, C. D., & Korenstein, D. (2015). Harnessing the power of peer pressure to reduce health care waste and improve clinical outcomes. *Mayo Clinic Proceedings, 90*(3), 311–312. doi:10.1016/j.mayocp.2015.01.011

Smith, G. C. S., & Pell, J. P. (2003). Parachute use to prevent death and major trauma related to gravitational challenge: Systematic review of randomised controlled trials. *British Medical Journal, 327,* 1459–1461. doi:10.1136/bmj.327.7429.1459

Smith, J. B., Lacey, S. R., Williams, A. R., Teasley, S. L., Olney, A., Hunt, C., . . . Kemper, C. (2011). Developing and testing a clinical information system evaluation tool: Prioritizing modifications through end-user input. *Journal of Nursing Administration, 41*(6), 252–258. doi:10.1097/NNA.0b013e31821c4634

Smith, J. M. (2014). *Meaningful graphs: Converting data into informative Excel® charts.* United States of America: Author.

Smith, S. W., Nazione, S., Laplante, C., Kotowski, M. R., Atkin, C., Skubisz, C. M., . . . Stohl, C. (2009). Topics and sources of memorable breast cancer messages and their impact on prevention and detection behaviors. *Journal of Health Communication, 14*(3), 293–307. doi:10.1080/10810730902805903

Smitz Naranjo, L. L., & Viswanatha Kaimal, P. (2011). Applying Donabedian's theory as a framework for bariatric surgery accreditation. *Bariatric Nursing and Surgical Patient Care, 6*(1), 33–37. doi:10.1089/bar.2011.9979

Snipelisky, D., Duello, K., Gallup, S., Myrick, J., Taylor, V., Yip. D., . . . Burton, M. C. (2016). Feasibility of canine therapy among hospitalized pre-heart transplant patients. *Southern Medical Journal, 109*(3), 154–157. doi:10.14423/SMJ.0000000000000420

Son, C., Chuck, T., Childers, T., Usiak, S., Dowling, M., Andiel, C., . . . Sepkowitz, K. (2011). Practically speaking: Rethinking hand hygiene improvement programs in health care settings. *American Journal of Infection Control, 39*(9), 716–724. doi:10.1016/j.ajic.2010.12.008

Song, E. H., Shirazian, A., Binns, B., Fleming, Y., Ferreira, L. M., Rohrich, R. J., & Azari, K. (2012). Benchmarking academic plastic surgery services in the United States. *Plastic and Reconstructive Surgery, 129*(6), 1407–1418.

Sonstein, L., Clark, C., Seidensticker, S., Zeng, L., & Sharma, G. (2014). Improving adherence for management of acute exacerbation of chronic obstructive pulmonary disease. *American Journal of Medicine, 127*(11), 1097–1104. doi:10.1016/j.amjmed.2014.05.033

Soo, S., Berta, W., & Baker, G. R. (2009). Role of champions in the implementation of patient safety practice change [Special issue]. *Healthcare Quarterly, 12,* 123–128. doi:10.12927/hcq.2009.20979

Soumerai, S. B., & Avorn, J. (1990). Principles of educational outreach ('academic detailing') to improve clinical decision making. *Journal of the American Medical Association, 263*(4), 549–556. doi:10.1001/jama.1990.03440040088034

Sparger, K., Selgas, M., Collins, P. M., Lindgren, C. L., Massieu, M., & Castillow, A. S. (2012). The EBP rollout process. *Nursing Management, 43*(5), 14–20. doi:10.1097/01.NUMA.0000413650.72966.f4

Spence, A. D., Derbyshire, S., Walsh, I. K., & Murray, J. M. (2016). Does video feedback analysis improve CPR performance in Phase 5 medical students? *BMC Medical Education, 16*(203), 1–7. doi:10.1186/s12909-016-0726-x

Sprakes, K., & Tyrer, J. (2010). Improving wound and pressure area care in a nursing home. *Nursing Standard, 25*(10), 43–49. doi:10.7748/ns2010.11.25.10.43.c8092

Spurlock, D., Jr., & Wonder, A. H. (2015). Validity and reliability evidence for a new measure: The Evidence-Based Practice Knowledge Assessment in Nursing. *Journal of Nursing Education, 54*(11), 605–613. doi:10.3928/01484834-20151016-01

Spyridonidis, D., & Calnan, M. (2011). Opening the black box: A study of the process of NICE guidelines implementation. *Health Policy, 102*(2–3), 117–125. doi:10.1016/j.healthpol.2011.06.011

Squires, J. E., Moralejo, D., & Lefort, S. M. (2007). Exploring the role of organizational policies and procedures in promoting research utilization in registered nurses. *Implementation Science, 2,* (17), 1–11. doi:10.1186/1748-5908-2-17

Srigley, J. A., Corace, K., Hargadon, D. P., Yu, D., MacDonald, T., Fabrigar, L., & Garberg, G. (2015). Applying psychological frameworks of behaviour change to improve healthcare worker hand hygiene: A systematic review. *Journal of Hospital Infection, 91*(3), 202–210. doi:10.1016/j.jhin.2015.06.019

Stacey, D., Légaré, F., Col, N. F., Bennett, C. L., Barry, M. J., Eden, K. B., . . . Wu, J. H. (2014). Decision aids for people facing health treatment or screening decisions. *Cochrane Database of Systematic Reviews, 28*(1), 1–335. doi:10.1002/14651858.CD001431.pub4

Stacey, D., Légaré, F., Lewis, K., Barry, M. J., Bennett, C. L., Eden, K. B., . . . Trevena, L. (2017). Decision aids for people facing health treatment or screening decisions. *Cochrane Database of Systematic Reviews* (4). doi:10.1002/14651858.CD001431.pub5

Standards for Quality Improvement Reporting Excellence (SQUIRE). (2015). SQUIRE 2.0. Retrieved from http://www.squire-statement.org/index.cfm?fuseaction=Page.ViewPage&PageID=471

Statistics How To. (2013). Make a histogram in easy steps. Retrieved from http://www.statisticshowto.com/make-histogram

Stebral, L. L., & Steelman, V. M. (2006). Double gloving for surgical procedures: An evidence-based practice project. *Perioperative Nursing Clinics, 1*(3), 251–260.

Stenberg, M., & Wann-Hansson, C. (2011). Health care professionals' attitudes and compliance to clinical practice guidelines to prevent falls and fall injuries. *Worldviews on Evidence-Based Nursing, 8*(2), 87–95. doi:10.1111/j.1741-6787.2010.00196.x

Stetler, C. B., Legro, M. W., Rycroft-Malone, J., Bowman, C., Curran, G., Guihan, M., . . . Wallace, C. M. (2006). Role of "external facilitation" in implementation of research findings: A qualitative evaluation of facilitation experiences in the Veterans Health Administration. *Implementation Science, 1*(23), 1–15.

Stetler, C. B., Ritchie, J. A., Rycroft-Malone, J., & Charns, M. P. (2014). Leadership for evidence-based practice: Strategic and functional behaviors for institutionalizing EBP. *Worldviews on Evidence-Based Nursing, 11*(4), 219–226. doi:10.1111/wvn.12044

Stevens, K. R. (2009). *Essential competencies for evidence-based practice in nursing* (2nd ed.). San Antonio, TX: Academic Center for Evidence-Based Practice (ACE) of The University of Texas Health Science Center at San Antonio.

Stichler, J. F. (2007). Leadership roles for nurses in healthcare design. *Journal of Nursing Administration, 37*(12), 527–530. doi:10.1097/01.NNA.0000302390.29485.7a

Stillwell, S. B., Fineout-Overholt, E., Melnyk, B. M., & Williamson, K. M. (2010). Evidence-based practice, step by step: Asking the clinical question: A key step in evidence-based practice. *American Journal of Nursing, 110*(3), 58–61. doi:10.1097/01.NAJ.0000368959.11129.79

Stone, P. W., Glied, S. A., McNair, P. D., Matthes, N., Cohen, B., Landers, T. F., & Larson, E. L. (2010). CMS changes in reimbursement for HAIs: Setting a research agenda. *Medical Care, 48*(5), 433–439. doi:10.1097/MLR.0b013e3181d5fb3f

Summerfield, M. R., & Feemster, A. A. (2015). Composing effective and efficient e-mails: A primer for pharmacy practitioners. *Hospital Pharmacy, 50*(8), 683–689. doi:10.1310/hpj5008-683

Sung, H.-C., Chang, A. M., & Abbey, J. (2008). An implementation programme to improve nursing home staff's knowledge of and adherence to an individualized music protocol. *Journal of Clinical Nursing, 17*(19), 2573–2579. doi:10.1111/j.1365-2702.2007.02010.x

Sveinsdóttir, H., Ragnarsdóttir, E. D., & Blöndal, K. (2016). Praise matters: The influence of nurse unit managers' praise on nurses' practice, work environment and job satisfaction: A questionnaire study. *Journal of Advanced Nursing, 72*(3), 558–568. doi:10.1111/jan.12849

Szilagyi, P. G., Serwint, J. R., Humiston, S. G., Rand, C. M., Schaffer, S., Vincelli, P., . . . Curtis, C. R. (2015). Effect of provider prompts on adolescent immunization rates: A randomized trial. *Academic Pediatrics, 15*(2), 149–157. doi:10.1016/j.acap.2014.10.006

Tandon, S. D., Phillips, K., Bordeaux, B. C., Bone, L., Brown, P. B., Cagney, K. A., . . . Bass, E. B. (2007). A vision for progress in community health partnerships. *Progress in Community Health Partnerships, 1*(1), 11–30. doi:10.1353/cpr.0.0007

Tannenbaum, D., Doctor, J. N., Persell, S. D., Friedberg, M. W., Meeker, D., Friesema, E. M., . . . Fox, C. R. (2015). Nudging physician prescription decisions by partitioning the order set: Results of a vignette-based study. *Journal of General Internal Medicine, 30*(3), 298–304. doi:10.1007/s11606-014-3051-2

Taxman, F. S., & Belenko, S. (2011). Incorporating clinician and other staff input. In F.S. Taxman & S. Belenko (Eds.), *Implementing evidence-based practices in community corrections and addiction treatment* (p. 222). New York, NY: Springer Publishing.

Taylor, N., Clay-Williams, R., Hogden, E., Braithwaite, J., & Groene, O. (2015). High performing hospitals: A qualitative systematic review of associated factors and practical strategies for improvement. *BMC Health Services Research, 15*(244), 1–22. doi:10.1186/s12913-015-0879-z

Teela, K. C., De Silva, D. A., Chapman, K., Synnes, A. R., Sawchuck, D., Basso, M., . . . Magee, L. A. (2015). Magnesium sulphate for fetal neuroprotection: Benefits and challenges of a systematic knowledge translation project in Canada. *BMC Pregnancy and Childbirth, 15*(347), 1–13. doi:10.1186/s12884-015-0785-8

ten Ham, W., Minnie, K., & van der Walt, C. (2016). Integrative review of benefit levers' characteristics for system-wide spread of best healthcare practices. *Journal of Advanced Nursing, 72*(1), 33–49. doi:10.1111/jan.12814

Tessier, D., Sarrazin, P., Nicaise, V., & Dupont, J. P. (2015). The effects of persuasive communication and planning on intentions to be more physically active and on physical activity behaviour among low-active adolescents. *Psychology & Health, 30*(5), 583–604. doi:10.1080/08870446.2014.996564

The Joint Commission. (2017a). National patient safety goals. Retrieved from https://www.jointcommission.org/standards_information/npsgs.aspx

The Joint Commission. (2017b). What is certification? Retrieved from https://www.jointcommission.org/certification/certification_main.aspx

Thompson, C., McCaughan, D., Cullum, N., Sheldon, T. A., Mulhall, A., & Thompson, D. R. (2001a). The accessibility of research-based knowledge for nurses in United Kingdom acute care settings. *Journal of Advanced Nursing, 36*(1), 11–22. doi:10.1046/j.1365-2648.2001.01938.x

Thompson, C., McCaughan, D., Cullum, N., Sheldon, T. A., Mulhall, A., & Thompson, D. R. (2001b). Research information in nurses' clinical decision-making: What is useful? *Journal of Advanced Nursing, 36*(3), 376–388. doi:10.1046/j.1365-2648.2001.01985.x

Thought leader. (n.d.). Retrieved from https://en.wikipedia.org/wiki/Thought_leader

Titler, M. G. (2008). The evidence for evidence-based practice implementation. In R. Hughes (Ed.), *Patient safety & quality: An evidence-based handbook for nurses* (pp. 126–173). Rockville, MD: Agency for Healthcare Research and Quality. Retrieved from https://archive.ahrq.gov/professionals/clinicians-providers/resources/nursing/resources/nurseshdbk/nurseshdbk.pdf

Titler, M. G. (2010). Translation science and context. *Research and Theory for Nursing Practice, 24*(1), 35–55. doi:10.1891/1541-6577.24.1.35

Titler, M. G., Conlon, P., Reynolds, M. A., Ripley, R., Tsodikov, A., Wilson, D. S., & Montie, M. (2016). The effect of a translating research into practice intervention to promote use of evidence-based fall prevention interventions in hospitalized adults: A prospective pre-post implementation study in the U.S. *Applied Nursing Research, 31,* 52–59. doi:10.1016/j.apnr.2015.12.004

Titler, M. G., & Drahozal, R. (1997). Family pet visiting, animal-assisted activities, and animal-assisted therapy in critical care. In M. Chulay & N. C. Molter (Eds.), *Protocols for practice: Creating a healing environment series* (pp. 1–64). Aliso Viejo, CA: American Association of Critical-Care Nurses.

Titler, M. G., Kleiber, C., Steelman, V., Goode, C., Rakel, B., Barry-Walker, J., . . . Buckwalter, K. (1994). Infusing research into practice to promote quality care. *Nursing Research, 43*(5), 307–313. doi:10.1097/00006199-199409000-00009

Titler, M. G., Kleiber, C., Steelman, V. J., Rakel, B. A., Budreau, G., Everett, L. Q., . . . Goode, C. J. (2001). The Iowa Model of Evidence-Based Practice to promote quality care. *Critical Care Nursing Clinics of North America, 13*(4), 497–509.

Titler, M. G., Herr, K., Brooks, J. M., Xie, X. J., Ardery, G., Schilling, M. L., . . . Clarke, W. R. (2009). Translating research into practice intervention improves management of acute pain in older hip fracture patients. *Health Services Research, 44*(1), 264–287. doi:10.1111/j.1475-6773.2008.00913.x

Tolley, K., Marks-Maran, D., & Burke, L. (2010). The snapshot tool: A new form of practice assessment. *British Journal of Nursing, 19*(14), 905–911. doi:10.12968/bjon.2010.19.14.49049

Tomatis, C., Taramona, C., Rizo-Patrón, E., Hernández, F., Rodríguez, P., Piscoya, A., . . . Estrada, C. A. (2011). Evidence-based medicine training in a resource-poor country, the importance of leveraging personal and institutional relationships. *Journal of Evaluation in Clinical Practice, 17*(4), 644–650. doi:10.1111/j.1365-2753.2011.01635.x

Toole, N., Meluskey, T., & Hall, N. (2016). A systematic review: Barriers to hourly rounding. *Journal of Nursing Management, 24*(3), 283–290. doi:10.1111/jonm.12332

Treadwell, J. R., Lucas, S., & Tsou, A. Y. (2014). Surgical checklists: A systematic review of impacts and implementation. *BMJ Quality & Safety, 23*(4), 299–318. doi:10.1136/bmjqs-2012-001797

Tucker, S. (2011, August). *Journal article review and evidence-based practice: How to begin.* Presented at Ambulatory Surgery Center Nurse Enrichment Series, University of Iowa Hospitals and Clinics, Iowa City, IA.

Tucker, S. J., Bieber, P. L., Attlesey-Pries, J. M., Olson, M. E., & Dierkhising, R. A. (2012). Outcomes and challenges in implementing hourly rounds to reduce falls in orthopedic units. *Worldviews on Evidence-Based Nursing, 9*(1), 18–29. doi:10.1111/j.1741-6787.2011.00227.x

Turck, C. J., Silva, M. A., Tremblay, S. R., & Sachse, S. L. (2014). A preliminary study of health care professionals' preferences for infographics versus conventional abstracts for communicating the results of clinical research. *Journal of Continuing Education in the Health Professions, 34*(Suppl. 1), S36–S38. doi:10.1002/chp.21232

Ubbink, D. T., Guyatt, G. H., & Vermeulen, H. (2013). Framework of policy recommendations for implementation of evidence-based practice: A systematic scoping review. *BMJ Open, 3*. doi:10.1136/bmjopen-2012-001881

Ubel, P. A., & Asch, D. A. (2015). Creating value in health by understanding and overcoming resistance to de-innovation. *Health Affairs, 34*(2), 239–244. doi:10.1377/hlthaff.2014.0983

Upenieks, V. V., & Sitterding, M. (2008). Achieving Magnet redesignation: A framework for cultural change. *Journal of Nursing Administration, 38*(10), 419–428. doi:10.1097/01.NNA.0000338154.25600.e0

Urquhart, R., Porter, G. A., & Grunfeld, E. (2011). Reflections on knowledge brokering within a multidisciplinary research team. *Journal of Continuing Education in the Health Professions, 31*(4), 283–290. doi:10.1002/chp.20128

U.S. Department of Health & Human Services (USDHHS). (n.d.-a). Office for Human Research Protections. Retrieved from https://www.hhs.gov/ohrp/

U.S. Department of Health & Human Services (USDHHS). (n.d.-b). Quality improvement activities FAQs. Retrieved from https://www.hhs.gov/ohrp/regulations-and-policy/guidance/faq/quality-improvement-activities/index.html

U.S. National Library of Medicine. (2008). Home. Retrieved from http://www.nlm.nih.gov

U.S. National Library of Medicine. (2016). Medical Subject Headings. Retrieved from https://www.nlm.nih.gov/mesh/meshhome.html

U.S. Preventive Services Task Force (USPSTF). (2016a). Home. Retrieved from https://www.uspreventiveservicestaskforce.org

U.S. Preventive Services Task Force (USPSTF). (2016b). Grade definitions. Retrieved from http://www.uspreventiveservicestaskforce.org/Page/Name/grade-definitions

Vaccaro, A. R., Fisher, C. G., Whang, P., Patel, A., Prasad, S., Mulpuri, K., . . . Thomas, K. (2010). Evidence and impact: Should these articles change the practice of spine care? An evidence-based medicine process. *Spine, 35*(6), E176–E177. doi:10.1097/BRS.0b013e3181d938df

Vachon, B., Désorcy, B., Gaboury, I., Camirand, M., Rodrigue, J., Quesnel, L., . . . Grimshaw, J. (2015). Combining administrative data feedback, reflection and action planning to engage primary care professionals in quality improvement: Qualitative assessment of short term program outcomes. *BMC Health Services Research, 15*(391), 1–8. doi:10.1186/s12913-015-1056-0

van Bodegom-Vos, L., Davidoff, F., & Marang-van de Mheen, P. J. (2016). Implementation and de-implementation: Two sides of the same coin? *BMJ Quality & Safety, 26*(6), 495–501. doi:10.1136/bmjqs-2016-005473

van der Voort, P. H., van der Veer, S. N., & de Vos, M. L. (2012). The use of indicators to improve the quality of intensive care: Theoretical aspects and experiences from the Dutch intensive care registry. *Acta Anaesthesiologica Scandinavica, 56*(9), 1084–1091. doi:10.1111/j.1399-6576.2012.02687.x

van der Zijpp, T. J., Niessen, T., Eldh, A. C., Hawkes, C., McMullan, C., Mockford, C., . . . Seers, K. (2016). A bridge over turbulent waters: Illustrating the interaction between managerial leaders and facilitators when implementing research evidence. *Worldviews on Evidence-Based Nursing, 13*(1), 25–31. doi:10.1111/wvn.12138

VanDeusen Lukas, C., Engle, R. L., Holmes, S. K., Parker, V. A., Petzel, R. A., Nealon Seiberg, M., . . . Sullivan, J. L. (2010). Strengthening organizations to implement evidence-based clinical practices. *Health Care Management Review, 35*(3), 235–245. doi:10.1097/HMR.0b013e3181dde6a5

Van Hoof, T. J., Harrison, L. G., Miller, N. E., Pappas, M. S., & Fischer, M. A. (2015). Characteristics of academic detailing: Results of a literature review. *American Health & Drug Benefits, 8*(8), 414–422.

van Riet Paap, J., Vernooij-Dassen, M., Sommerbakk, R., Moyle, W., Hjermstad, M. J., Leppert, W., . . . IMPACT Research Team (2015). Implementation of improvement strategies in palliative care: An integrative review. *Implementation Science, 10*(103), 1–9. doi:10.1186/s13012-015-0293-2

Veness, M. (2010). Strategies to successfully publish your first manuscript. *Journal of Medical Imaging and Radiation Oncology, 54*(4), 395–400. doi:10.1111/j.1754-9485.2010.02186.x

Veniegas, R. C., Kao, U. H., Rosales, R., & Arellanes, M. (2009). HIV prevention technology transfer: Challenges and strategies in the real world. *American Journal of Public Health, 99*(Suppl. 1), S124–S130. doi:10.2105/AJPH.2007.124263

Venkatasalu, M. R., Kelleher, M., & Shao, C. H. (2015). Reported clinical outcomes of high-fidelity simulation versus classroom-based end-of-life care education. *International Journal of Palliative Nursing, 21*(4), 179–186. doi:10.12968/ijpn.2015.21.4.179

Vigorito, M. C., McNicoll, L., Adams, L., & Sexton, B. (2011). Improving safety culture results in Rhode Island ICUs: Lessons learned from the development of action-oriented plans. *Joint Commission Journal on Quality & Patient Safety, 37*(11), 509–514. doi:10.1016/S1553-7250(11)37065-1

Vollman, K. M. (2013). Interventional patient hygiene: Discussion of the issues and a proposed model for implementation of the nursing care basics. *Intensive & Critical Care Nursing, 29*(5), 250–255. doi:10.1016/j.iccn.2013.04.004

Wade, T. J., & Webb, T. P. (2013). Tackling technical skills competency: A surgical skills rating tool. *Journal of Surgical Research, 181*(1), 1–5. doi:10.1016/j.jss.2012.05.052

Wagner, M., Matthews, G., & Cullen, L. (2013). Promoting evidence-based nursing procedures by partnering with a vendor. *Journal of PeriAnesthesia Nursing, 28*(5), 300–309. doi:10.1016/j.jopan.2013.07.003

Walker, E. M., Mwaria, M., Coppola, N., & Chen, C. (2014). Improving the replication success of evidence-based interventions: Why a preimplementation phase matters. *Journal of Adolescent Health, 54*(Suppl. 3), S24–S28. doi:10.1016/j.jadohealth.2013.11.028

Walston, S. L., & Chou, A. F. (2006). Healthcare restructuring and hierarchical alignment: Why do staff and managers perceive change outcomes differently? *Medical Care, 44*(9), 879–889.

Wang, A., Grayburn, P., Foster, J. A., McCulloch, M. L., Badhwar, V., Gammie, J. S., . . . Martin, R. P. (2016). Practice gaps in the care of mitral valve regurgitation: Insights from the American College of Cardiology mitral regurgitation gap analysis and advisory panel. *American Heart Journal, 172,* 70–79. doi:10.1016/j.ahj.2015.11.003

Wang, M.-Y., Kao, C.-C., & Lin, C.-F. (2015). The EPCOR model: A model for promoting the successful implementation of evidence-based nursing in hospital-based settings. *Journal of Nursing Research, 23*(1), 15–24. doi:10.1097/jnr.0000000000000061

Ware, L. J., Herr, K. A., Booker, S. S., Dotson, K., Key, J., Poindexter, N., . . . Packard, A. (2015). Psychometric evaluation of the Revised Iowa Pain Thermometer (IPT-R) in a sample of diverse cognitively intact and impaired older adults: A pilot study. *Pain Management Nursing, 16*(4), 475–482. doi:10.1016/j.pmn.2014.09.004

Waring, J., Currie, G., Crompton, A., & Bishop, S. (2013). An exploratory study of knowledge brokering in hospital settings: Facilitating knowledge sharing and learning for patient safety? *Social Science and Medicine, 98,* 79–86. doi:10.1016j.socscimed.2013.08.037

Warren, J. I., Montgomery, K. L., & Friedmann, E. (2016). Three-year pre-post analysis of EBP integration in a Magnet-designated community hospital. *Worldviews on Evidence-Based Nursing, 13*(1), 50–58. doi:10.1111/wvn.12148

Watson, C. A., Bulechek, G. M., & McCloskey, J. C. (1987). QAMUR: A quality assurance model using research. *Journal of Nursing Quality Assurance, 2*(1), 21–27.

Watson, R., Stimpson, A., Topping, A., & Porock, D. (2002). Clinical competence assessment in nursing: A systematic review of the literature. *Journal of Advanced Nursing, 39*(5), 421–431. doi:10.1046/j.1365-2648.2002.02307.x

Web of Science. (2016). InCites journal citation reports. Retrieved from https://jcr.incites.thomsonreuters.com

Web Sites and Sound Bites. (2011). Sound bites. Retrieved from http://www.websitesandsoundbites.com/soundbites.htm

Weddig, J., Baker, S. S., & Auld, G. (2011). Perspectives of hospital-based nurses on breastfeeding initiation best practices. *Journal of Obstetric, Gynecologic, and Neonatal Nursing, 40*(2), 166–178. doi:10.1111/j.1552-6909.2011-01232.x

Weisner, T. S., & Cameron Hay, M. (2015). Practice to research: Integrating evidence-based practices with culture and context. *Transcultural Psychiatry, 52*(2), 222–243. doi:10.1177/1363461514557066

Weled, B. J., Adzhigirey, L. A., Hodgman, T. M., Brilli, R. J., Spevetz, A., Kline, A. M., . . . Wheeler, D. S. (2015). Critical care delivery: The importance of process of care and ICU structure to improved outcomes: An update from the American College of Critical Care Medicine Task Force on models of critical care. *Critical Care Medicine, 43*(7), 1520–1525. doi:10.1097/CCM.0000000000000978

Wensing, M., Bosch, M., & Grol, R. (2010). Developing and selecting interventions for translating knowledge to action. *Canadian Medical Association Journal, 182*(2), E85–E88. doi:10.1503/cmaj.081233

Wenzel, V., Dünser, M. W., & Lindner, K. H. (2011). A step-by-step guide to writing a scientific manuscript. Retrieved from http://www.anrianovara.org/file/stepbystepguide1.pdf

Whitehill King, K., Freimuth, V., Lee, M., & Johnson-Turbes, C. A. (2013). The effectiveness of bundled health messages on recall. *American Journal of Health Promotion, 27*(Suppl. 3), S28–S35. doi:10.4278/ajhp.120113-QUAN-27

Wieck, K. L., Dols, J., & Northam, S. (2009). What nurses want: The nurse incentives project. *Nursing Economic$, 27*(3), 169–177, 201.

Wigder, H. N., Cohan Ballis, S. F., Lazar, L., Urgo, R., & Dunn, B. H. (1999). Successful implementation of a guideline by peer comparisons, education, and positive physician feedback. *Journal of Emergency Medicine, 17*(5), 807–810.

Willems, M., Schröder, C., van der Weijden, T., Post, M. W., & Visser-Meily, A. M. (2016). Encouraging post-stroke patients to be active seems possible: Results of an intervention study with knowledge brokers. *Disability and Rehabilitation, 38*(17), 1748–1755. doi:10.3109/09638288.2015.1107644

Williams, B., Perillo, S., & Brown, T. (2015). What are the factors of organisational culture in health care settings that act as barriers to the implementation of evidence-based practice? A scoping review. *Nurse Education Today, 35*(2), e34–e41. doi:10.1016/j.nedt.2014.11.012

Williams, J. L., & Cullen, L. (2016). Evidence into practice: Disseminating an evidence-based practice project as a poster. *Journal of PeriAnesthesia Nursing, 31*(5), 440–444. doi:10.1016/j.jopan.2016.07.002

Williams, J. R., Caceda-Castro, L. E., Dusablon, T., & Stipa, M. (2016). Design, development, and evaluation of printed educational materials for evidence-based practice dissemination. *International Journal of Evidence-Based Healthcare, 14*(2), 84–94. doi:10.1097/XEB.0000000000000072

Wilson, M., Ice, S., Nakashima, C. Y., Cox, L. A., Morse, E. C., Philip, G., & Vuong, E. (2015). Striving for evidence-based practice innovations through a hybrid model journal club: A pilot study. *Nurse Education Today, 35*(5), 657–662. doi:10.1016/jnedt.2015.01.026

Wilson, M., Sleutel, M., Newcomb, P., Behan, D., Walsh, J., Wells, J. N., & Baldwin, K. M. (2015). Empowering nurses with evidence-based practice environments: Surveying Magnet, Pathway to Excellence, and non-Magnet facilities in one healthcare system. *Worldviews on Evidence-Based Nursing, 12*(1), 12–21. doi:10.1111/wvn.12077

Wiltsey Stirman, S., Kimberly, J., Cook, N., Calloway, A., Castro, F., & Charns, M. (2012). The sustainability of new programs and innovations: A review of the empirical literature and recommendations for future research. *Implementation Science, 7*(17), 1–19. doi:10.1186/1748-5908-7-17

Windsor, C., Douglas, C., & Harvey, T. (2012). Nursing and competencies—A natural fit: The politics of skill/competency formation in nursing. *Nursing Inquiry, 19*(3), 213–222. doi:10.1111/j.1440-1800.2011.00549.x

Windt, K. (2016). Development of online learning modules as an adjunct to skills fairs and lectures to maintain nurses' competency and comfort level when caring for pediatric patients requiring continuous renal replacement therapy (CRRT). *Nephrology Nursing Journal, 43*(1), 39–46.

Wingfield, T., Boccia, D., Tovar, M. A., Huff, D., Montoya, R., Lewis, J. J., . . . Evans, C. A. (2015). Designing and implementing a socioeconomic intervention to enhance TB control: Operational evidence from the CRESIPT project in Peru. *BMC Public Health, 15*(810), 1–16. doi:10.1186/s12889-015-2128-0

Winters, B. D., Gurses, A. P., Lehmann, H., Sexton, J. B., Rampersad, C. J., & Pronovost, P. J. (2009). Clinical review: Checklists—Translating evidence into practice. *Critical Care, 13*(6), 210. doi:10.1186/cc7792

Wishart, G. C., Warwick, J., Pitsinis, V., Duffy, S., & Britton, P. D. (2010). Measuring performance in clinical breast examination. *British Journal of Surgery, 97*(8), 1246–1252. doi:10.1002/bjs.7108

Wood, G. J., & Morrison, R. S. (2011). Writing abstracts and developing posters for national meetings. *Journal of Palliative Medicine, 14*(3), 353–359. doi:10.1089/jpm.2010.0171

Woolf, S., Schünemann, H. J., Eccles, M. P., Grimshaw, J. M., & Shekelle, P. (2012). Developing clinical practice guidelines: Types of evidence and outcomes; values and economics, synthesis, grading, and presentation and deriving recommendations. *Implementation Science, 7*(61), 1–12. doi:10.1186/1748-5908-7-61

World Health Organization [WHO]. (n.d.). Safe surgery. Retrieved from http://www.who.int/patientsafety/safesurgery/en

World Health Organization [WHO]. (2000). The world health report 2000—Health systems: Improving performance (p. 61). Geneva, Switzerland: World Health Organization.

World Health Organization [WHO]. (2008). Implementation manual surgical safety checklist (1st ed.). Geneva: World Health Organization. Retrieved from http://www.who.int/patientsafety/safesurgery/tools_resources/SSSL_Manual_finalJun08.pdf

World Health Organization [WHO]. (2009). WHO surgical safety checklist. Retrieved from http://www.who.int/patientsafety/safesurgery/checklist/en

World Health Organization [WHO]. (2010). Using audit and feedback to health professionals to improve the quality and safety of health care. Retrieved from http://www.euro.who.int/__data/assets/pdf_file/0003/124419/e94296.pdf

Wuchner, S. S. (2014). Integrative review of implementation strategies for translation of research-based evidence by nurses. *Clinical Nurse Specialist, 28*(4), 214–223. doi:10.1097/NUR.0000000000000055

Wyatt, K. D., Branda, M. E., Anderson, R. T., Pencille, L. J., Montori, V. M., Hess, E. P., . . . Leblanc, A. (2014). Peering into the black box: A meta-analysis of how clinicians use decision aids during clinical encounters. *Implementation Science, 9*(26), 1–10. doi:10.1186/1748-5908-9-26

Wylie, A. (2009). Create snappy sound bites: How to write compelling quotes and memorable quips. *Public Relations Tactics, 16*(4), 10.

Xian, Y., Pan, W., Peterson, E. D., Heidenreich, P. A., Cannon, C. P., Hernandez, A. F., & Fonarow, G. C. (2010). Are quality improvements associated with the Get With the Guidelines—Coronary Artery Disease (GWTG-CAD) program sustained over time? A longitudinal comparison of GWTG-CAD hospitals versus non-GWTG-CAD hospitals. *American Heart Journal, 159*(2), 207–214.

Xu, Y., Ren, X., Shi, W., & Jiang, H. (2013). Implementation of the best practice in nasogastric tube feeding of critically ill patients in a neurosurgical intensive care unit. *International Journal of Evidence-Based Healthcare, 11*(2), 128–133. doi:10.1111/1744-1609.12020

Xyrichis, A., & Lowton, K. (2008). What fosters or prevents interprofessional teamworking in primary and community care? A literature review. *International Journal of Nursing Studies, 45*(1), 140–153. doi:10.1016/j.ijnurstu.2007.01.015

Yackel, E., McKennan, M., & Fox-Deise, A. (2010). A nurse-facilitated depression screening program in an Army primary care clinic: An evidence-based project. *Nursing Research, 59*(Suppl. 1), S58–S65. doi:10.1097/NNR.0b013e3181c3cab6

Yam, P., Fales, D., Jemison, J., Gillum, M., & Bernstein, M. (2012). Implementation of an antimicrobial stewardship program in a rural hospital. *American Journal of Health-System Pharmacy, 69*(13), 1142–1148. doi:10.2146/ajhp110512

Yanke, E., Zellmer, C., Van Hoof, S., Moriarty, H., Carayon, P., & Safdar, N. (2015). Understanding the current state of infection prevention to prevent *Clostridium difficile* infection: A human factors and systems engineering approach. *American Journal of Infection Control, 43*(3), 241–247. doi:10.1016/j.ajic.2014.11.026

Yaqub, R. (2014, September). How my (literal) elevator pitch landed our first big contract. *Inc., 36*(7), 130.

Yeh, J. S., Van Hoof, T. J., & Fischer, M. A. (2016). Key features of academic detailing: Development of an expert consensus using the Delphi method. *American Health & Drug Benefits, 9*(1), 42–50.

Young, T., Rohwer, A., van Schalkwyk, S., Volmink, J., & Clarke, M. (2015). Patience, persistence and pragmatism: Experiences and lessons learnt from the implementation of clinically integrated teaching and learning of evidence-based health care—A qualitative study. *PLoS ONE, 10*(6), e0131121. doi:10.1371.journal.pone.0131121

Yudkin, M. (2011). *The sound bite workbook: How to generate snappy tag lines, scintillating interview quotes, captivating book or article titles, and irresistible marketing or publicity handles.* Creative Ways Publishing.

Zachariah, P., Reagan, J., Furuya, E. Y., Dick, A., Hangsheng, L., Herzig, C. T. A., . . . Saiman, L. (2014). The association of state legal mandates for data submission of central line-associated bloodstream infections in neonatal intensive care units with process and outcome measures. *Infection Control & Hospital Epidemiology, 35*(9), 1133–1139. doi:10.1086/677635

Zhang, Y., Padman, R., & Levin, J. E. (2014). Paving the COWpath: Data-driven design of pediatric order sets. *Journal of the American Medical Informatics Association, 21*(e2), e304–e311. doi:10.1136/amiajnl-2013-002316

Zorger, J. (2009, February). Take your elevator pitch to the next level. *Wearables, 13*(5), 38–38.

Zwarenstein, M., Shiller, S. K., Croxford, R., Grimshaw, J. M., Kelsall, D., Paterson, J. M., . . . Hux, J. E. (2014). Printed educational messages aimed at family practitioners fail to increase retinal screening among their patients with diabetes: A pragmatic cluster randomized controlled trial. *Implementation Science, 9*(87), 1–9. doi:10.1186/1748-5908-9-87

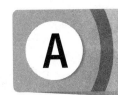

# THE IOWA MODEL REVISED: EVIDENCE-BASED PRACTICE TO PROMOTE EXCELLENCE IN HEALTH CARE

# The Iowa Model Revised: Evidence-Based Practice to Promote Excellence in Health Care

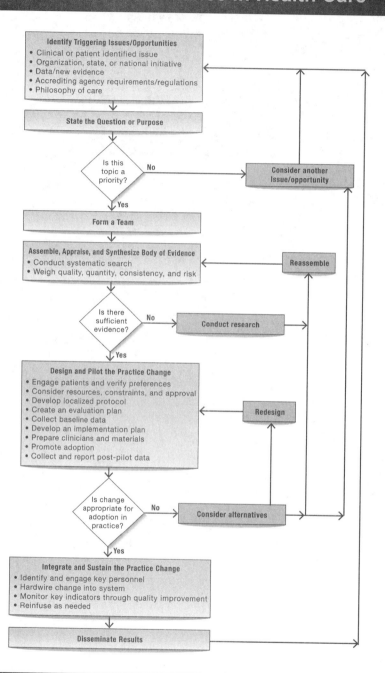

**Identify Triggering Issues/Opportunities**
- Clinical or patient identified issue
- Organization, state, or national initiative
- Data/new evidence
- Accrediting agency requirements/regulations
- Philosophy of care

**State the Question or Purpose**

*Is this topic a priority?* — No → **Consider another Issue/opportunity**

↓ Yes

**Form a Team**

**Assemble, Appraise, and Synthesize Body of Evidence**
- Conduct systematic search
- Weigh quality, quantity, consistency, and risk

← **Reassemble**

*Is there sufficient evidence?* — No → **Conduct research**

↓ Yes

**Design and Pilot the Practice Change**
- Engage patients and verify preferences
- Consider resources, constraints, and approval
- Develop localized protocol
- Create an evaluation plan
- Collect baseline data
- Develop an implementation plan
- Prepare clinicians and materials
- Promote adoption
- Collect and report post-pilot data

← **Redesign**

*Is change appropriate for adoption in practice?* — No → **Consider alternatives**

↓ Yes

**Integrate and Sustain the Practice Change**
- Identify and engage key personnel
- Hardwire change into system
- Monitor key indicators through quality improvement
- Reinfuse as needed

**Disseminate Results**

©University of Iowa Hospitals and Clinics, Revised June 2015
To request permission to use or reproduce, go to http://www.uihealthcare.org/nursing-research-and-evidence-based-practice

Iowa Model Collaborative. (2017). Iowa Model of Evidence-Based Practice: Revisions and validation. *Worldviews on Evidence-Based Nursing, 14*(3), 175–182. doi:10.1111/wvh.12223

# IMPLEMENTATION STRATEGIES FOR EVIDENCE-BASED PRACTICE

## Implementation Strategies for Evidence-Based Practice

Create Awareness & Interest → Build Knowledge & Commitment → Promote Action & Adoption → Pursue Integration & Sustained Use

### Connecting with Clinicians, Organizational Leaders, and Key Stakeholders

| Create Awareness & Interest | Build Knowledge & Commitment | Promote Action & Adoption | Pursue Integration & Sustained Use |
|---|---|---|---|
| ▪ Highlight advantages* or anticipated impact*<br>▪ Highlight compatibility*<br>▪ Continuing education programs*<br>▪ Sound bites*<br>▪ Journal club*<br>▪ Slogans & logos<br>▪ Staff meetings<br>▪ Unit newsletter<br>▪ Unit inservices<br>▪ Distribute key evidence<br>▪ Posters and postings/fliers<br>▪ Mobile 'show on the road'<br>▪ Announcements & broadcasts | ▪ Education (e.g., live, virtual, or computer-based)*<br>▪ Pocket guides<br>▪ Link practice change & power holder/stakeholder priorities*<br>▪ Change agents (e.g., change champion*, core group*, opinion leader*, thought leader, etc.)<br>▪ Educational outreach or academic detailing*<br>▪ Integrate practice change with other EBP protocols*<br>▪ Disseminate credible evidence with clear implications for practice*<br>▪ Make impact observable*<br>▪ Gap assessment/gap analysis*<br>▪ Clinician input*<br>▪ Local adaptation* & simplify*<br>▪ Focus groups for planning change*<br>▪ Match practice change with resources & equipment<br>▪ Resource manual or materials (i.e., electronic or hard copy)<br>▪ Case studies | ▪ Educational outreach/academic detailing*<br>▪ Reminders or practice prompts*<br>▪ Demonstrate workflow or decision algorithm<br>▪ Resource materials and quick reference guides<br>▪ Skill competence*<br>▪ Give evaluation results to colleagues*<br>▪ Incentives*<br>▪ Try the practice change*<br>▪ Multidisciplinary discussion & troubleshooting<br>▪ "Elevator speech"<br>▪ Data collection by clinicians<br>▪ Report progress & updates<br>▪ Change agents (e.g., change champion*, core group*, opinion leader*, thought leader, etc.)<br>▪ Role model*<br>▪ Troubleshooting at the point of care/bedside<br>▪ Provide recognition at the point of care* | ▪ Celebrate local unit progress*<br>▪ Individualize data feedback*<br>▪ Public recognition*<br>▪ Personalize the messages to staff (e.g., reduces work, reduces infection exposure, etc.) based on actual improvement data<br>▪ Share protocol revisions with clinician that are based on feedback from clinicians, patient, or family<br>▪ Peer influence<br>▪ Update practice reminders |

### Building Organizational System Support

| Create Awareness & Interest | Build Knowledge & Commitment | Promote Action & Adoption | Pursue Integration & Sustained Use |
|---|---|---|---|
| ▪ Knowledge broker(s)<br>▪ Senior executives announcements<br>▪ Publicize new equipment | ▪ Teamwork*<br>▪ Troubleshoot use/application*<br>▪ Benchmark data*<br>▪ Inform organizational leaders*<br>▪ Report within organizational infrastructure*<br>▪ Action plan*<br>▪ Report to senior leaders | ▪ Audit key indicators*<br>▪ Actionable and timely data feedback*<br>▪ Non-punitive discussion of results*<br>▪ Checklist*<br>▪ Documentation*<br>▪ Standing orders*<br>▪ Patient reminders*<br>▪ Patient decision aids*<br>▪ Rounding by unit & organizational leadership*<br>▪ Report into quality improvement program*<br>▪ Report to senior leaders<br>▪ Action plan*<br>▪ Link to patient/family needs & organizational priorities<br>▪ Unit orientation<br>▪ Individual performance evaluation | ▪ Audit and feedback*<br>▪ Report to senior leaders*<br>▪ Report into quality improvement program*<br>▪ Revise policy, procedure, or protocol*<br>▪ Competency metric for discontinuing training<br>▪ Project responsibility in unit or organizational committee<br>▪ Strategic plan*<br>▪ Trend results*<br>▪ Present in educational programs<br>▪ Annual report<br>▪ Financial incentives*<br>▪ Individual performance evaluation |

* Implementation strategy is supported by at least some empirical evidence in healthcare.

For permission to use, go to https://uihc.org/implementation-strategies-evidence-based-practice-evidence-based-practice-implementation-guide

Cullen, L., & Adams, S. L. (2012). Planning for implementation of evidence-based practice. *Journal of Nursing Administration, 42*(4), 222–230. doi:10.1097/NNA.0B013E31824CCD0A

# UI HOSPITALS AND CLINICS EVIDENCE-BASED PRACTICE PUBLICATIONS REPORTING USE OF THE IOWA MODEL

This appendix contains select evidence-based practice (EBP) exemplars on a variety of clinical topics that were completed using the Iowa Model (Iowa Model Collaborative, 2017; Titler et al., 2001) at the University of Iowa Hospitals and Clinics. Reading some of these articles may increase understanding of the EBP process or may be helpful when thinking about potential topics for an EBP project.

Abbott, L., & Hooke, M. C. (in press). Energy Through Motion: An activity intervention for cancer-related fatigue in an ambulatory infusion center. *Clinical Journal of Oncology Nursing.*

*Block, J., Lilienthal, M., Cullen, L., & White, A. (2012). Evidence-based thermoregulation for adult trauma patients. *Critical Care Nursing Quarterly, 35*(1), 50–63. doi:10.1097/CNQ.0b013e31823d3e96

*Bowman, A., Greiner, J. E., Doerschug, K. C., Little, S. B., Bombei, C. L., & Comried, L. M. (2005). Implementation of an evidence-based feeding protocol and aspiration risk reduction algorithm. *Critical Care Nursing Quarterly, 28*(4), 324–333. doi:10.1097/00002727-200510000-00004

Cullen, L., Baumler, S., Farrington, M., Dawson, C. J., Folkmann, P., & Brenner, L. (in press). Oral care for symptom management in head and neck cancer. *American Journal of Nursing.*

Cullen, L., Dawson, C. J., Hanrahan, K., & *Dole, N. (2014). Evidence-based practice: Strategies for nursing leaders. In D. L. Huber (Ed.), *Leadership & nursing care management* (5th ed., pp. 274–290, 495–501). St Louis, MO: Elsevier Saunders.

Cullen, L., Dawson, C. J., & *Williams, K. (2010). Evidence-based practice: Strategies for nursing leaders. In D. L. Huber (Ed.), *Leadership and nursing care management* (4th ed., pp. 367–386, 851–855). Maryland Heights, MO: Elsevier Saunders.

Cullen, L., *Greiner, J., Greiner, J., Bombei, C., & Comried, L. (2005). Excellence in evidence-based practice: Organizational and unit exemplars. *Critical Care Nursing Clinics of North America, 17*(2), 127–142. doi:10.1016/j.ccell.2005.01.002

Cullen, L., Hanrahan, K., *Neis, N., Farrington, M., Laffoon, T. A., & Dawson, C. J. (in press). Evidence-based practice: Strategies for nursing leaders. In D. L. Huber (Ed.), *Leadership and nursing care management* (6th ed.). Philadelphia, PA: Elsevier.

Dolezal, D., Cullen, L., Harp, J., & Mueller, T. (2011). Implementing preoperative screening of undiagnosed obstructive sleep apnea. *Journal of PeriAnesthesia Nursing, 26*(5), 338–342. doi:10.1016/j.jopan.2011.07.003

Farrington, M., Bruene, D., & Wagner, M. (2015). Pain management prior to nasogastric tube placement: Atomized lidocaine. *ORL – Head and Neck Nursing, 33*(1), 8–16.

Farrington, M., Cullen, L., & Dawson, C. (2010). Assessment of oral mucositis in adult and pediatric oncology patients: An evidence-based approach. *ORL – Head and Neck Nursing, 28*(3), 8–15.

Farrington, M., Cullen, L., & Dawson, C. (2013). Evidence-based oral care for oral mucositis. *ORL – Head and Neck Nursing, 31*(3), 6–15.

Farrington, M., *Hanson, A., Laffoon, T., & Cullen, L. (2015). Low-dose ketamine infusions for post-operative pain in opioid-tolerant orthopedic spine patients. *Journal of PeriAnesthesia Nursing, 30*(4), 338–345. doi:10.1016/j.jopan.2015.03.005

Farrington, M., Laffoon, T., Dawson, C., & Kealey, C. (2017). Pain management interventions for needle stick procedures: An ambulatory EBP project. *ORL – Head and Neck Nursing, 35*(2), 6–12.

*Farrington, M., Lang, S., Cullen, L., & Stewart, S. (2009). Nasogastric tube placement verification in pediatric and neonatal patients. *Pediatric Nursing, 35*(1), 17–24.

Gordon, M., Bartruff, L., Gordon, S., Lofgren, M., & Widness, J. A. (2008). How fast is too fast? A practice change in umbilical arterial catheter blood sampling using the Iowa Model for Evidence-Based Practice. *Advances in Neonatal Care, 8*(4), 198–207. doi:10.1097/01.ANC.0000333707.37776.08

Hanrahan, K. (2013). Hyaluronidase for treatment of intravenous extravasations: Implementation of an evidence-based guideline in a pediatric population. *Journal for Specialists in Pediatric Nursing, 18*(3), 253–262. doi:10.1111/jspn.12035

Hanrahan, K., Wagner, M., Matthews, G., Stewart, S., Dawson, C., Greiner, J.,…Williamson, A. (2015). Sacred cow gone to pasture: A systematic evaluation and integration of evidence-based practice. *Worldviews on Evidence-Based Nursing, 12*(1), 3–11. doi:10.1111/wvn.12072

*Hiller, A., Farrington, M., Forman, J., McNulty, H., & Cullen, L. (in press). Evidence-based nurse-driven algorithm for intrapartum bladder care. *Journal of PeriAnesthesia Nursing*.

Huether, K., Abbott, L., Cullen, L., Cullen, L., & Gaarde, A. (2016). Energy Through Motion: An evidence-based exercise program to reduce cancer-related fatigue and improve quality of life. *Clinical Journal of Oncology Nursing, 20*(3), E60–E70. doi:10.1188/16.CJON.E60-E70

*Madsen, D., Sebolt, T., Cullen, L., Folkedahl, B., Mueller, T., Richardson, C., & Titler, M. (2005). Listening to bowel sounds: An evidence-based practice project. *American Journal of Nursing, 105*(12), 40–49. doi:10.1097/00000446-200512000-00029

Smith, A., Farrington, M., & Matthews, G. (2014). Monitoring sedation in patients receiving opioids for pain management. *Journal of Nursing Care Quality, 29*(4), 345–353. doi:10.1097/NCQ.0000000000000059

*Stebral, L. L., & Steelman, V. M. (2006). Double gloving for surgical procedures: An evidence-based practice project. *Perioperative Nursing Clinics, 1*(3), 251–260.

Stenger, K., Montgomery, L., & Briesemeister, E. (2007). Creating a culture of change through implementation of a safe patient handling program [corrected] [published erratum appears in *Critical Care Nursing Clinics of North America* (2009, December), *21*(4), 595]. *Critical Care Nursing Clinics of North America, 19*(2), 213–222. doi:10.1016/j.ccell.2007.02.007

*Van Waning, N. R., Kleiber, C., & Freyenberger, B. (2005). Development and implementation of a protocol for transfers out of the pediatric intensive care unit. *Critical Care Nurse, 25*(3), 50–55.

*EBP Staff Nurse Interns

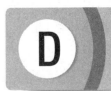

# SELECT EVIDENCE-BASED PRACTICE PROCESS MODELS

| MODEL | CITATION | SAMPLE REPORT |
|---|---|---|
| Iowa Model Revised: Evidence-Based Practice to Promote Excellence in Health Care | Iowa Model Collaborative. (2017). Iowa Model of Evidence-Based Practice: Revisions and validation. *Worldviews on Evidence-Based Nursing, 14*(3), 175–182. doi:10.1111/wvn.12223 | Farrington, M., Hanson, A., Laffoon, T., & Cullen, L. (2015). Low-dose ketamine infusions for postoperative pain in opioid-tolerant orthopaedic spine patients. *Journal of PeriAnesthesia Nursing, 30*(4), 338–345. doi:10.1016/j.jopan.2015.03.005 |
| Iowa Model of Evidence-Based Practice to Promote Quality Care | Titler, M. G., Kleiber, C., Steelman, V. J., Rakel, B. A., Budreau, G., Everett, L. Q.,…Goode, C. J. (2001). The Iowa Model of Evidence-Based Practice to Promote Quality Care. *Critical Care Nursing Clinics of North America, 13*(4), 497–509. | |
| Johns Hopkins Nursing Evidence-Based Practice (JHNEBP) Model | Newhouse, R. P., & Johnson, K. (2009). A case study in evaluating infrastructure for EBP and selecting a model. *Journal of Nursing Administration, 39*(10), 409–411. doi:10.1097/NNA.0b013e3181b920b7 | Mori, C. (2015). Implementing evidence-based practice to reduce infections following arthroplasty. *Orthopaedic Nursing, 34*(4), 188–194. doi:10.1097/NOR.0000000000000157 |
| Stetler Model of Evidence-Based Practice | Stetler, C. B. (2001). Updating the Stetler Model of Research Utilization to facilitate evidence-based practice. *Nursing Outlook, 49*(6), 272–279. doi:10.1067/mno.2001.120517 | Velez, R. P., Becker, K. L., Davidson, P., & Sloand, E. (2015). A quality improvement intervention to address provider behaviour as it relates to utilisation of CA-MRSA guidelines. *Journal of Clinical Nursing, 24*(3–4), 556–562. doi:10.1111/jocn.12684 |
| Advancing Research and Clinical Practice Through Close Collaboration (ARCC) Model | Melnyk, B. M. (2012). Achieving a high-reliability organization through implementation of the ARCC model for systemwide sustainability of evidence-based practice. *Nursing Administration Quarterly, 36*(2), 127–135. doi:10.1097/NAQ.0b013e318249fb6a | Melnyk, B. M., & Fineout-Overholt, E. (2011). *Implementing evidence-based practice: Real life success stories.* Indianapolis, IN: Sigma Theta Tau International. |
| ACE Star Model of Knowledge Transformation | Stevens, K. R. (2013, May 31). The impact of evidence-based practice in nursing and the next big ideas. *OJIN: The Online Journal of Issues in Nursing, 18*(2), 4. | Farra, S. L., Miller, E. T., & Hodgson, E. (2015). Virtual reality disaster training: Translation to practice. *Nurse Education in Practice, 15*(1), 53–57. doi:10.1016/j.nepr.2013.08.017 |
| Promoting Action on Research Implementation in Health Services (PARIHS) Framework | Harvey, G., & Kitson A. (2016). PARIHS revisited: From heuristic to integrated framework for the successful implementation of knowledge into practice. *Implementation Science, 11*(1), 1–13, 33. doi:10.1186/s13012-016-0398-2 | Powrie, S. L., Danly, D., Corbett, C. F., Purath, J., & Dupler, A. (2014). Using implementation science to facilitate evidence-based practice changes to promote optimal outcomes for orthopaedic patients. *Orthopaedic Nursing, 33*(2), 109–114. doi:10.1097/NOR.0000000000000036 |

Modified from Cullen, L., Hanrahan, K., Neis, N., Farrington, M., Laffoon, T., & Dawson, C. (in press). Evidence-based practice: Strategies for nursing leaders. In D. Huber (Ed.), *Leadership and nursing care management* (6th ed.). Philadelphia, PA: Elsevier.

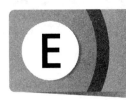

# GLOSSARY

**Academic detailing:** Structured presentations with specific elements (e.g., evidence summary, actionable goals, unattractive alternatives) designed to influence provider adoption of a recommended practice.

**Action plan:** Document outlining steps for project management with objectives, specific activities to accomplish the objectives, an estimated timeline, assignment of responsibility, and tracking progress.

**Adaptation/reinvention:** Modification of an evidence-based intervention by a user when designing the EBP protocol to suit the needs of the setting or to improve the fit to local conditions.

**Adoption:** Decision about and use of a clinical practice recommendation.

**AGREE II (Appraisal of Guidelines, for Research, & Evaluation II):** Established instrument that provides a framework for assessing the quality and reporting of clinical practice guidelines (CPGs).

**Anecdotal evidence:** Informal evidence supported by local experts, local data, theory, or scientific principles.

**Anticipated impact:** The expected benefit of the new EBP over the usual care or traditional practice.

**Audit:** A routine method for collecting evaluative data from key indicators that provide a summary of clinical performance or provision of evidence-based healthcare over a specific time period; serves as a proxy for identifying actual practice patterns.

**Baseline data collection:** Data collected before implementation of the practice change, focused on key indicators related to the proposed practice change, to guide implementation and post-implementation evaluation.

**Benchmarking:** Comparing outcome measures with top performers to evaluate performance.

**Body of evidence:** The relevant research, synthesis reports, patient preferences, case reports, local data, and/or expert opinion that answers clinical questions and guides development of practice recommendations.

**Case report:** Retrospective account of an individual or select individuals with unusual or pertinent diseases, interventions, or therapies.

**Case study:** The collection and presentation of detailed information about a particular individual or small group, including accounts for how EBP was helpful or would have been helpful for patient care.

**Case-control study:** Retrospective design where subjects with a certain outcome or disease (cases) are grouped and then exposures/risks compared to matched controls.

**Change agent:** Influential person who, based on his or her role, expertise, or leadership style, can impact implementation.

**Change champion:** Change agent who works in the clinical area, uses social influence, commits to promoting a specific practice change, develops expertise on key aspects of the evidence, guides designing the practice change based on his/her understanding of the evidence and the local context, assists with creating resources for implementation, and trains peers.

**Clinical decision support:** Point-of-care reminders to improve recall, influence decision-making, and improve use of clinical practice recommendations.

**Clinical practice guidelines (CPGs):** Document including recommendations for or against related assessments, procedures, tests, or interventions, based on a systematic review of evidence and analysis of benefits versus harms intending to change clinician practices and to optimize patient care.

**Clinical significance:** Effect of the intervention showing a difference between usual care and evidence-based intervention.

**Clinician input:** The process of obtaining clinicians' suggestions through shared decision-making from nurses and other professionals to improve the design of the EBP protocol, implementation plan, or integration into clinical workflow.

**Cohort study:** Design in which prospective subjects are grouped by exposure (cohort) and followed over time to determine outcomes.

**Compatibility:** The degree to which an EBP protocol is perceived to be consistent with existing values, past experiences, and needs of potential patients or clinician users.

**Competency metric:** An indicator that refers to successful learning and performance of essential skills at a preset goal.

**Consensus statement:** Report of a panel of experts based on their evaluation of the state of scientific knowledge available at the time with a determination for practice.

**Consistency of evidence:** The degree to which studies report similar results or have similar implications for practice.

**Context:** Setting within which an EBP intervention is designed to be used; includes the social, regulatory, norms, and cultures of the setting.

**Core group:** Small group of change agents from representative shifts or work days who review key evidence, train colleagues, serve as role models, reinforce desired practices, and troubleshoot issues to expand the reach of a team.

**Cross-sectional study:** The prospective observational design that examines health status, behavior, and other risk factors of a subpopulation measured at a given time.

**Decision algorithm:** Flowchart that guides sequential actions using patient data or risk as a cue to determine a course of action or interventions based on specific patient circumstances related to a clinical condition.

**Diffusion:** Passive spread of an intervention or practice change.

**Dissemination:** Active approach to spreading EBP to target audience of patients, families, and/or clinician users.

**Documentation:** Electronic or paper record of assessments, findings, and care given to a patient by members of the interprofessional healthcare team.

**EBP facilitator/mentor:** Individual with advanced EBP knowledge and skills, who provides leadership and guides others throughout the EBP process.

**Educational outreach:** The use of structured presentations designed to influence use of a recommended practice; may be provided by a clinician or lay leader from within the community.

**Effectiveness:** Evaluation of difference between usual care and EBP intervention impact, considering typical patients and families in the healthcare setting.

**Efficacy:** Evaluation of whether an intervention works in ideal circumstances such as research trials.

**Electronic alert:** Clinical decision support, provided to clinicians at the point of care to direct decisions or action, using a prompt from the electronic documentation system or another electronic device.

**Elevator speech:** Persuasive "pitch" that can be shared in less than a minute to secure funding or "sell" the idea that the work is special; includes a compelling goal, key evidence, benefits to audience or organization, current progress, and action request.

**Evidence-based practice (EBP):** Systematic process of shared decision-making with clinician-led discussion engaging the patient and others significant to them based on the best evidence; the patient's experiences, preferences, and values; clinical expertise; and other available robust sources of information.

**Executive summary:** A concise and convenient way to summarize work completed for key stakeholders.

**External validity:** Findings are generalizable, applicable to other populations and settings.

**Face validity:** Degree a test or tool measures the desired concept, as established by topic experts.

**Feedback:** Reporting on clinical performance using data to demonstrate desired actions taken or needed to achieve the goal.

**Fidelity:** EBP protocol carried out as intended such that practices match the most critical elements from research and other best evidence.

**Focus group:** Small-group interviews may be used to identify how EBP adoption has happened previously, guide design of the EBP protocol, and inform selection of implementation strategies and planning.

**Gap assessment/analysis:** Demonstrates the difference between current practice or outcomes and the desired practice or outcome compared with the goal, best evidence, high performers, or benchmarks.

**Generalizable:** Findings that are applicable to patients or groups beyond those participating in the current study.

**Grading of Recommendations Assessment, Development and Evaluations (GRADE) Working Group:** A group who developed a systematic and transparent approach to rate the body of evidence indicating quality and strength of the recommendation.

**Health technology assessment:** Systematic review to determine the effectiveness of a health technology, drug, device, or intervention for a condition or topic, to make recommendations for practice or policy.

**Histogram:** A diagram consisting of graphic bars where the area is proportional to the frequency of an indicator vertically on the y-axis and the x-axis horizontally represents the reference (e.g., time).

**Human subjects research determination:** Institutional Review Board decision following U.S. Department of Health and Human Services regulations that the proposed work fits the definition of research (i.e., involves obtaining data through intervention or interaction with a living individual or from identifiable information about the individual).

**Implementation:** Putting clinical practice recommendations into use in a clinical setting.

**Implementation science:** Scientific investigation of methods that promote adoption and/or integration of clinical practice recommendations by patients and families, clinicians, and/or organizations.

**Incentive:** Any factor (financial or nonfinancial) that provides motivation for a particular course of action.

**Incident:** Number of new conditions, events, or occurrences in a defined group or population.

**Indicator:** Topic-specific measure showing extent a practice is used; clinician or patient/family input, or quality is achieved; includes knowledge, attitudes, practices, outcomes, and associated risks.

**Individual performance evaluation:** Systematic, standardized process that compares work behavior to a preset standard that is completed at least annually by an employee's supervisor; may be used to identify contribution to EBP priorities.

**Individualized data feedback:** Communication of data reported back to the individual and/or the team to demonstrate individual compared to group performance.

**Integration:** Continuous use or delivery of recommended clinical practice, as the standard approach to care delivery.

**Integrative review:** Method used to synthesize research on a topic or condition to establish extent of or gap in scientific knowledge.

**Internal validity:** Methods designed to control for risk of bias such that findings provide a precise and unprejudiced answer to the clinical question.

**Journal club:** Sessions organized for clinicians to review and discuss strengths and limitations of research articles published in scientific journals and to facilitate understanding and use of research findings and promote evidence-based care delivery.

**Just-in-time:** Precise timing or delivery of needed information or supplies.

**Key evidence distribution:** Disbursement that provides strategic articles or evidence reports to inform the intended audience of clinicians, leaders, or stakeholders.

**Knowledge broker:** Change agent from outside the organization serving as a trusted intermediary who increases knowledge sharing and local use of best evidence by assessing facilitators and barriers, locates best evidence, trains, establishes learning networks, mentors clinicians and leaders, and reports results.

**Knowledge-focused trigger:** Clinical questions stemming from new information or new scientific findings, standards, regulations, or reports.

**Leadership rounds:** Routine, proactive visits to clinical areas to provide visible, continuous support for adopting and sustaining practice recommendations while recognizing individual and team activities to achieve the goal.

**Literature review:** Written summary of knowledge on a topic.

**Meta-analysis:** Statistical analysis that synthesizes findings from small, less powered individual studies, creating a pooled effect to improve precision in reported findings.

**Metasynthesis:** Analysis of qualitative studies with findings intended to describe a phenomenon or inform theory development.

**Observable impact:** Visible or tangible effect that is clinically meaningful as a result of an EBP intervention.

**Operational definition:** Statement of how a variable or indicator will be measured to reflect the presence, absence, or extent the concept of interest is present.

**Opinion leader:** Change agent who is informally influential and provides energy to motivate participation by reviewing evidence and judging the local fit, educating peers, and positively influencing the practice of others.

**Patient decision aids:** Learning tools to help patients participate in decisions that involve weighing the benefits and harms of treatment options while considering best evidence, preferences, and values.

**Peer influence:** Interpersonal communication used by trusted, respected, credible colleagues to motivate incorporation of practice recommendations as the new "norm" or standard for care.

**PICO (Patient population/problem/pilot area, Intervention, Comparison, Outcome):** Tool that helps clearly articulate and narrow the scope of a proposed practice change and guides formation of a focused, clear purpose statement.

**PICOT (Patient population/problem/pilot area, Intervention, Comparison, Outcome, Time frame):** Method that helps clearly articulate and narrow the scope of a proposed practice change, guides formation of the purpose statement, and provides a timeline for short-term projects.

**Pilot:** Small-scale and short-term trial of an EBP to determine feasibility, incorporate patient/family or clinician input, inform the implementation planning, and show effect on outcomes prior to larger rollout or scale-up.

**Pocket guide:** Concise and simple information describing critical steps or key decision points for hard-to-remember details in EBP recommendations; designed to fit into a pocket.

**Practice prompt:** Just-in-time cue to clinicians, provided at the point of care, to encourage use of EBP recommendations and perform or avoid specific action.

**Prevalence:** Portion of a group or population with a condition or attribute at a given point in time or period of time.

**Problem-focused trigger:** Clinical questions stemming from existing data, known risks, or clinical issues.

**Process indicator:** Clinicians' knowledge, attitude, or practices related to a clinical practice recommendation.

**Qualitative research:** Focuses on observational or investigative techniques that seek to systematically examine and explain phenomena in real-world setting, build theory, and inform practice.

**Quality care:** Healthcare delivery that is safe, effective, patient-centered, timely, efficient, and equitable.

**Quality improvement (QI):** Process or program that analyzes and changes the structures, processes, and outcomes related to a continuous practice improvement that may be evidence-based with the intent of increasing the likelihood of effective, timely, efficient, equitable, patient-centered care within the local setting.

**Quality of evidence:** Determination or rating of the extent to which we can be confident in findings based on the study design and analyses to minimize systematic bias and control confounding variables that may affect findings.

**Quantitative research:** Deductive approach to study design with statistical or mathematical techniques used to test hypotheses and measure variables to establish relationships among variables (e.g., correlation or cause-effect).

**Quantity of evidence:** Extent or magnitude of treatment effect, number of studies, or overall sample size across studies.

**Quasi-experimental study:** Design to determine causality testing one intervention, therapy, or test compared to another in real-world settings when complete control is not possible.

**Randomized controlled trial (RCT):** Study design to determine cause-effect relationship testing one intervention versus another under ideal circumstances with random assignment to groups, controlling for other influencing factors.

**Return on investment:** Amount of improvement achieved with a certain investment; may be calculated by determining costs avoided (e.g., reduced length of stay) minus implementation costs (e.g., personnel and materials).

**Risk:** Balance between desirable and undesirable effects and costs, comparing current practice with proposed change.

**Run chart:** Graph used to depict change in observed data that includes multiple data points and a line representing the median for comparison over time.

**Sacred cow:** Old practice habits that are particularly resistant to change despite evidence of the need to change.

**Scoping review:** A rapid collection of evidence related to a given topic or condition to map concepts, establish gaps in scientific knowledge, and/or determine if evidence is sufficient to develop a systematic review.

**Sensitivity:** Probability of correct identification of a patient condition (e.g., fall risk assessment correctly identifies a patient who will go on to fall).

**Sigma:** Calculated estimate of variance, similar to standard deviation in a bell-shaped curve, creating zones on either side of the mean to assist interpretation of special or common cause variation using trended data; each zone represents one sigma or approximately one standard deviation from the mean.

**Skill competence:** The combination of the ability to perform a task, action, or function and knowledge, attitudes, values, and abilities using minimum expenditure of time and energy.

**Specificity:** Probability of correct identification of the patients who will not have a specified condition (e.g., fall risk assessment correctly identifies a patient who will not go on to fall).

**Sound bite:** Short and memorable phrase of three important points that are relevant to the target audience, the need for change, expected outcome, and required practice change.

**Stakeholders:** Individuals invested in the practice who may contribute resources, influence, or support for EBP.

**Statistical process control chart:** Graph used to depict process stability or statistically significant changes that includes multiple data points and a line representing the average/mean for comparison over time, sigma as zones (similar to standard deviations), and lines displaying an upper and lower control limit to aid interpretation.

**Strategic plan:** Document outlining the plan for actualizing the organization's mission, vision, and values.

**Strength of evidence:** Combination of research studies (study design minimizing bias and precision of analysis) and other evidence used as a whole to guide practice recommendations, often from systematic reviews.

**Sustainability:** Continuous use or delivery of recommended clinical practice as the standard approach to care delivery.

**Synthesis of evidence:** Systematic process combining research, other robust evidence, and local information in new ways to balance bias, increase understanding, guide design of an EBP protocol, and define the limits or boundaries of the evidence.

**Systematic review:** Synthesis of research findings related to a specific question, using a standardized, transparent, and reproducible method to locate, combine, and describe the state of the science for a practice recommendation.

**Thought leader:** Change agent who provides persuasive information.

**Trend results:** Routine and consistent display of results and outcomes from a practice change over time.

**Translation research:** Evaluation of interventions used to promote the rate and extent of adoption of a clinical practice recommendation by individuals, groups, or organizations.

**Trigger:** Stimulus for the identification of questions.

**Umbrella review:** Report using methods for reviewing systematic reviews related to a topic, issue, or condition that is broader than addressing a single question about the topic of interest.

**U.S. Preventive Services Task Force (USPSTF):** Panel of experts under the Agency for Healthcare Research and Quality (AHRQ) of the U.S. Department of Health and Human Services that makes evidence-based recommendations about clinical preventive services such as screenings, counseling services, and preventive medications.

**Workflow demonstration:** Method of mapping the flow of steps while performing a procedure to guide integration of EBP recommendations into work routines.

# INDEX

# T